HCO_3	Bicarbonate
H_2CO_3	Carbonic acid
Hct	Hematocrit
Hgb	Hemoglobin
HR	Heart rate
IF	Inspiratory force
Ig	Immunoglobulin
IMV	Intermittent mandatory ventilation
IPPB	Intermittent positive pressure breathing
LDH	Lactate dehydrogenase
LPM	Liters per minute
MLT	Minimal leak technique
MOV	Minimal occlusion volume
OT	Old tuberculin
PA	Posteroanterior
$P(A-a)o_2$	Alveolar-arterial oxygen gradient
$Paco_2$	Partial pressure of arterial carbon dioxide
Pao_2	Partial pressure of arterial oxygen
PAP	Pulmonary artery pressure
PCWP	Pulmonary capillary wedge pressure
PE	Pleural effusion, pulmonary edema, or pulmonary embolism
PEEP	Positive end-expiratory pressure
PEFR	Peak expiratory flow rate
PMN	Polymorphonuclear neutrophil
PPD	Purified protein derivative
PT	Prothrombin time
PTT	Partial thromboplastin time
R_{AW}	Airway resistance
RBCs	Red blood cells
RV	Reserve volume
Sao_2	Saturation of arterial hemoglobin with oxygen
SGOT	Serum glutamic oxaloacetic transaminase
SIMV	Synchronized intermittent mandatory ventilation
SOB	Shortness of breath
SRS	Slow-reacting substance of anaphylaxis
SSKI	Saturated solution of potassium iodide
Svo_2	Saturation of venous hemoglobin with oxygen
TB	Tuberculosis
TLC	Total lung capacity
TPN	Total parenteral nutrition
TT	Thrombin time
V_D	Anatomic dead space
V_T	Tidal volume
VC	Vital capacity
$\dot{V}/\dot{Q}$	Ventilation/perfusion ratio
WBCs	White blood cells

RESPIRATORY DISORDERS

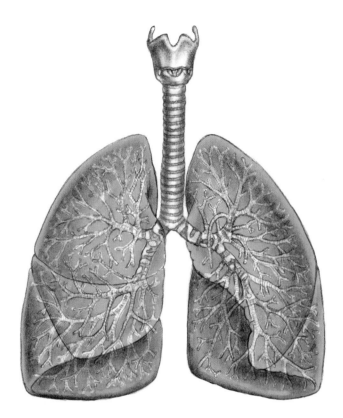

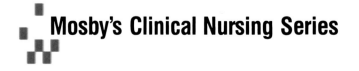

Mosby's Clinical Nursing Series

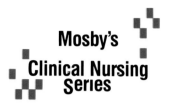

Mosby's Clinical Nursing Series

Cardiovascular Disorders

by Mary Canobbio

Respiratory Disorders

by Susan Wilson and June Thompson

Infectious Diseases

by Deanna Grimes

Immunologic Disorders

by Christine Mudge-Grout

Neurologic Disorders

by Victor Campbell

Musculoskeletal Disorders

by Leona Mourad

Gastrointestinal Disorders

by Debra Broadwell

Renal and Genitourinary Disorders

by Dorothy Brundage and Mikel Gray

Neoplastic and Hematologic Disorders

by Anne Belcher

Eye, Ear, Nose, and Throat Disorders

by Jane Hirsch

RESPIRATORY DISORDERS

SUSAN F. WILSON, RN, PhD

Associate Professor
Texas Christian University
Harris College of Nursing
Fort Worth, Texas

JUNE M. THOMPSON, RN, MS

Assistant Professor
Prairie View A & M University
Houston, Texas

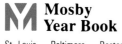 **Mosby Year Book**

St. Louis   Baltimore   Boston   Chicago   London   Philadelphia   Sydney   Toronto

Mosby
Year Book
Dedicated to Publishing Excellence

Editor: William Grayson Brottmiller
Senior developmental editor: Sally Adkisson
Developmental writer: Daphna Gregg
Project manager: Mark Spann
Designer: Liz Fett

The author wishes to acknowledge the significant contributions of two
agencies in the development of this book. . .

  Irving Healthcare System in Irving, Texas, particularly Skip Wilson,
  Vice President; Sandy Dunn, Director, Respiratory Therapy; and Sharon
  Peters, Director, Public Relations

  and

  Jeff Smith of Lincare, Inc. of Grand Prairie, Texas

Mosby–Yearbook, Inc.
11830 Westline Industrial Drive, St. Louis, Missouri 63146
ISBN 0-8016-5087-9

Library of Congress Cataloging-in-Publication Data

Wilson, Susan Fickertt.
    Respiratory disorders / Susan F. Wilson, June M. Thompson.
        p.   cm.—(Mosby's clinical nursing series)
    Includes bibliographical references.
    Includes index.
    ISBN 0-8016-5087-9
    1. Respiratory Organs—Diseases—Nursing.   I. Thompson, June M.,
1946– . II. Title. III. Series.
    [DNLM: 1. Respiratory Tract Diseases—nursing.   WY   163 W753r]
RC735.5.W54   1990
616.2—dc20
DNLM/DLC
for Library of Congress   90-6228
                                                                                CIP

        The authors and publisher have made a conscientious effort
        to ensure that the drug information and recommended dosages
        in this book are accurate and in accord with accepted standards
        at the time of publication. However, pharmacology is a
        rapidly changing science, so readers are advised to check
        the package insert provided by the manufacturer before
        administering any drug.

C/CD/VH 9 8 7 6 5 4 3 2

Chapter 8, "Respiratory Drugs," contributed by
Mark Hamelink, MSN, CRNA, CCRN
Nurse Anesthetist
Morpheus Anesthesia Servies, P.C.
South Haven, Michigan

Original illustrations prepared by
George J. Wassilchenko
Tulsa, Oklahoma
and
Donald P. O'Connor
St. Peters, Missouri

Photography by
Patrick Watson
Poughkeepsie, New York

PREFACE

Respiratory Disorders is the second volume in *Mosby's Clinical Nursing Series*, a new kind of resource for practicing nurses.

The *Series* is the result of the most elaborate market research ever undertaken by The C.V. Mosby Company. We first surveyed hundreds of working nurses to determine what kind of resources practicing nurses want in order to meet their advanced information needs. We then approached clinical specialists—proven authors and experts in 10 practice areas, from cardiovascular to ENT—and asked them to develop a common format that would meet the needs of nurses in practice, as specified by the survey respondents. This plan was then presented to 9 focus groups composed of working nurses over a period of 18 months. The plan was refined between each group, and in the later stages we published a 32-page full-color sample so that detailed changes could be made to improve the physical layout and appearance of the book, section by section and page by page.

The result is a new genre of professional books for nursing professionals.

Respiratory Disorders begins with an innovative Color Atlas of Respiratory Structure and Function. This is not a mere review of anatomy and physiology taught in undergraduate curriculums; it is actually a collection of highly detailed full-color drawings designed to explain how respiratory problems develop. Every effort was made to explain pulmonary structure and function in a way that rationalizes nursing interventions.

Chapter 2 is a pictorial guide to the nurse's assessment of the respiratory system. Clear, full-color photographs show proper position and technique in sharp detail, aided by concise instructions, rationales, and tips.

Chapter 3 presents the latest in diagnostic tests, again using full-color photographs of equipment, techniques, monitors, and output. A consistent format for each diagnostic procedure gives nurses information about the purpose of the test, indications and contraindications, and nursing care associated with each test, including patient teaching.

Chapters 4, 5, and 6 present the nursing care of patients experiencing noninfectious respiratory disorders, infectious respiratory diseases, and major surgical and therapeutic interventions, respectively. Each disease is presented in a format that you invented to meet your advanced practice needs. Information on pathophysiology answers questions nurses often have. A unique box alerting nurses to possible complications provides this information to health professionals in the best position to observe, respond to, and report dangerous changes in patient conditions. Definitive diagnostic tests and the physician's treatment plan are briefly reviewed to promote collaborative care among members of the health care team.

The heart of the book is the nursing care, presented according to the nursing process. These pages are bordered in blue to make them easy to find and use on the unit. The nursing care is structured to integrate the five steps of the nursing process, centered around appropriate nursing diagnoses accepted by the North American Nursing Diagnostic Association (NANDA). The material can be used to develop individualized care plans quickly and accurately, and it meets the standards of nursing care required by the Joint Commission on the Accreditation of Hospitals (JCAH). By facilitating the development of individualized and authoritative care plans, this book can actually save you time to spend on direct patient care.

In response to requests from scores of nurses participating in our research, a distinctive feature of this book is its use in patient teaching. Background information on diseases and medical interventions enables nurses to answer with authority questions patients often ask. The illustrations in the book, particularly those in the Color Atlas and the chapter on Diagnostic Studies, are specifically designed to support patient teaching. Chapter 7 consists of 14 Patient Teaching Guides written at a ninth-grade level so they can be copied, distributed to patients and their families, and used for self-care after discharge. Patient teaching sections in each care plan provide nurses with checklists of concepts to teach, promoting this increasingly vital aspect of nursing care.

The book concludes with a concise guide to respiratory drugs and, inside the back cover, a resource section, printed on yellow paper, that directs you to organizations and other resources on respiratory health for nurses and patients.

This book is intended for medical-surgical nurses, who invariably care for patients with acute respiratory disorders. Critical care nurses in our survey and focus groups also expressed a need for the book. We expect that students will find the book an indispensable help in developing clinical skills and judgment in caring for patients with respiratory disorders, as it will also be for nurses returning to practice after a hiatus, nurses seeking advanced certification, and nurses transferring to medical-surgical or critical care settings.

We hope this book contributes to the advancement of professional nursing by serving as a first step toward a body of professional literature for nurses to call their own.

Contents

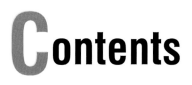

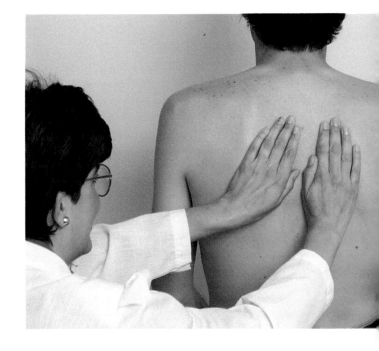
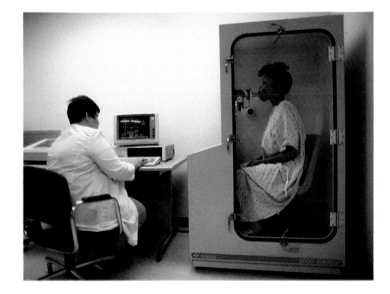

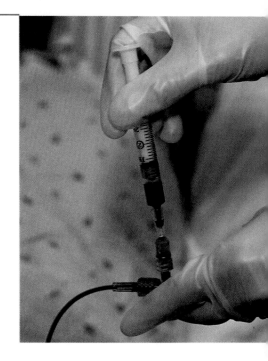

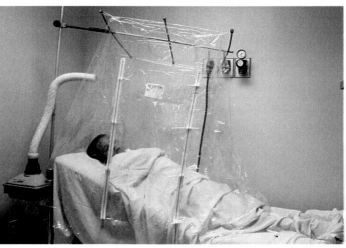

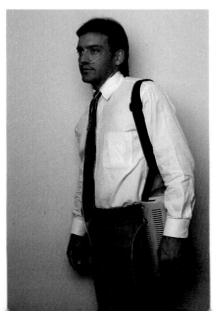

7 Patient teaching guides, 275

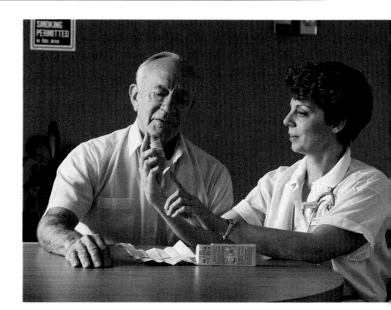

8 Respiratory drugs, 290

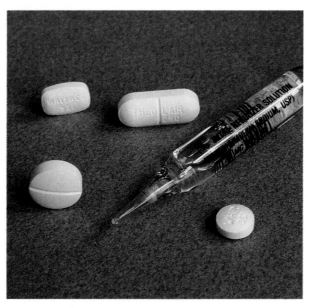

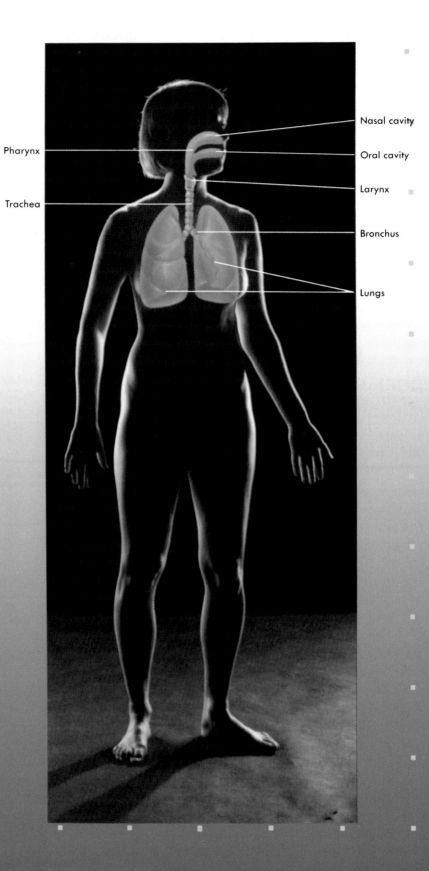

Pharynx

Nasal cavity

Oral cavity

Larynx

Trachea

Bronchus

Lungs

CHAPTER 1

Color Atlas of Respiratory Structure and Function

The respiratory system continually obtains oxygen from the environment, delivers oxygen to the body's cells, removes carbon dioxide from the cells, and expels carbon dioxide into the environment. During quiet activities, the average adult keeps this cycle going with about 15 respirations per minute. With each breath, an adult moves about 500 ml in and out of the lungs (tidal volume) for a total of about 18,925 liters of air every day. However, this half-liter is only about 12% of the maximum breathing capacity. With strenuous activity, respirations double and the volume of air with each breath increases more than five times.

The respiratory system is intimately related to the cardiovascular system. Respiration transpires on two levels: external and internal. *External respiration* is the exchange of gases between the alveoli and the pulmonary capillaries. *Internal respiration* is gas exchange between peripheral capillaries and the cells.

Although respiration is considered the work of the airways and lungs, every living cell is engaged in respiration. The cells require oxygen, which combines with adenosine diphosphate (ADP) and simple sugars (CHO) to produce energy in the form of adenosine triphosphate (ATP). The chemical byproducts of cellular metabolism are carbon dioxide and water. Respiratory physiology is, consequently, a complex event that involves four distinct phases:

- *Ventilation*—movement of air between body and environment and distribution of air within the tracheobronchial tree to alveoli
- *Alveolar diffusion and perfusion*—gas exchange across the alveolar-capillary membrane into the pulmonary blood supply
- *Transportation of respiratory gases*—the movement of oxygen and carbon dioxide through the circulatory system to peripheral tissues, and back across the alveolar-capillary membrane
- *Control of ventilation*—the neuromuscular and chemical regulation of air movement to maintain adequate gas exchange in response to changing metabolic demands

Each of these four phases is addressed in this chapter.

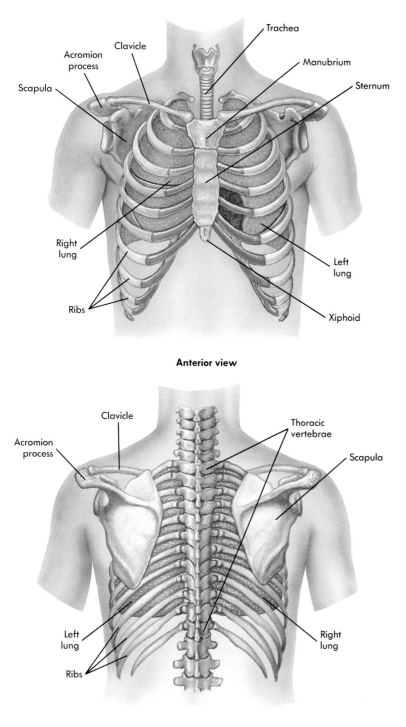

Anterior view

Posterior view

FIGURE 1-1
Skeletal structures of the chest.

VENTILATION

Ventilation is the mechanical process of moving air into and out of the lungs to deliver oxygen to the alveoli, where gas exchange occurs, and to expel carbon dioxide. The muscles of respiration must exert enough force to overcome resistance in the respiratory system to move the chest wall and expand the lungs. The volume of air entering the respiratory system is determined by anatomic properties of the chest wall, thoracic cavity, upper airways, and lower airways.

CHEST WALL

The bony structures of the chest form a protective, expandable cage around the lungs and heart (Figure 1-1). The ribs attach to the sternum with costal cartilage, allowing the rib cage to expand and providing a substantial degree of elasticity to the chest wall.

In adults the transverse diameter of the chest is normally greater than the anteroposterior diameter (see Figure 2-3, page 24). At birth these two dimensions are roughly the same, giving the newborn's chest a round appearance. The chest and head circumference are about equal until age 2 years. The chest wall is more cartilaginous in infants and young children, often with a more prominent xiphoid process. The anteroposterior diameter of the chest wall is often increased in older adults, even those who have normal respiratory function. This change evolves from loss of muscle strength in the thorax and diaphragm and an increased dorsal curve of the thoracic spine.

The muscles of ventilation are shown in Figure 1-2. Inspiration, the active phase of ventilation, is initiated by contractions of the primary muscles of ventilation—the diaphragm and intercostal muscles. When the work of breathing increases, accessory muscles—the scalene, sternocleidomastoid, and abdominal muscles—actively assist respiration.

Expiration during quiet breathing is a passive event resulting from lung recoil. When movement of air out of the lungs is impeded, expiration becomes active. Table 1-1 describes the muscle physiology of ventilation.

• • •

Respiratory distress is often immediately evident from the appearance of the chest wall and exaggerations or aberrations in respiratory patterns. Chronic hyperinflation causes a barrel chest appearance characterized by enlarged anteroposterior diameter, a rib angle that is more horizontal, a prominent sternal angle, and a kyphotic spine. It is the hallmark of long-standing pulmonary disorders, particularly asthma, emphysema, and cystic fibrosis, and is accompanied by prolonged expiration and diaphragmatic depression.

Use of accessory muscles during rest is associated with several acute and chronic pulmonary disorders. Marked retraction of the intercostal muscles and prominent contraction of the sternocleidomastoid muscles are often seen in acute respiratory distress.

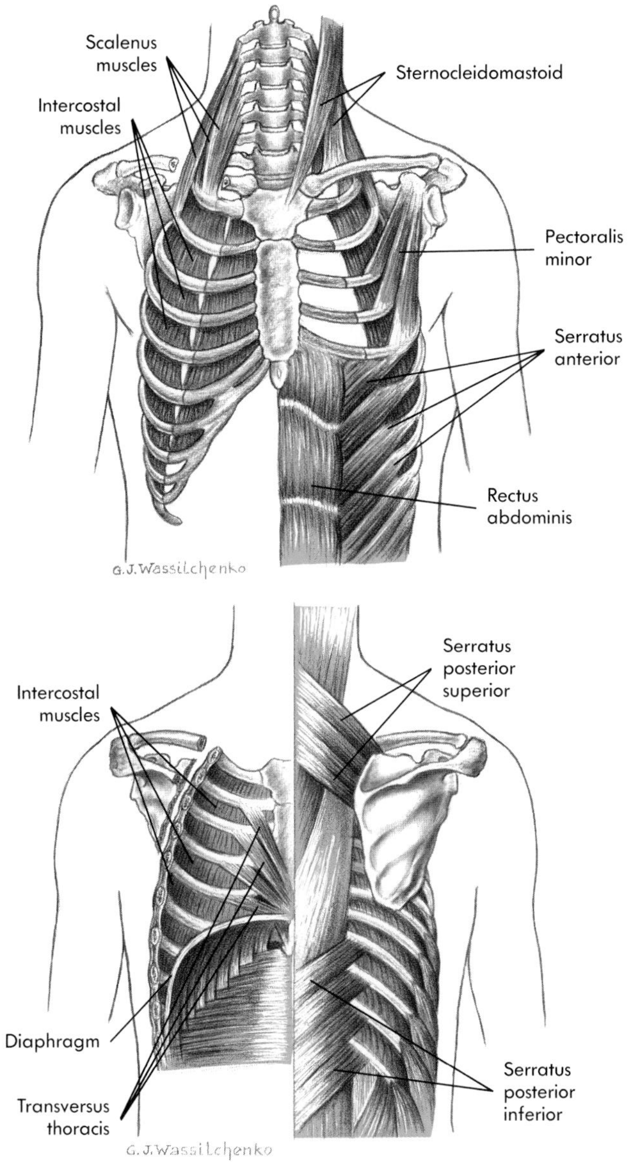

FIGURE 1-2
Muscles of the chest.

Table 1-1 ⎯⎯

MUSCLES OF RESPIRATION

	Action	Result
Quiet Breathing	Diaphragm begins contraction	Lower ribs rise up and out to increase transverse and lateral intrathoracic space.
	Diaphragm completes contraction	Diaphragm moves downward 3-5 cm (from 10th-12th rib) and compresses abdomen.
	External intercostals contract	Increases anteroposterior diameter of thoracic cavity.
	Internal intercostals contract	Decreases transverse diameter of rib cage.
Increased Effort Breathing	Scalene muscles contract	Elevates 1st and 2nd ribs during inspiration to enlarge upper thorax and stabilize chest wall.
	Sternocleidomastoid muscles contract	Elevates sternum during inspiration and slightly enlarges thoracic cavity.
	Abdominal muscles contract	Compresses lower ribs to assist forced expiration.

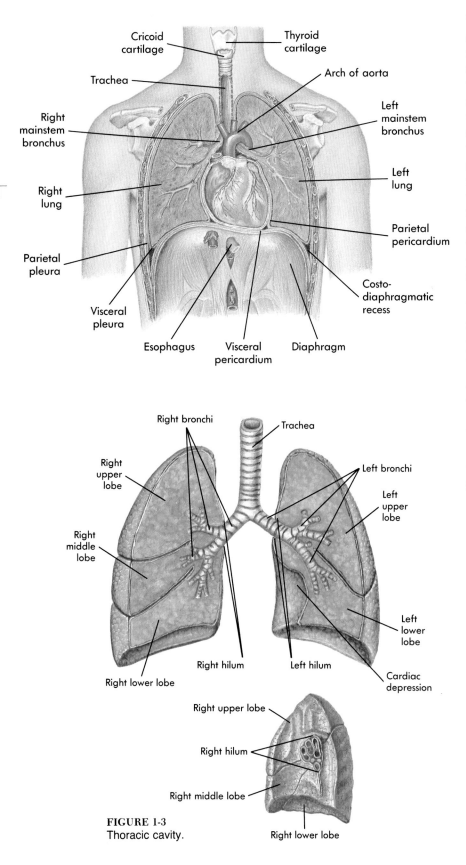

Cricoid cartilage
Thyroid cartilage
Trachea
Arch of aorta
Right mainstem bronchus
Left mainstem bronchus
Right lung
Left lung
Parietal pleura
Parietal pericardium
Visceral pleura
Costo-diaphragmatic recess
Esophagus
Visceral pericardium
Diaphragm

Right bronchi
Trachea
Right upper lobe
Left bronchi
Left upper lobe
Right middle lobe
Right hilum
Left hilum
Right lower lobe
Left lower lobe
Cardiac depression

Right upper lobe
Right hilum
Right middle lobe
Right lower lobe

FIGURE 1-3
Thoracic cavity.

THORACIC CAVITY

The thoracic cavity is divided into right and left pleural cavities separated by the mediastinum (Figure 1-3). The **mediastinum** is the centrally located area, containing the heart, aorta, major blood vessels, lower trachea, large bronchi, part of the esophagus, thymus, lymph nodes, and numerous major nerves, including the phrenic nerve, the cardiac and splanchnic branches of the sympathetic nervous system, and the laryngeal and vagus branches of the parasympathetic nervous system. At the center of the mediastinum are the right and left **hilum** where the mainstem bronchi and the pulmonary vessels enter the lungs (Figure 1-3).

Lining each pleural cavity is a two-layered membrane, the **pleura**, that forms a closed protective sac surrounding each lung. The visceral, or pulmonary, layer lines the outer wall of each lung, and the parietal pleura lines the chest wall and upper surface of the diaphragm. The visceral and parietal pleurae join at the hilum to form a sheath around the bronchi. Serous lubricating film in the space between the pleural layers permits them to slide together without friction, facilitating lung movement.

The lungs fill the pleural cavities, extending to about 4 cm above the first rib anteriorly and to the level of the first thoracic vertebra (T1) posteriorly. Their medial surface is concave, forming a cradle around the mediastinum. On deep inspiration the lower lung borders descend to about T12 and on forced expiration rise to about T10 (Figure 1-4).

• • •

Increased pressure within the thoracic cavity can interfere with lung expansion. This can result from pleural effusion, hemothorax or pneumothorax, empyema, pulmonary edema, or space-occupying lesions within the thoracic cavity.

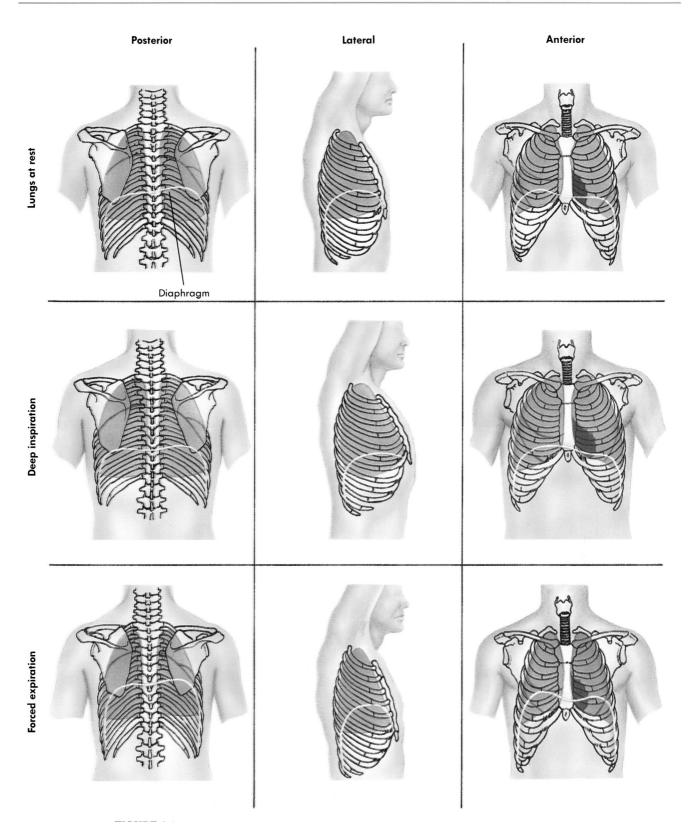

Posterior   Lateral   Anterior

Lungs at rest

Diaphragm

Deep inspiration

Forced expiration

FIGURE 1-4
Movement of the lungs during rest, deep inspiration, and forced expiration. The lung tissue is drawn as transparent here to show the movement of the diaphragm (white line) during the three phases of respiration. As the diaphragm moves the inner portion of the lung tissue follows the movement of the diaphragm, while the outer portion of the lung falls below the diaphragm.

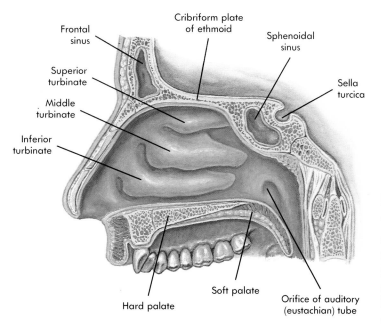

FIGURE 1-5
Cross-section of the nose and nasopharynx.

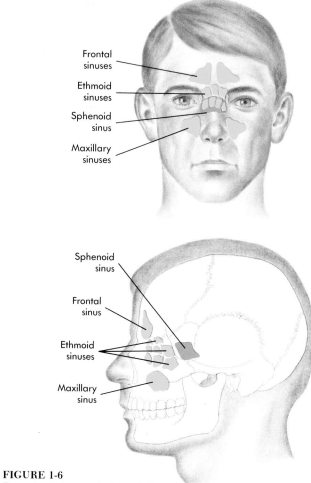

FIGURE 1-6
Paranasal sinuses in the adult.

UPPER AIRWAY STRUCTURES

Nasal passages
Sinuses
Pharynx
Larynx
Upper trachea

UPPER AIRWAY

The upper airway consists of the nasal passages and sinuses, pharynx, larynx, and upper trachea. In addition to conducting air to the lower airway, the primary functions of the upper airway are to protect the lower airway from foreign material and to warm, filter, and humidify inspired air. Both tasks are aided by a mucous membrane made of pseudostratified ciliated epithelium that lines all upper airway structures. In the nose, sinuses, and part of the pharynx this membrane is primarily columnar, changing to squamous cells in the pharynx. Goblet cells throughout the epithelium produce debris-trapping mucus, which drains into the nasopharynx for swallowing or expectoration (see Figure 1-11).

Nasal Passages

Air enters the nares, passes over the coarse nasal hairs (vibrissae) lining the vestibules, and enters the nasopharynx. The cribriform plate at the roof of the nose houses sensory endings of the olfactory nerve. Numerous small, fragile arteries and veins intertwine through the mucous membrane.

The curved **turbinates,** which form the lateral walls of the nasal passages, provide a larger surface area in which to warm, humidify, and filter inspired air (Figure 1-5). Each turbinate has a meatus for drainage into the nose. The nasolacrimal duct drains into the inferior turbinate meatus, while the paranasal sinuses drain into the medial and superior turbinate meatus.

In addition to the olfactory nerve, the nose is innervated by sensory fibers of the trigeminal nerve.

Paranasal Sinuses

The hollow, paired, but rarely symmetric sinuses (Figure 1-6) produce additional mucus for the nasal passages. Drainage from the maxillary and frontal sinuses is through the medial meatuses. The ethmoid sinuses open into both the medial and superior meatus, and the sphenoid sinuses drain into the superior meatus. The paranasal sinuses also provide resonance during vocalization and lighten the weight of the skull.

At birth the maxillary and ethmoid sinuses are present but are quite small. Frontal sinuses form by age 7 or 8 years, and the sphenoid sinuses develop completely by puberty.

Only the maxillary and frontal sinuses are directly accessible for examination, because the ethmoid sinuses lie behind the frontal sinuses, and the sphenoid sinuses are posterior to the ethmoids.

Pharynx

The pharynx is about 13 cm long and is divided into three parts (Figure 1-7). The entire area contains numerous sensory fibers from the glossopharyngeal and facial nerves.

The **nasopharynx** lies directly behind the nasal cavities and is connected to the nose by two posterior nares. Two eustachian tubes lead from the middle ear into the nasopharynx. Near these openings are clusters of lymphoid tissue that make up the adenoids, or pharyngeal tonsils. At birth the nasopharynx is covered with columnar ciliated epithelium, but after age 10 years the epithelial cells become stratified and squamous.

The **oropharynx** is the posterior portion of the oral cavity that is visible when the tongue is depressed. Its primary landmarks are the uvula and the soft palate. The oropharynx houses two sets of tonsils: the palatine tonsils in the lateral wall and the lingual tonsils at the base of the tongue.

The **laryngopharynx** opens into the larynx and esophagus. Its main boundaries are the root of the tongue and the hyoid bone. The epiglottis projects upward into the laryngopharynx.

Larynx

The larynx connects the upper airway to the trachea and houses the vocal cords (see Figure 1-7). It is a rigid tube formed by nine cartilages held together with striated muscles and ligaments. The narrowest point in children is the cricoid cartilage, the only portion of the larynx that forms a closed circle.

The leaf-shaped epiglottis cartilage resting atop the hyoid bone is attached in a hinge-like manner to the thyroid cartilage, which is the structure in the larynx. This permits the epiglottis to close over the trachea during swallowing to prevent aspiration of food.

The mucosa lining the larynx is very sensitive to stimulation by foreign particles. Two branches of the vagus nerve innervate the larynx, with the recurrent laryngeal nerve providing motor innervation and the superior laryngeal nerve supplying some motor and all sensory innervation. Stimulation of this latter nerve initiates the cough reflex.

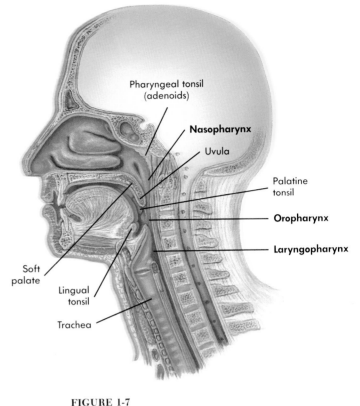

FIGURE 1-7
Cross-section of the pharynx and larynx.

• • •

The hallmark antigenic response in the upper respiratory tract is mucosal edema with increased tissue sensitivity and copious mucus production. This occurs in response to invasion by pathogenic organisms or hypersensitivity to environmental agents. Blockage of the turbinate meatus, particularly the medial meatus, can lead to sinusitis.

Infants and young children are especially susceptible to complications from upper respiratory tract infections. The shorter, more vertical placement of the eustachian tubes in early childhood encourages bacterial transit to the middle ear, resulting in otitis media. Tonsillitis is also most common in young children. Significant edema of the larynx can completely block the airway in children.

Neurologic disorders affecting pharyngeal or laryngeal innervation can interfere with cough, swallow, or gag reflexes and lead to aspiration of food or secretions into the lungs.

The right lung conducts 55% and the left lung 45% of normal lung function.

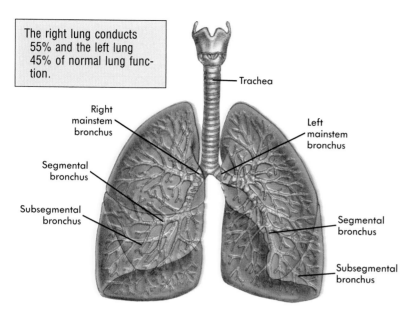

FIGURE 1-8
Trachea and lungs.

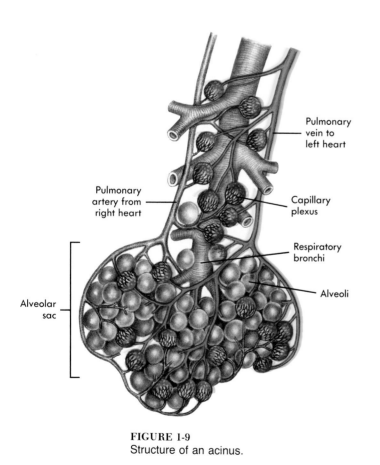

FIGURE 1-9
Structure of an acinus.

LOWER AIRWAY

The lungs are spongy, highly elastic organs. They are paired but not symmetric. The right lung is composed of three lobes and ten bronchopulmonary segments, whereas the left lung has two lobes and nine bronchopulmonary segments.

> **LOWER AIRWAY STRUCTURES**
>
> The lower airway is formed by serial branching, giving it a tree-like shape. The trachea, mainstem bronchi, segmental bronchi, subsegmental bronchioles, terminal bronchioles, and gas exchange units form the lower airway.

Trachea and Bronchi

The trachea and bronchi are made up of C-rings of cartilage held together with fibromuscular tissue (Figure 1-8). Lined with ciliated epithelium interspersed with mucus-producing goblet cells, the cilia sweep foreign particles upward toward the pharynx (see Figure 1-11). The **carina,** located at about the level of T5, marks the point where the trachea divides to form the two mainstem bronchi.

The right mainstem bronchus is about 5 cm shorter than the left bronchus and nearly vertical. In contrast, the left bronchus lies more horizontally. The mainstem bronchi divide into lobar bronchi, 3 on the right and 2 on the left. Within a short distance the lobar bronchi branch into 19 segmental bronchi, 10 on the right and 9 on the left. The segmental bronchi divide to form numerous subsegmental bronchioles.

Bronchioles

The structure of bronchioles differs considerably from that of the larger airways. The bronchioles have no cartilage and the mucosa has no goblet cells or submucosal glands. Rather, the bronchiole comprises a concentric ring of smooth muscle with two sets of muscle fibers. The inner walls are lined with mucosa.

Subsegmental bronchioles end in terminal bronchioles, which conduct air to the alveolar ducts. Terminal bronchioles are lined with epithelium and Clara cells (see Figure 1-11). Together, both lungs contain about 35,000 terminal bronchioles, which further divide into terminal respiratory units (acini) where gas exchange occurs.

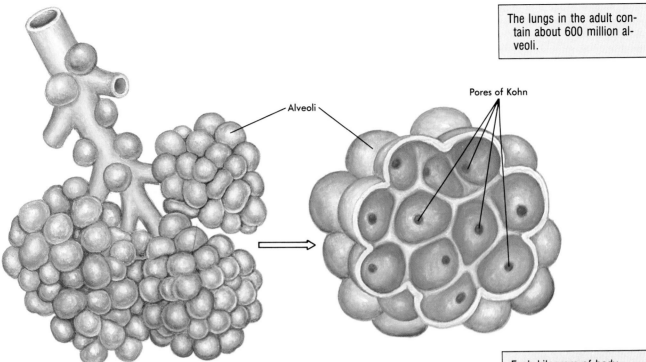

The lungs in the adult contain about 600 million alveoli.

FIGURE 1-10
Structure of alveoli and the pores of Kohn.

Each kilogram of body weight requires about 1 square meter of lung surface to meet the body's metabolic needs. In the average adult, this translates to a lung surface equivalent to a regulation size tennis court.

Gas Exchange Units

Acini, arranged in clusters throughout the lungs, are composed of respiratory bronchioles, alveolar sacs, and alveoli (terminal air sacs) (Figure 1-9). Each acinus has a network of pulmonary arteries and veins. A flattened, one-cell-thick layer of epithelium covers the surface of the acini.

The **alveolar sacs** (Figure 1-10) are formed by a five-layered epithelial membrane containing type II cells. These specialized cells secrete **surfactant**, a lipoprotein that coats the membrane surface to decrease the surface tension of the alveoli so the lungs can inflate easily. The alveolar membrane forms the division between the alveolar space and the pulmonary capillary.

Tiny openings called the **pores of Kohn** connect the alveoli (Figure 1-10). These pores allow even air distribution throughout the acinus so all alveoli have the same gas concentration. Consequently, these pores also provide collateral ventilation if a small airway becomes obstructed.

• • •

Aspiration of foreign particles into the right lung is more common, owing to the nearly vertical position of the right mainstem bronchus. The smaller airways of the lower respiratory tract are easily obstructed by accumulations of mucus or foreign particles. Constriction of the bronchioles, as occurs in asthma, narrows the airways and compromises ventilation. If production of surfactant is insufficient or absent, as occurs in hyaline membrane disease and adult respiratory distress syndrome, the alveolar sacs fail to inflate.

HISTOLOGY OF THE RESPIRATORY TRACT

The epithelium of the respiratory tract has different characteristics (Figure 1-11). Mucosa lining most of the upper respiratory tract and large airways of the lower respiratory tract consists of three layers—the epithelium, the basement membrane, and the lamina propria.

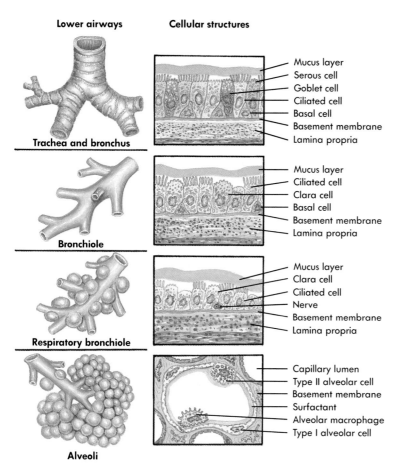

Lower airways

Trachea and bronchus

Bronchiole

Respiratory bronchiole

Alveoli

Cellular structures

Mucus layer
Serous cell
Goblet cell
Ciliated cell
Basal cell
Basement membrane
Lamina propria

Mucus layer
Ciliated cell
Clara cell
Basal cell
Basement membrane
Lamina propria

Mucus layer
Clara cell
Ciliated cell
Nerve
Basement membrane
Lamina propria

Capillary lumen
Type II alveolar cell
Basement membrane
Surfactant
Alveolar macrophage
Type I alveolar cell

FIGURE 1-11
Cellular anatomy of the respiratory airway.

The **epithelial layer** contains several cell types, most notably ciliated pseudostratified epithelial cells, goblet cells, and Clara cells. The ciliated cells, which propel secretions out of the respiratory tract, appear in the large airways on columnar epithelium and in small airways on cuboidal epithelium. Goblet cells, found on columnar epithelium in larger airways, synthesize and secrete mucus. Clara cells are located in cuboidal epithelium of distal small airways. Although their exact purpose is uncertain, they are thought to be at least one source of fluid lining the small airways.

The **basement membrane** (mucociliary membrane) traps airborne particles between 2 and 10 μm in diameter, transporting them to the pharynx for expulsion. Particles making it to the smaller airways are trapped on a ciliated mucus blanket that is 95% water and coats the airway surface. The bottom watery layer is in direct contact with the epithelium and cleans the cilia. The top gel layer consists of streams of mucus that trap the particles. The mucus blanket propels debris upward at a velocity of 10 to 20 mm per minute.

The **lamina propria** contains lymphocytes, plasma cells, occasional polymorphonuclear leukocytes, and numerous mast cells. Mast cells release histamine in antigen-antibody reactions seen in asthma and allergic reactions. Lymphoid nodules scattered at intervals throughout the tracheobronchial tree are thought to be involved in a number of immune responses occurring in the lung, including the production of immunoglobulin A (IgA).

THE PROCESS OF VENTILATION

In addition to mechanical properties of ventilation, two other processes affect ventilation: (1) respiratory pressures and surface tension and (2) lung compliance.

Respiratory Pressures and Surface Tension

Thoracic expansion occurs normally as a result of muscle contraction and rib cage expansion. To facilitate lung expansion, pressure inside the pleural cavity is maintained below 760 mm Hg, the normal atmospheric pressure. Intrapleural pressure between respirations is approximately 755 mm Hg, dropping to about 751 mm Hg with thoracic expansion. This slightly negative atmospheric pressure is enough to draw air into the lungs.

The alveoli must maintain a high surface tension to promote gas exchange (Figure 1-12). However, the alveoli have a tendency to collapse and pull away from the chest wall at high surface tensions. To counteract this, **surfactant** between the membrane and air inside the alveolar sacs decreases the surface tension and promotes even gas distribution throughout the alveoli. As a result, lung inflation is accomplished with greater ease.

Lung Compliance

Compliance is the degree of elasticity or expansibility of the lungs and thorax. It is measured by plethysmography, in which the inspired or expired gas volume and the intrapleural pressure are determined. Generally, when the intrapleural pressure is increased by 1 cm of water, the lung volume increases 130 ml. Any condition that impedes lung contraction and expansion causes a decrease in compliance. (See Plethysmography, page 40, for details.)

• • •

A break in the pleural layers, as occurs in pneumothorax, increases respiratory pressure and leads to poor pulmonary inflation or lung collapse. Increased surface tension from inadequate production

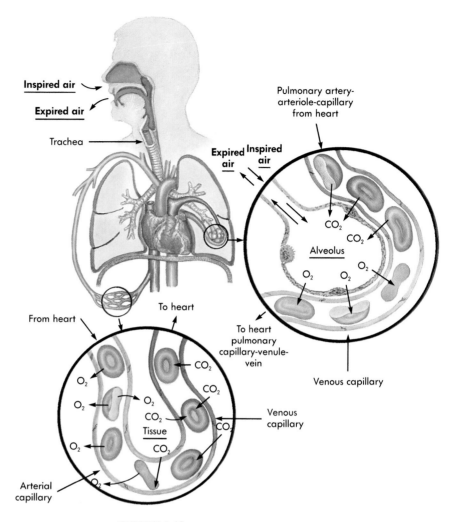

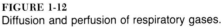

FIGURE 1-12
Diffusion and perfusion of respiratory gases.

of surfactant also causes poor lung inflation.

Decreased lung compliance may occur from poor lung contraction or expansion, such as occurs in disorders that destroy lung tissue, causing it to become fibrotic or edematous or to block the bronchioles. Reduced thoracic cage expansibility from kyphosis, severe scoliosis, fibrotic pleurisy, or muscle paralysis also reduces lung compliance. Increased lung compliance occurs with chronic obstructive pulmonary disease when alveoli lose their elasticity.

ALVEOLAR DIFFUSION AND PULMONARY PERFUSION

Once inspired air reaches the alveoli, gas exchange occurs at the alveolar-capillary membrane: oxygen from the alveolar space crosses the membrane and enters the pulmonary arterial system, and carbon dioxide from the pulmonary veins crosses the membrane and enters the alveolar space.

Exchange of respiratory gases involves two components: alveolar diffusion and pulmonary perfusion. Pulmonary function tests measure various aspects of diffusion and perfusion. Arterial blood gas measurements provide information on the efficiency of ventilation, diffusion, and perfusion.

NORMAL VALUES FOR ARTERIAL BLOOD GASES

PO_2	90 ± 10 mm Hg
O_2 saturation	96% + 1%
PCO_2	40 + 3 mm Hg
pH	7.4 + 0.03
Bicarbonate	22-26 mEq/L

ALVEOLAR DIFFUSION

Diffusion is defined as a movement of molecules from an area of higher concentration to one of lower concentration. It is the process by which gas transfer occurs between the alveolus and the capillary. Alveolar diffusion is determined by several variables:

- Total surface area of alveolar-capillary membranes in the lung
- Thickness of the alveolar-capillary membrane
- Alveolar-capillary gradient, which is the difference in partial pressures of the gases on either side of the membrane
- Diffusion coefficient, which is the measure of a gas's ability to diffuse and depends on the properties of a particular gas

The rate of gas transfer is affected by changes in these variables. Gas transfer slows if the alveolar-capillary membrane surface area is decreased, if the thickness of this membrane is increased, if the alveolar-capillary gradient is decreased, or if the concentration of one gas (such as oxygen) is decreased.

Surface Area

The total alveolar surface for a normal adult is approximately 80 square meters. Pulmonary capillaries cover 85% to 90% of this surface, giving a 70 square meter surface area that is available for gas diffusion. Any reduction in the surface area, as occurs with emphysema or removal of a lobe, reduces the overall diffusing capacity of the lung.

Membrane Thickness

The alveolar-capillary interface is normally a one-cell-thick, semipermeable membrane. This membrane becomes thickened and less permeable when the lung tissues become fibrotic as a result of chronic pulmonary conditions. Consequently, gas exchange is inhibited and diffusing capacity is decreased.

Partial Pressures

Partial pressure of a gas is the relationship between the concentration of that gas in a mixture and the total pressure of the mixture. Since gas diffuses from an area of high pressure to an area of low pressure, respiratory gases cross the alveolar-capillary membrane when partial pressures on the opposite side of the membrane drop (see Figure 1-12).

Diffusion Coefficients

Respiratory gases are present in different concentrations. The concentration of a gas in a mixture affects its rate of diffusion. Diffusion coefficients are the relative number of gas molecules capable of diffusing in a given amount of time compared with other gases in the mixture. It should be stressed that diffusion coefficients are relative values against which other respiratory gases are compared. Diffusion coefficients for respiratory gases are:

Oxygen: 1.0
Carbon dioxide: 20.3
Nitrogen: 0.53

As can be seen by these diffusion coefficients, carbon dioxide has a diffusing capacity 20 times that of oxygen. The standard way of determining diffusing capacity is to measure carbon dioxide diffusing capacity (DL_{CO}).

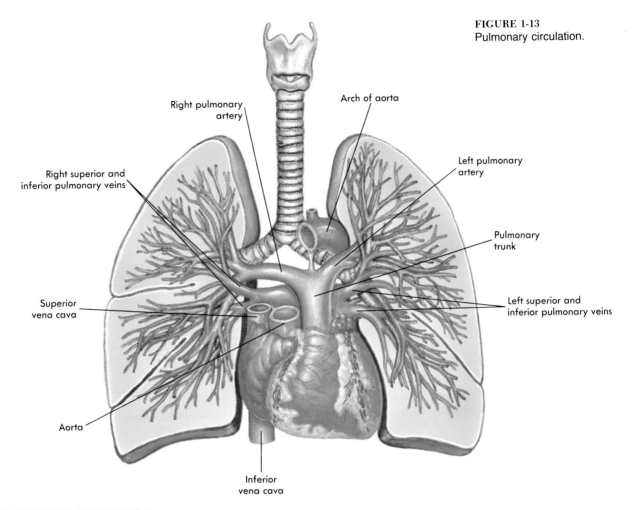

FIGURE 1-13
Pulmonary circulation.

Right pulmonary artery

Arch of aorta

Right superior and inferior pulmonary veins

Left pulmonary artery

Superior vena cava

Pulmonary trunk

Left superior and inferior pulmonary veins

Aorta

Inferior vena cava

PULMONARY PERFUSION

Perfusion is the process of dispersing respiratory gases to a wide area. This is accomplished by the pulmonary circulation, which delivers blood in a thin film to the alveoli so oxygen uptake and carbon dioxide elimination can transpire.

The pulmonary vascular system operates as a high volume, low pressure system. This means a large amount of blood flows through the pulmonary circulation with very low capillary resistance.

Pulmonary circulation (Figure 1-13) begins when carbon dioxide–laden blood is pumped from the right ventricle of the heart into the right and left pulmonary arteries. These arteries quickly branch into the 6 billion alveolar capillaries where gas exchange occurs. After the blood is oxygenated, it enters the four pulmonary veins and returns to the left atrium of the heart.

Pulmonary vascular pressure is very low, only about one-fifth the pressure within systemic vessels. The mean pulmonary artery pressure (PAP), as measured by a pulmonary artery catheter, is normally about 15 mm Hg.

Under normal resting conditions, only about 25% of the pulmonary capillaries are actively perfused. Even with increased cardiac output, PAP remains fairly constant because of two compensatory mechanisms:

- Recruitment—this mechanism decreases pulmonary vascular resistance to accommodate increased blood flow.
- Capillary dilation—this mechanism directly increases capillary size via stimulation of the autonomic nervous system.

Should either of these mechanisms fail, pulmonary hypertension may result.

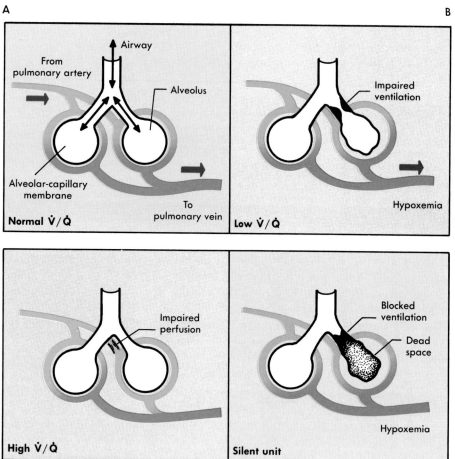

A

B

FIGURE 1-14
Pathologic alterations in ventilation and perfusion.

A, In normal pulmonary function, ventilation matches perfusion.

B, Physiologic shunting occurs when the pulmonary circulation is adequate, but not enough air is available to the alveoli for normal diffusion. As a result, a portion of the blood flowing through the pulmonary vessels does not become oxygenated. This occurs in atelectasis and pneumonia.

C, Alveolar dead space occurs when ventilation is normal, but perfusion of a number of alveoli is reduced or absent. This may occur from inadequate pulmonary circulation to a portion of the lung or from an obstruction that prevents blood from reaching the alveoli. Pulmonary emboli are a common cause of alveolar dead space.

D, Silent units occur in the absence of ventilation and perfusion; neither blood nor oxygen can reach the alveoli. Pulmonary embolism that results in adult respiratory distress syndrome can cause silent unit.

C

D

Ventilation-Perfusion Ratio

Actual gas composition can be determined by the ventilation-perfusion ratio ($\dot{V}/\dot{Q}$). $\dot{V}$ is the volume (liters) of gas per minute, and $\dot{Q}$ is the blood flow volume (liters) per minute. The ideal match between all alveoli and all pulmonary capillaries would yield a $\dot{V}/\dot{Q}$ ratio of 1.0. However, gravity affects perfusion. In the upright position, the lung bases receive a greater volume of blood while the apex receives a greater airflow. Therefore the normal $\dot{V}/\dot{Q}$ ratio is 0.8.

Alveolar dead space, physiologic shunting, and silent unit are common abnormalities in $\dot{V}/\dot{Q}$ ratios and result from defects in ventilation and/or perfusion (Figure 1-14).

TRANSPORT OF RESPIRATORY GASES

Once respiratory gases diffuse across the alveolar membrane, they must be trans-ported to the tissues. In order to understand the importance of blood gas analysis in evaluating respiratory function, one must first understand the basics of oxygen and carbon dioxide transport.

Oxygen

Oxygen is carried in the blood in two ways. A small proportion is dissolved in blood plasma, but most oxygen combines chemically with hemoglobin and serves as a reserve.

The amount of oxygen dissolved in plasma is directly proportional to the partial pressure of oxygen. Exactly 0.003 ml of oxygen dissolves in 100 ml of blood plasma for each 1 mm Hg of partial pressure. Therefore at the ideal Pa_{O_2} of 100 mm Hg, only 0.3 ml of oxygen is present in 100 ml of plasma. The reserve oxygen supply carried by hemoglobin continuously replenishes the plasma oxygen supply, which is used to meet metabolic demands.

In contrast, 60 times that much oxygen is transported by hemoglobin in the average healthy person. The oxygen-hemoglobin bond is loose and reversible. When Po_2 is high, as in the pulmonary capillaries, oxygen combines readily with hemoglobin. At low Po_2, as in the tissue capillaries, oxygen is easily released from the hemoglobin and diffuses into the tissues.

The amount of oxygen in the blood carried by hemoglobin depends on the hemoglobin concentration. The average person has about 15 g of hemoglobin per 100 ml of blood, and each gram of hemoglobin has a maximum oxygen capacity (100% saturation) of 1.34 ml of oxygen. Thus a hemoglobin of 15 g/100 ml has a 100% saturation of 20.1 ml of oxygen.

Actual saturation varies, however, according to the partial pressure. The **oxyhemoglobin dissociation curve** (Figure 1-15) shows the ease with which oxygen dissociates, or leaves, the blood at different partial pressures. There are three important points along this curve: (1) as blood leaves the lungs the Pao_2 is about 100 mm Hg and saturation is 97.5%; (2) on the midpoint where the Pao_2 is 50 mm Hg, saturation is about 84%; (3) normal mixed venous blood (Pvo_2) is about 40 mm Hg with a 75% saturation. Note that between points 1 and 2 there is a 10% saturation change for every 10 mm Hg Po_2 change, whereas between points 2 and 3 a 50 mm Hg change in Po_2 produces only a 13% change in saturation.

The dissociation curve reflects oxygen extraction from the blood. Consequently, shifts in pH, $PaCo_2$, body temperature or 2, 3 DPG cause a shift in the oxyhemoglobin dissociation curve. Figure 1-14 details the shift potential.

CARBON DIOXIDE

The amount of carbon dioxide in transit is one of the major determinants of acid-base balance. Carbon dioxide is carried in the blood in three forms: 7% is dissolved in plasma, 23% is combined with hemoglobin, and 70% is combined with water as carbonic acid. On entering the capillary, carbon dioxide initiates the

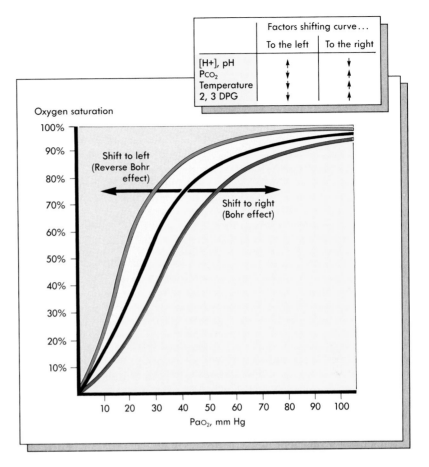

FIGURE 1-15

Oxyhemoglobin dissociation curve. **Shift to the right** indicates the hemoglobin's intrinsic ability to hold on to oxygen has weakened and higher partial pressures are needed for binding. O_2 escapes hemoglobin more easily and is more available to the tissues. This shift is produced by decreased pH, rise in $Paco_2$, and increased temperature or by prolonged hypoxia. **Normal curve** occurring at blood pH 7.4, normal $Paco_2$, and body temperature at 37° C. **Shift to the left** indicates hemoglobin and oxygen are bound too tightly and, although less pressure is needed for binding, the molecules separate with difficulty at the cellular level. O_2 is less available to the tissues. This shift is produced by increased pH, decreased $PaCO_2$, and decrease in temperature. It can also occur with prolonged hypoxia in which 2, 3-diphosphoglycerate (DPG) increases inside the red blood cells.

following variety of physical and chemical reactions:

- CO_2 dissolved in the plasma and red blood cell reacts with water to form carbonic acid (H_2CO_3). This reaction is catalyzed by the enzyme carbonic anhydrase.
- H_2CO_3 within the red blood cell dissociates into hydrogen (H^+) and bicarbonate (HCO_3^-).
- H^+ then combines with hemoglobin (Hgb), a powerful acid-base buffer, in the red cell.
- Many of the HCO_3^- ions diffuse into the plasma in exchange for chloride (Cl^-)

ions. This exchange is possible because of a bicarbonate-chloride carrier protein in the red cell membrane that moves the two ions in opposite directions.

- CO_2 loosely bonds to Hgb to form carbamino hemoglobin ($HgbCO_2$). This reaction is quickly reversible so that CO_2 is easily released in the alveoli.

As with oxygen, carbon dioxide extraction is expressed in a dissociation curve. The carbon dioxide dissociation curve is the relationship between $Paco_2$ and the entire blood content of CO_2. Because it is influenced by oxygen saturation (SO_2) changes from arterial to venous blood, carbon dioxide dissociation is shown as two curves. The true physiologic dissociation curve probably lies somewhere between these two curves.

ACID-BASE BALANCE

Acid-base balance is the ratio between carbonic acid and bicarbonate. For normal function, body fluid must maintain a hydrogen ion concentration, or pH, within a very narrow range. Normal blood pH relies on a bicarbonate to dissolved carbon dioxide ratio of 20:1. A pH lower than the normal range of 7.35 to 7.45 causes the blood to become more acidic, leading to acidemia, and a higher pH causes alkalemia.

Acid-base balance is maintained by respiration, renal function, and a set of buffering mechanisms that prevent an excessive rise or fall in the H^+ concentration. The respiratory system regulates H^+ by determining the carbon dioxide concentration. Several intracellular buffering systems regulate the rate of breakdown of protein and phosphates, which in turn regulate H^+. However, the most important buffering system is the bicarbonate-carbonic acid system of the plasma. Since the extracellular bicarbonate-carbonic buffer is in equilibrium with the intracellular systems, arterial blood gas pH provides adequate information about all buffers in the body.

• • •

Four distinct abnormalities can arise when the acid-base balance is upset: respiratory acidosis, respiratory alkalosis, metabolic acidosis, and metabolic alkalosis. The first two disorders are caused by ventilatory dysfunction. In the latter two disorders, the respiratory system attempts to compensate for the altered pH.

ACID-BASE ABNORMALITIES

Disorder	pH	Initiating event	Compensatory effect
Respiratory acidosis	↓	↑ $Paco_2$	↑ HCO_3^-
Respiratory alkalosis	↑	↓ $Paco_2$	↓ HCO_3^-
Metabolic acidosis	↓	↓ HCO_3^-	↓ Pco_2
Metabolic alkalosis	↑	↑ HCO_3^-	↑ Pco_2

Respiratory acidosis is caused by alveolar hypoventilation secondary to cardiopulmonary, neuromuscular, skeletal, or obstructive lung disease; to acute infections; or to drug-induced respiratory depression. In attempting to compensate for the elevated $Paco_2$, excess H^+ is excreted in the urine in exchange for bicarbonate ions. Plasma bicarbonate levels rise to help restore normal blood pH. For this reason, $Paco_2$ may continue to be elevated after the pH returns to normal.

Respiratory alkalosis is caused by alveolar hyperventilation as a result of hyperventilation from anxiety, brain injury or brain tumors, gram-negative sepsis, or improper management of patients on a ventilator. Compensatory mechanisms are aimed at increasing renal excretion of bicarbonate and retention of hydrogen ions. These mechanisms lower blood bicarbonate levels and restore normal pH.

Metabolic acidosis is caused by either increased levels of metabolic acids or excessive excretion of bicarbonate in body fluids. Elevated metabolic acids can result from salicylate poisoning, renal failure, diabetic ketoacidosis, or circulatory failure that produces a build-up of lactic acids. Chronic persistent diarrhea can produce excessive bicarbonate loss. Regardless of the cause, the body enlists bicarbonate ions as an intracellular buffer, thus depleting bicarbonate levels in plasma. The compensatory mechanisms are increased ventilation and renal retention of bicarbonate.

Metabolic alkalosis is caused by increased levels of bicarbonate resulting from excessive base intake (as may occur if too much bicarbonate is given during cardiopulmonary resuscitation) or from excessive H^+ loss through vomiting or gastric suction. The respiratory system compensates by decreasing ventilation to conserve CO_2 and raise $Paco_2$. The kidneys increase excretion of bicarbonate ions to conserve H^+.

THE ACIDOSIS AND ALKALOSIS PROCESSES

	Initial Cause	Buffering	Compensation
ACIDOSIS		$(CO_2 + H_2O = H_2CO_3 = H^+ + HCO_3^-)$	

Respiratory acidosis	↑P_{CO_2}	Reaction moves to right to handle excess CO_2* ↑HCO_3^-	Lungs
			   Elimination of CO_2
			Kidneys
			   Elimination of H^+; HCO_3^- conserved (the higher the P_{CO_2}, the more HCO_3^- reabsorbed)

Metabolic acidosis	↓ Base
	↑ Fixed acids
		Reaction moves to the left to handle excess H^+ ↓HCO_3^-	Lungs
			   Elimination of CO_2
			Kidneys
			   Conserve HCO_3^- (the lower the H_2CO_3, the more HCO_3^- conserved)

ALKALOSIS		$(CO_2 + H_2O = H_2CO_3 = H^+ + HCO_3^-)$	
Respiratory alkalosis	↓P_{CO_2}	Movement to left to form more CO_2† ↓HCO_3^-	Kidneys Conservation of H^+ HCO_3^- excretion (the lower the P_{CO_2}, the less HCO_3^- reabsorbed)

Metabolic alkalosis	↑ Base
	↓ Fixed acids
		Movement to right to form more H^+ to offset increased base HCO_3^- ↑	Lungs
			   ↓ Ventilation to ↑P_{CO_2}
			Kidneys
			   Conserve H^+ by excreting HCO_3^- (the higher the plasma HCO_3^-, the greater

From Harper.[37]

*Movement to the right refers to moving from left side of the above equation to the right side, therefore decreasing CO_2 production.

†Movement to the left refers to moving from the right side of the above equation to the left side, therefore increasing CO_2 production.

NEURAL CONTROL OF VENTILATION

The mechanisms that control ventilation are complex and not well understood. Because much of the present knowledge is derived from experience with central nervous system abnormalities, some aspects of normal control of ventilation are speculative. Figure 1-16 shows the basic respiratory control pathways.

Ventilation is conducted primarily by the autonomic nervous system. Higher areas of the cerebral cortex can override autonomic ventilatory control, but only to a limited extent. Although breathing can be regulated consciously, safety mechanisms are in place that will interrupt detrimental patterns. For example, holding the breath too long results in loss of consciousness, allowing the autonomic system to reinstate control.

The brain houses at least three primary respiratory centers, one in the medulla oblongata and two in the pons. Chemoreceptors are located in the medulla and among peripheral stimulators. Neural reflexes transmit impulses in an organized manner to coordinate and respond to neural signals.

MEDULLARY CENTER

The respiratory center in the medulla functions as "control central" for ventilation and is the final determinant of breathing patterns. It receives data continuously from sensory, gas exchange, and chemical units throughout the body. It coordinates this information to determine respiratory needs. Finally, it sends nerve impulses to two subcenters within the medulla. The medullary inspiratory subcenter and the medullary expiratory subcenter are responsible for forwarding nerve impulses to the muscles that control breathing.

PONS CENTERS

The two respiratory areas of the pons are the apneustic and the pneumotaxic centers. The apneustic, or pontine, center is located in the lower portion of the pons. Apneusis is a condition of stopping ventilation in the inspiratory position. The apneustic center is controlled by the pneumotaxic center and the inflation reflexes (Figure 1-16). Diseases of the pons may lead to abnormal stimulation of this center, causing apneustic breathing.

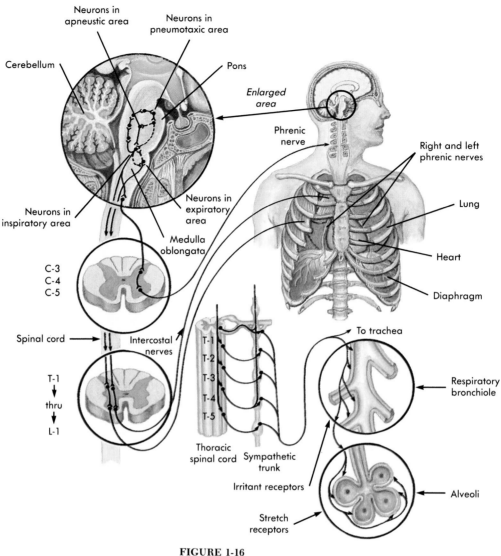

FIGURE 1-16
Neural control of ventilation.

The pneumotaxic center is thought to receive impulses from the medullary inspiratory subcenter and transmit these impulses to the medullary expiratory subcenter, thus limiting inspiration.

CHEMORECEPTORS

Respiratory chemoreceptors are groups of nerve cells that can distinguish between concentrations of hydrogen ions and oxygen. As either gas crosses their membranes and the concentration changes, chemoreceptors send impulses to the medullary center. Chemoreceptors exert the greatest influence on the autonomic nervous system's control of ventilation by correlating acid-base balance with gas exchange requirements.

The medullar, or central, chemoreceptors are the primary receptors involved in the control of ventilation. Peripheral chemoreceptors are located in the various areas, including the carotid arteries and the arch of the aorta.

INFLATION REFLEXES

Neuroreceptors in the lung include stretch and irritant receptors that detect mechanical changes in the lung. Stimulation of the bronchiolar or alveolar walls initiates the inflation reflex, commonly called the **Hering-Breuer reflex.** The inflation reflex sends impulses from the lung to the apneustic center via the vagus nerve. This reflex limits inhalation and aids the medullary center in establishing a smooth combination of ventilation rate and tidal volume. The right and left phrenic nerves innervate the diaphragm, the primary muscles of respiration. The intercostal nerves innervate the intercostal muscles that provide lateral movement of the thorax. These are shown in Figure 1-16.

CHAPTER 2

Assessment

Evaluation of the patient with respiratory problems begins with the patient's history and proceeds to a systematic examination of the upper airways, lungs, and respiratory patterns. Both the patient and the examiner should be relaxed; taking time to allow the patient to relax helps ensure a comprehensive assessment.

HISTORY

The nursing interview serves three purposes: (1) to determine the patient's chief complaint, (2) to discover elements in the patient's history that relate to the present problem, and (3) to observe the patient for clues to his or her health and emotional status. The interview also provides an excellent opportunity to establish rapport with the patient. Awareness of nonverbal communication during the interview process can expand the nurse's understanding of the patient considerably.

Obtaining a complete history from patients who are in respiratory distress often requires patience. The nurse may need to collect data during several visits or allow for periods of rest for patients who become dyspneic during the interview.

The patient's chief complaint is best elicited by asking direct questions such as "What has brought you here?" or "What is bothering you?" The response should be recorded in the patient's own words. The examiner should then determine when the symptoms first started. The nature of the complaint will direct the nurse's line of questioning. Complete information should be requested by specific questions to determine the exact nature of the symptoms, including cough, sputum production, aggravating symptoms, shortness of breath, and location, quality, and intensity of pain. A complete history should be obtained, with particular attention to potential causes or aggravating factors, medical history relating to respiratory problems, and related family history.

HEALTH HISTORY

Chief complaint
Cough

Onset and duration
  Sudden or gradual
  Episodic or continuous
Characteristics
  Dry or wet
  Hacking, hoarse, barking, or congested
  Productive or nonproductive
Sputum
  Present or absent
  Frequency of production
  Appearance—color (clear, mucoid, purulent, blood-
    tinged, mostly bloody), foul odor, frothy, amount
Pattern
  Paroxysmal
  Related to time of day, weather, activities, talking, or
    deep breathing
  Change over time
Severity
  Causes fatigue
  Disrupts sleep or conversation
  Produces chest pain
Associated symptoms
  Shortness of breath
  Chest pain or tightness with breathing
  Fever
  Upper respiratory tract signs (sore throat, congestion,
    increased mucus production)
  Noisy respirations or hoarseness
  Gagging or choking
  Anxiety, stress, or panic reactions
Efforts to treat
  Prescription or nonprescription drugs
  Vaporizers
  Effective or ineffective

Shortness of breath (SOB) or dyspnea on exertion (DOE)

Onset and duration
  Sudden or gradual
  Gagging or choking episode a few days before onset
Pattern
  Related to position—improves when sitting up or with
    head elevated; number of pillows used to alleviate
    problem
  Related to activity—exercise or eating; extent of activ-
    ity that produces dyspnea
  Related to other factors—time of day, season, or expo-
    sure to something in the environment
  Harder to inhale or harder to exhale
Severity
  Extent activity is limited
  Breathing itself causes fatigue
  Anxiety about getting enough air
Associated symptoms
  Pain or discomfort—exact location in respiratory tree
  Cough, diaphoresis, swelling of ankles, or cyanosis
Efforts to treat
  Prescription or nonprescription drugs
  Oxygen
  Effective or ineffective

HEALTH HISTORY

Chief complaint—cont'd

Chest pain

Onset and duration
  Gradual or sudden
  Associated with trauma, coughing, or lower respiratory
    tract infection
Associated symptoms
  Shallow breathing
  Uneven chest expansion
  Fever
  Cough
  Radiation of pain to neck or arms
  Anxiety about getting enough air
Efforts to treat
  Heat, splinting, or pain medication
  Effective or ineffective

Patient's perception of the problem

Degree of concern about the symptoms
Opinion of its cause

Patient history: factors relating to respiratory disorders
(causes or aggravating factors)

Tobacco use—both present and past
  Type of tobacco—cigarettes, cigars, pipes, or smoke-
    less
  Duration and amount—age started, inhale when smok-
    ing, amount used in the past and present
  Pack years—number of packs per day multiplied by
    number of years patient has smoked
  Efforts to quit—previous attempts and current interest
Work environment
  Nature of work
  Environmental hazards: chemicals, vapors, dust, pul-
    monary irritants, or allergens
  Use of protective devices
Home environment
  Location
  Possible allergens: pets, house plants, plants and trees
    outside the home, or other environmental hazards
  Type of heating
  Use of air conditioning or humidifier
  Ventilation
  Stairs to climb

Medical history

Infectious respiratory diseases
  Strep throat
  Mumps
  Tonsillitis
Thoracic trauma or surgery
Previous diagnosis of pulmonary disorders—dates of hos-
  pitalization
Chronic pulmonary diseases—date, treatment, and com-
  pliance with therapy
  Tuberculosis
  Bronchitis
  Emphysema
  Bronchiectasis
  Asthma
  Cystic fibrosis
  Sinus infection
Other chronic disorders—cardiovascular, cancer, muscu-
  loskeletal, neurologic
  Nasal surgery or injury
  Obstruction of one or both nares
  Mouth breathing often necessary (especially at night)
  History of nasal discharge
Nosebleeds
  Affects one or both nostrils
  Aggravated by crusting
Previous tests
  Allergy testing
  Pulmonary function tests
  Tuberculin and fungal skin tests
  Chest x-rays

Family history

Tuberculosis
Cystic fibrosis
Emphysema
Allergies
Asthma
Atopic dermatitis
Smoking by household members
Malignancy

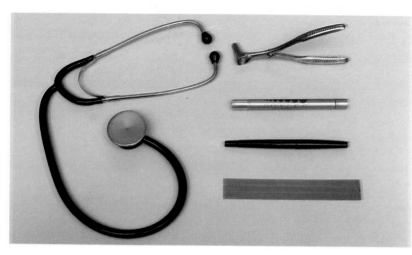

FIGURE 2-1
Equipment for examination of the respiratory system.

THE ENVIRONMENT AND EQUIPMENT

Before starting the physical examination, it is important to ensure the examining room is well-lit, quiet, and private. Natural lighting is necessary to assess subtleties of color and breathing patterns, and a minimal noise level allows the examiner to detect respiratory sounds. Every effort should be made to ensure patient privacy with no interruptions. This encourages the patient to relax and increases the patient's confidence and the examiner's concentration.

Figure 2-1 shows the necessary equipment for conducting an examination of the respiratory system—a stethoscope, nasal speculum, penlight (or small flashlight), marker, and centimeter ruler. The diaphragm of the stethoscope should be covered with the manufacturer's cover, not a piece of x-ray film, and the bell should have a rubber or plastic ring to ensure a secure fit against the chest wall. Thick, stiff, heavy tubing that is between 30.5 and 46 cm (12 to 18 inches) long conducts sound best. The earpiece should fit snugly to occlude ambient sound. For examining infants or small children, a pediatric stethoscope with a small-diameter diaphragm is recommended.

GENERAL EXAMINATION

The physical examination actually begins with the initial interview by observing the patient's general state of health and degree of respiratory distress. Signs of inadequate nutrition or physical abnormalities should be noted. The patient's mental development and emotional state are often obvious by the manner in which the patient responds to the interview.

For evaluation of the chest and lungs, the patient should wear a gown that can be dropped to the waist. Bras and undershirts must be removed.

The examiner should explain at each step in the examination ("Now I am going to look inside your nose") and give clear directions when needed ("Breathe in deeply and hold it"). A calm, matter-of-fact manner can often allay anxiety, even for patients who are in distress.

The examination should be conducted in an organized manner. It includes visual inspection and proceeds to palpation, percussion, and auscultation of the thoracic cage. The upper airway should also be inspected. Any abnormal findings should be described in relation to anatomic and topographic landmarks (Figure 2-2).

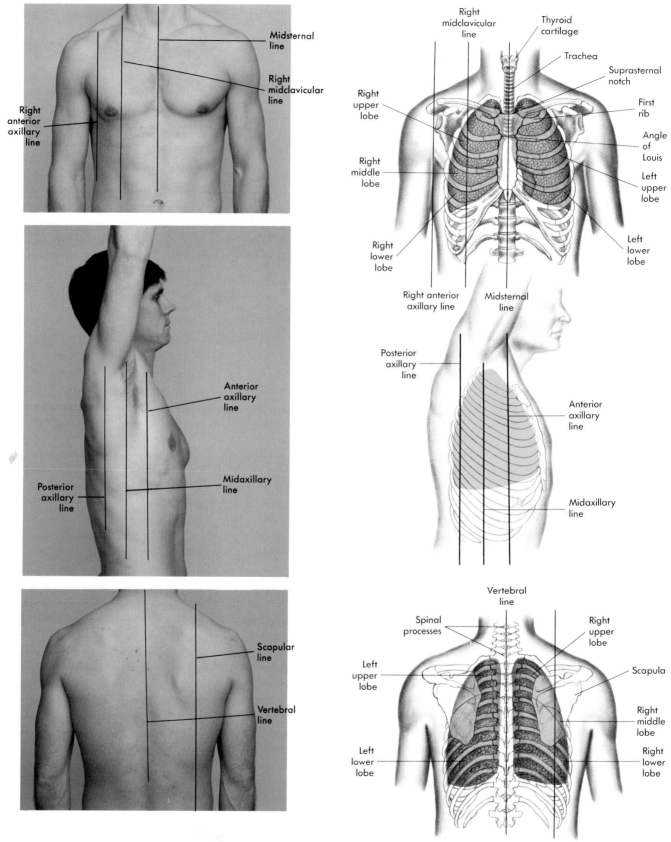

FIGURE 2-2
Anatomic and topographic landmarks of the thorax.

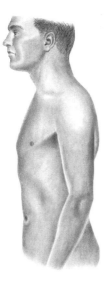

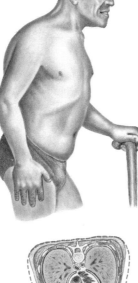

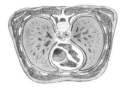

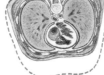

Normal chest of healthy man. Note AP to transverse ratio.

Barrel chest with increased AP diameter.

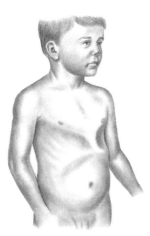

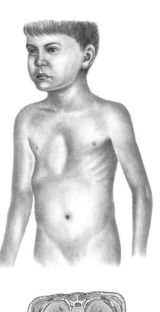

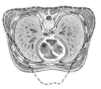

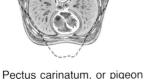

Pectus carinatum, or pigeon chest. Note prominent sternum.

Pectus excavatum, or funnel chest. Note sternum is indented above xiphoid.

FIGURE 2-3
Normal and abnormal chest structures.

INSPECTION

During inspection, the patient should be sitting on the edge of the examination table with the upper body exposed. Stand back and observe the patient's posture and breathing style, noting any breathing difficulties. Inspect the patient from both the front and the back.

> **INSPECTION: NL. FINDINGS**
>
> Symmetric chest expansion, regular respirations
> Men—primarily diaphragmatic breathing
> Women—primarily thoracic or costal breathing
> School-age children—diaphragmatic breathing
> Infants and young children—barrel chest up to age 2 years, Cheyne-Stokes breathing during sleep, abdominal breathing common up to age 7 years

Note the configuration of the thorax and the ratio of anteroposterior (AP) and transverse diameters of the chest. The normal chest is symmetric with bilateral muscular development, although slightly greater muscle development may be present on the patient's dominant side. In adults, the normal AP to transverse ratio is 1:2 to 5:7. The rib cartilages should curve slightly out from the sternum. The spinal processes of C7 and T1 through T7 should be straight, and the scapulae should be symmetric. Figure 2-3 shows normal and abnormal chest structures.

Expansion during breathing should be symmetric without obvious use of accessory muscles. Asymmetry with lung expansion results from a collapsed lung or inhibited lung expansion from extrapleural air, fluid, or solid mass. Unilateral or bilateral bulging, during either inspiration or expiration, indicates retraction of the ribs and interspaces from respiratory obstruction. Bulging during expiration suggests an outflow obstruction or thoracic space compression. Unilateral retraction may occur from a foreign body in the bronchi. An obstruction of the trachea or larynx is characterized by stridor and a caved-in appearance at the sternum, between the ribs, in the suprasternal notch, above the clavicles, and at the lowest costal margin.

Evaluate the patient's breathing patterns, watching for any factors that may reflect breathing difficulties, such as leaning forward to inhale. Lip pursing accompanies increased expiratory effort and is associated with chronic obstructive lung disease. Nostril flaring is a common sign of air hunger, particularly when the alveoli are extensively compromised.

Listen for audible breath sounds. The normal adult breathing pattern is smooth and regular with 12 to 20 breaths per minute. The ratio of respiratory to pulse rate

Counting ribs accurately is essential when assessing the respiratory system. For example, rib numbers are necessary for documenting the location of abnormal breath sounds. They are also useful when interpreting chest x-rays. Normally 8 ribs are seen anteriorly and 9 to 10 ribs are seen posteriorly. If you count fewer ribs there may be consolidation in the base of the lung fields, while counting more than 9 ribs may indicate an overinflated lung.

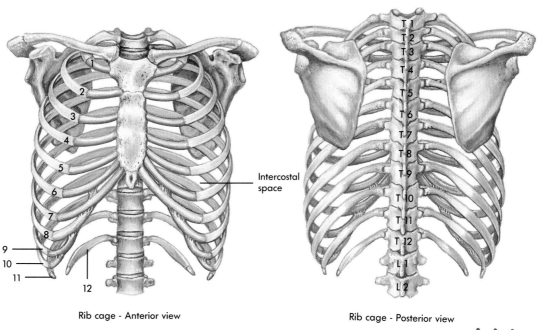

Rib cage - Anterior view

Rib cage - Posterior view

Table 2-1

BREATHING PATTERNS

Pattern	Description	Associated conditions
	Normal: smooth and even at a rate of 12-20 per minute	
	Tachypnea: shallow breathing at a rate of >20 per minute	Anxiety, pain, massive liver enlargement, abdominal ascites
	Bradypnea: <12 per minute	Neurogenic disorders, electrolyte imbalance, infection, protective response to pain or pleurisy or other discomfort aggravated by breathing
	Hyperpnea or hyperventilation: deep breathing at a rate of >20 per minute	Exercise, acute anxiety, panic reactions, metabolic disorders
	Central neurogenic hyperventilation: hyperpnea over a sustained period of time	Lesions in lower midbrain or upper pons, often from transtentorial herniation
	Air trapping: normal breathing pattern interspersed with forced expirations	Obstructive lung disease
	Kussmaul: fast (>20 per min), deep, sighing breaths without pauses; labored breathing	Renal failure, metabolic acidosis
	Cheyne-Stokes: alternating hyperpnea and apnea	In adults, bilateral lesions in cerebral hemisphere, basal ganglia, midbrain, pons, or cerebellum. In infants this pattern is normal
	Apneustic: end-inspiratory phase, often followed by expiratory phase	Injury to mid or lower pons
	Biot's or cluster: disorganized sequence of breaths with irregular periods of apnea	Lesions of lower pons or upper medulla
	Ataxic breathing: irregular breathing patterns with both deep and shallow breaths occurring randomly	Lesions of medulla

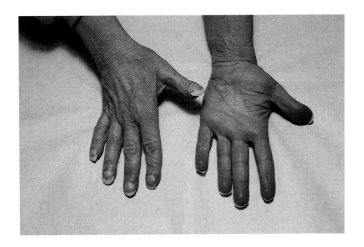

FIGURE 2-4
Clubbing and cyanosis of fingers.

is about 1:4. Women tend toward a pattern of thoracic breathing, while men are diaphragmatic breathers. Table 2-1 illustrates normal and abnormal breathing patterns.

Look for signs of central cyanosis in highly vascular areas. In light-skinned people, cyanosis can be detected in the lips, nail beds, tip of the nose, top of the ear, and underside of the tongue. Color changes can be more subtle in dark-skinned individuals. A bluish hue in the nail beds, lips, and gums is normal in people with very dark skin, so the buccal mucosa is the most reliable area to examine for cyanosis. The facial skin may also be pale gray in a dark-skinned person with central cyanosis.

Examine the fingers for signs of clubbing (Figure 2-4). Clubbing is associated with chronic fibrotic lung disease, cystic fibrosis, and congenital heart disease with cyanosis. It is not seen with other chronic lung disorders, such as asthma and emphysema.

> **PALPATION: NL. FINDINGS**
>
> Trachea—midline
> Thoracic expansion—
>   adequate; may be de-
>   creased in older adults
>   with normal respiratory
>   physiology
> Tactile fremitus—present

PALPATION

The palmar surface of both hands should be used during palpation, with one hand on the right chest wall and the other on the left (Figure 2-5). This allows the examiner to evaluate symmetry of the chest wall. Palpate the thoracic muscles and skeleton, feeling for pulsations, tenderness, bulges, depressions, and unusual movement with respirations. The chest wall should be stable and without masses or tenderness. Palpation that produces audible crackling or crepitus indicates subcutaneous emphysema, in which fine beads of air are trapped under the skin. Crepitation may result from pneumothorax. Evaluate the skin surface, which should feel warm and smooth and have elastic turgor. The spinal processes should be straight and nontender. The rib cage should feel somewhat elastic, but the sternum and xiphoid should be relatively inflexible.

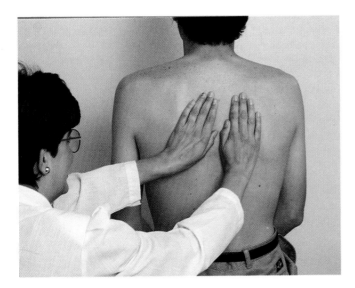

FIGURE 2-5
Palpation of the posterior chest wall.

THORACIC EXPANSION

Thoracic expansion is evaluated for both degree and symmetry by placing the hands on the patient's lower posterior thorax at about the 10th rib level, with thumbs almost touching at the spinal process and fingers wrapped around the rib cage (Figure 2-6). Instruct the patient to take several deep breaths. Expansion should be bilateral, and the examiner's thumbs should move an equal distance away from the spine. Repeat the process while facing the patient, with thumbs along the costal margin and xiphoid and palms on the anterolateral chest. Again, the examiner's thumbs should move an equal distance when the patient inhales.

Asymmetric thoracic expansion may occur with atelectasis, bronchiectasis, pleural effusion, pneumonia, or pneumonia with consolidation. Decreased thoracic expansion is associated with emphysema, but older adults may also exhibit diminished expansion from cartilage calcification and muscle weakness.

TACTILE FREMITUS

Fremitus is vibration of the chest wall produced during vocalization. Palpate both sides of the chest simultaneously while the patient repeats "one, two, three" or "how now brown cow." Although the intensity varies among individuals, fremitus should be bilaterally equal, with the most intense area of vibration occurring in the upper posterior chest wall medial to the scapula at about the second intercostal space.

Decreased or absent fremitus is caused by excess air in the lungs and suggests emphysema, pleural thickening or effusion, massive pulmonary edema, or bronchial obstruction. Increased fremitus suggests lung consolidation, a condition in which alveolar air is replaced by fluid or tissue, such as occurs in pneumonia, lung compression, tumor, or fibrosis. A gentle, tremulous fremitus occurs with some lung consolidations and inflammatory or infectious processes.

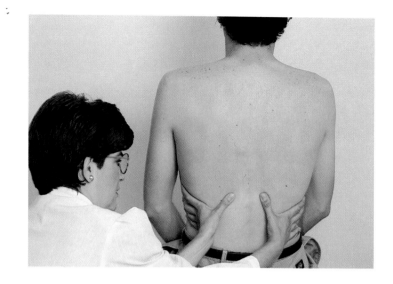

FIGURE 2-6
Assessment of thoracic expansion.

TRACHEAL POSITION

Place the thumbs on either side of the patient's trachea just above the clavicles (Figure 2-7) and gently move the trachea from side to side. Compare the space between the trachea and the sternocleidomastoid muscles on either side. Deviation from midline may result from a number of respiratory disorders, including atelectasis, pleural effusion, pulmonary fibrosis, unilateral emphysema, or tension pneumothorax. Other causes are thyroid and lymph node enlargement, neck tumor, and scoliosis.

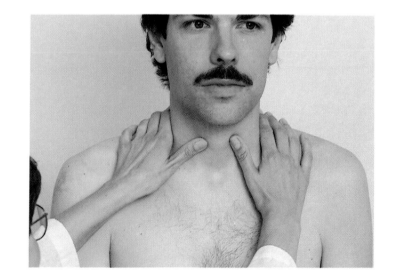

FIGURE 2-7
Assessment of tracheal position.

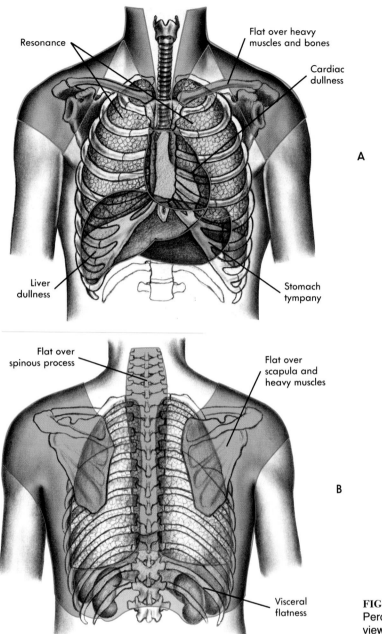

PERCUSSION

Percussion creates sound waves that help distinguish whether the underlying structures are solid, fluid-filled, or air-filled. Five percussion tones are produced, representing vibrations from 4 to 5 cm under the surface. Figure 2-8 shows the normal percussion tones of the chest wall. (See also Table 2-2.)

TECHNIQUE

In general, indirect percussion is the preferred technique for evaluating the chest wall. However, direct percussion with the fist may be required to evaluate heavily muscled or obese patients. Regardless of the technique used, avoid percussing breast tissue or bony surfaces.

PERCUSSION: NL. FINDINGS

Resonant over lung fields—in infants and young children increased resonance or hyperresonance common; in older patients hyperresonance sometimes present in absence of pathologic processs Diaphragmatic excursion—3 to 5 cm in adults; may be less in older adults with decreased chest expansion

---

FIGURE 2-8
Percussion tones of the thorax. **A**, Anterior view. **B**, Posterior view.

Table 2-2

PERCUSSION TONES OF THE CHEST

Area Percussed	Tone	Intensity	Pitch	Duration	Quality
Lungs	Resonant	Loud	Low	Long	Hollow
Bone and muscle	Flat	Soft	High	Short	Extremely dull
Viscera and liver borders	Dull	Medium	Medium-High	Medium	Thudlike
Stomach and gas bubbles in intestines	Tympanic	Loud	High	Medium	Drumlike
Air trapped in lung (abnormal in adults)	Hyperresonant	Very loud	Very low	Longer	Booming

Indirect percussion (Figure 2-9)

- Place the nondominant hand flat on the chest wall, fingers spread apart, with only the middle finger pressed firmly against the skin. The interphalangeal joint of the middle finger will be the striking surface or pleximeter.
- Using the middle finger of the dominant hand as a hammer, or plexor, tap the pleximeter sharply with a rapid stroke. Strike with the fingertip, not the finger pad. (Note that short fingernails are required.)
- The striking motion should be done with a sharp, downward snap of the wrist. Do not use elbow or shoulder motion.
- After the tap, the plexor should snap back up to ensure pure tone quality.

Tap each location several times to be sure of interpreting the sound correctly.

Direct percussion (Figure 2-10)

- Use the ulnar aspect of the fist to deliver a firm blow.
- The striking motion should come from the elbow, not the shoulder or wrist.
- Use direct percussion to elicit tenderness.

Compare all areas bilaterally for tone and intensity, percussing at 4 to 5 cm intervals and working systematically from side to side, superior to inferior, and medial to lateral. The lung fields should sound resonant, although infants and young children often display hyperresonance. Hyperresonance in older children and adults indicates hyperinflation from emphysema, pneumothorax, or asthma. Dullness or flatness over the lung fields suggests atelectasis, pleural effusion, or lung consolidation.

To percuss the posterior chest wall, have the patient sit with head bent forward and arms crossed in front. This pulls the scapulae to the sides and exposes a larger area for examination. Percuss down the chest wall, avoiding the spine and scapulae, and compare each side for tone and intensity. Ask the patient to raise his or her arms overhead to percuss the lateral (Figure 2-9) and anterior chest.

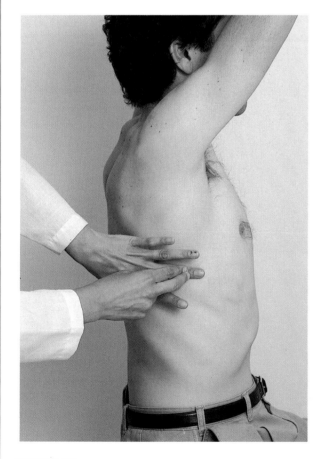

FIGURE 2-9
Indirect percussion of lateral chest wall.

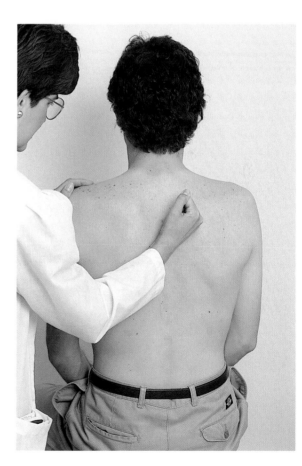

FIGURE 2-10
Direct percussion of posterior chest.

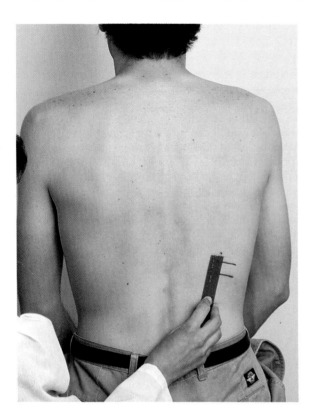

FIGURE 2-11
Measuring diaphragmatic excursion.

DIAPHRAGMATIC EXCURSION

Evaluate diaphragmatic excursion of the posterior lungs with the patient sitting upright. Instruct the patient to breathe deeply several times, take a deep breath, and hold it. Starting at the apex of the scapulae, percuss downward until the tone changes. Mark that point on the patient's skin with the marking pencil. Then instruct the patient to breathe several times, exhale completely, and hold it. Repeat the percussion from the scapula apex and mark the point where the tone changes. Do the same procedure on the other side of the posterior chest wall. With the centimeter ruler, measure and record the distance between the two lines. This determines the patient's lung expansion. Normal findings are equilateral marks with inhalation and expiration, with a 3 to 5 cm downward excursion, as shown in Figure 2-11.

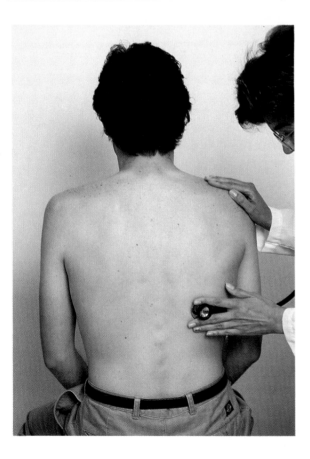

FIGURE 2-12
Auscultation of the posterior chest.

AUSCULTATION

Nearly all breath sounds are amplified by a stethoscope. The only exception is that, on rare occasions, a sound is readily audible to the ear but lost through the stethoscope, such as the click of an aspirated foreign body. The diaphragm of the stethoscope should be used to auscultate the chest wall because it covers a larger surface than the bell. Place the diaphragm firmly against the chest wall to avoid extraneous sounds.

Have the patient sit upright, if possible, and breathe slowly and deeply through the mouth to exaggerate normal respiration (Figure 2-12). Since hyperventilation can develop more quickly than one might think, make sure the patient does not breathe too fast. Keep in mind that exaggerated breathing can be exhausting for ill and older patients, so auscultation should be conducted quickly.

Auscultate the posterior, lateral, and anterior chest at 4 to 5 cm intervals, comparing the right and left sides (Figure 2-13). Have the patient assume the same positions as for percussion: head and shoulders bent forward during auscultation of the posterior chest, arms raised to auscultate the lateral walls, and shoulders back and spine straight during examination of the anterior chest.

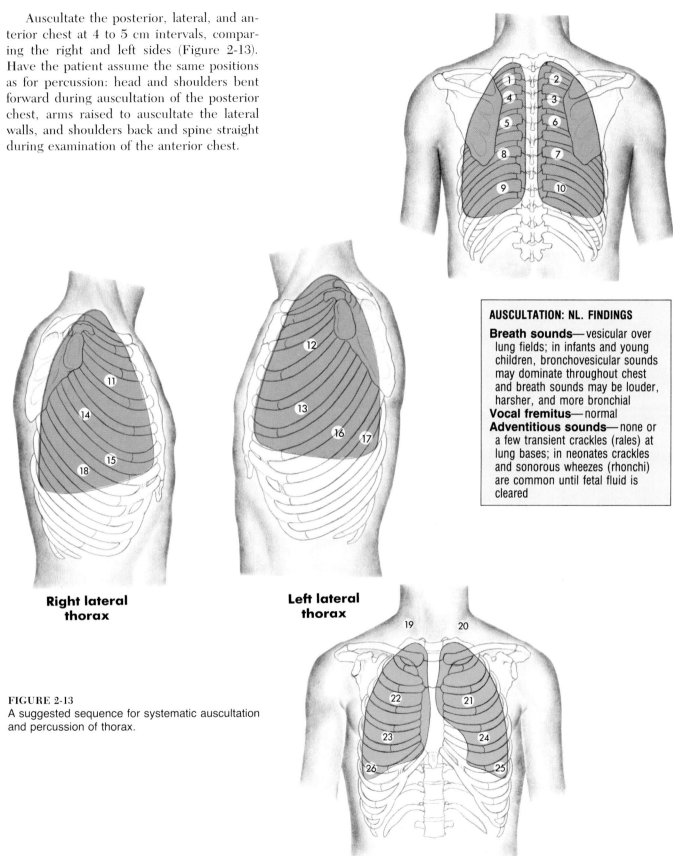

AUSCULTATION: NL. FINDINGS

Breath sounds—vesicular over lung fields; in infants and young children, bronchovesicular sounds may dominate throughout chest and breath sounds may be louder, harsher, and more bronchial
Vocal fremitus—normal
Adventitious sounds—none or a few transient crackles (rales) at lung bases; in neonates crackles and sonorous wheezes (rhonchi) are common until fetal fluid is cleared

Right lateral thorax

Left lateral thorax

Anterior thorax

FIGURE 2-13
A suggested sequence for systematic auscultation and percussion of thorax.

KEY:

☐ Bronchovesicular over main bronchi

☐ Vesicular over lesser bronchi, bronchioles, and lobes

☐ Bronchial over trachea

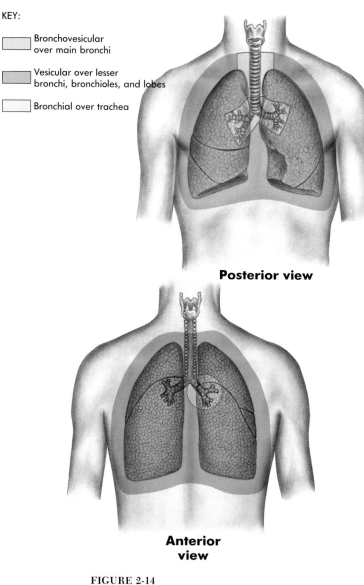

Posterior view

Anterior view

FIGURE 2-14
Normal auscultatory sounds.

BREATH SOUNDS

Normally, three distinct breath sounds are produced, each corresponding to specific areas in the respiratory tract, as demonstrated in Figure 2-14. **Bronchial** sounds are heard over the main bronchi anteriorly and the upper right lung field posteriorly (which is the left bronchus), and **bronchovesicular sounds** are present over all other areas of the lung. Both bronchial and bronchovesicular sounds are abnormal if they are detected over peripheral lung tissue. However, bronchovesicular sounds are typically heard throughout the lung fields in infants and young children because of their thinner chest walls.

Breath sounds can be diminished or absent if fluid or pus has accumulated in the pleural space, if the bronchi are obstructed by secretions or a foreign object, if the lungs are hyperinflated, or if breathing is shallow from splinting for pain. Solid tissue conducts sounds better than air-filled alveoli. Consequently, breath sounds that are unexpectedly easy to hear suggest lung consolidation.

Most of the unexpected sounds heard on auscultation are **adventitious**—that is, abnormal sounds superimposed on breath sounds. However, ambient sound (such as crinkling of chest hair against the diaphragm) must be carefully distinguished from adventitious sounds. These abnormal sounds are classified as crackles (rales), rhonchi, wheezes, and friction rub (Table 2-3). If adventitious sounds are detected, ask the patient to cough, noting any changes in the sound.

VOCAL RESONANCE

Vocal resonance is produced by the same mechanism as vocal fremitus. The sounds are loudest medially. Ask the patient to repeat "ninety-nine" during auscultation. The words should sound muffled and indistinct ("nines-nin"). Decreased intensity results from obstruction in the respiratory tree.

An increase in clarity and loudness is termed **bronchophony.** If bronchophony is present, ask the patient to whisper "ninety-nine." A whisper that can be heard distinctly through the stethoscope is termed **whispered pectoriloquy.** The patient should also be evaluated for **egophony.** Ask the patient to say *"e-e-e-e;"* if the sound is transmitted as *"a-a-a-a,"* egophony is present. Bronchophony with whispered pectoriloquy and egophony suggests consolidated lung tissue.

Table 2-3 ⌇⌇⌇

ADVENTITIOUS BREATH SOUNDS

Type	Characteristics	Comments
Crackles (rales)	Brief, not continuous, more common on inspiration; wet or dry crackling sound; not cleared by coughing	Caused by fluid, mucus, or pus in the small airways and alveoli
Fine crackles	As described above; high-pitched, sibilant crackling at end of inspiration	Found in diseases affecting bronchioles and alveoli
Medium crackles	As described above; medium pitch, more sonorous, moister sound during mid-inspiration	Associated with diseases of small bronchi
Coarse crackles	As described above; loud, bubbly sound in early inspiration	Associated with diseases of small bronchi
Sonorous wheezes (rhonchi)	Deep, rumbling sound that may be continuous; usually louder in early expiration	Caused by air moving through narrowed tracheobronchial passages (e.g., secretions, tumor, spasm); cough may alter sound if caused by mucus in trachea or large bronchi
Wheeze (sibilant rhonchi)	High-pitched, musical, whistle-like sound during inspiration or expiration; sound may consist of several notes or one, and may vary from one minute to the next	Caused by narrowed bronchioles; bilateral wheeze often result of bronchospasm; unilateral, sharply localized wheeze may result from foreign body or tumor compression
Pleural friction rub	Dry, creaking, grating, low-pitched sound with a machine-like quality during both inspiration and expiration; loudest over anterior chest	Sound originates outside respiratory tree, usually caused by inflammation; over the lung fields it suggests pleurisy; over the pericardium it suggests pericarditis; may have no significance if heard over liver or spleen

UPPER AIRWAY EXAMINATION

Upper airway disorders occur frequently, and the upper respiratory tract is the most common site of infection. Therefore a thorough assessment of the upper airway is necessary for patients who have symptoms of upper respiratory tract infection, chronic headache, or breathing obstruction.

EXTERNAL NOSE

Inspect the external nose for deviation in shape, size, or color. Observe the nares during respiration. Flaring of the nares indicates respiratory distress, whereas narrowing during inspiration suggests chronic nasal obstruction and mouth breathing.

The most common appearance of nose fracture is deviation to one side and a depression across the nasal bridge. Nose fractures are usually accompanied by epistaxis, often profuse because of the large number of small blood vessels in the nasal cavity.

A transverse nasal crease near the nose tip, at the juncture of the cartilage and bone, appears in patients with chronic nasal itching and allergies. It is seen especially in children, who are prone to wipe their noses with an upward sweep of the hand, which accounts for the name "adenoidal salute" to describe this crease.

If nasal discharge is present, note the character (watery, mucoid, purulent, crusty, or bloody), amount, odor, and whether it is unilateral or bilateral.

Gently palpate the ridge and soft tissues of the nose. Note any displacement of bone or cartilage, tenderness, or masses. The tissues should feel firm and stable with palpation.

Evaluate patency of each naris by placing a finger alongside the nose to occlude the naris. Ask the patient to breathe in and out, keeping the mouth closed. Repeat with the other naris. Nasal breathing should be easy and noiseless.

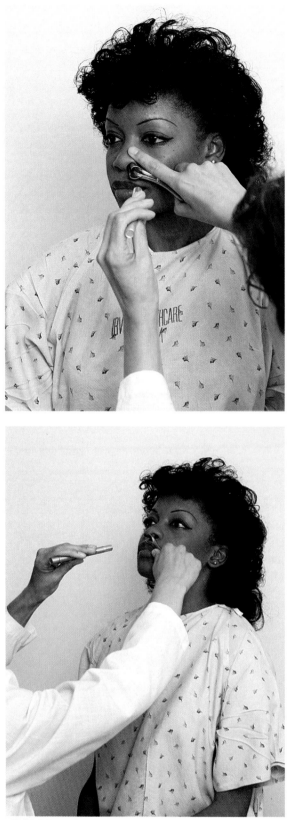

FIGURE 2-15
Inspection of the nasal cavity. The head may have to be moved in several directions to examine all the areas.

NASAL CAVITY

Use a nasal speculum and penlight to inspect the nasal cavity. (An otoscope with nasal speculum attachment may also be used.) Hold the speculum nestled in your palm, resting your index finger against the side of the patient's nose to stabilize the instrument. Use the other hand to position the patient's head and direct the penlight. Insert the speculum slowly and cautiously about 1 cm and dilate the outer naris as much as possible.

The nose floor and inferior turbinate are visible with the patient's head erect. By tilting the patient's head back, the middle meatus and middle turbinate become visible (Figures 2-15 and 2-16). Examine the posterior portion of the septum.

Note the color and condition of the mucosa. Its normal state is a deeper red than the oral mucosa, and it is coated with a small amount of clear fluid. Increased redness throughout the mucosa occurs with infection. In contrast, a localized redness and swelling in the vestibule suggests a furuncle.

The turbinates should be the same color as the surrounding mucosa and have a firm consistency. Turbinates that are bluish-grey or pale pink and have a swollen, boggy consistency suggest allergy. A rounded, elongated mass projecting into the nasal cavity may be a polyp.

The septum should be close to midline, fairly straight, thicker at the anterior end, and without perforation. Asymmetry in size of the nasal cavities suggests septal deviation. Although some deviation without compromising breathing is common, marked deviation invariably occludes the passage of air. Note any crusting or bleeding along the septum. Crusting on the anterior portion of the septum often follows epistaxis.

Other abnormal findings include discharge, lesions or masses, tenderness, yellow or green discharge, and sinus drainage from the middle meatus or middle turbinate.

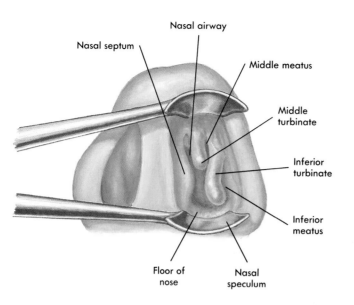

Nasal airway

Nasal septum

Middle meatus

Middle turbinate

Inferior turbinate

Inferior meatus

Floor of nose

Nasal speculum

FIGURE 2-16
Landmarks of the nasal cavity seen through the nasal speculum.

SINUSES

Inspect the frontal and maxillary sinuses for swelling. Palpate the frontal sinuses by placing your thumbs under the bony brow on each side of the patient's nose and pressing upward (Figure 2-17). The maxillary sinuses are palpated by pressing under the zygomatic processes (the cheek bones). No tenderness or swelling should be present over the soft tissues.

Percuss the areas over the sinuses to detect tenderness. Lightly tap directly over each sinus area with the index finger, using a sharp downward wrist motion. Swelling, tenderness, and pain over the sinuses suggest possible sinus infection or obstruction.

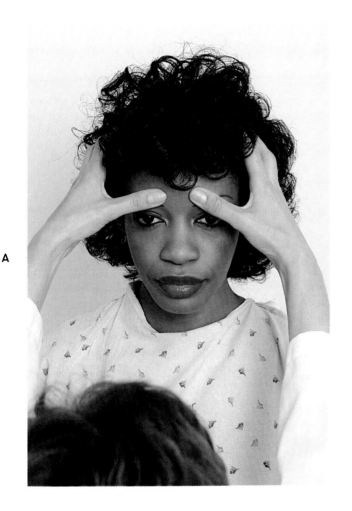

A

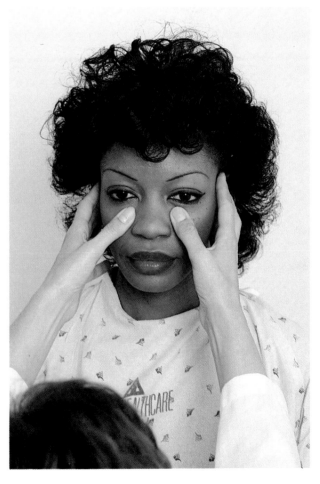

B

FIGURE 2-17
A, Palpation of the frontal sinuses. **B,** Palpation of the maxillary sinuses.

CHAPTER 3

Diagnostic Procedures

PULMONARY FUNCTION TESTS

Pulmonary function tests are performed to assess the presence and severity of disease in the large and small airways. Lung mechanics are tested by measuring the volume of air moving in and out of the lungs and then calculating various lung capacities. The relationship of lung volume and capacity is shown in Figure 3-1. Some tests also measure gas diffusion in the lungs.

Three types of equipment are used for different tests of pulmonary function: the simple spirometer, the spirometer with gas dilution, and body plethysmography. Table 3-1 details the various pulmonary function tests and their clinical significance.

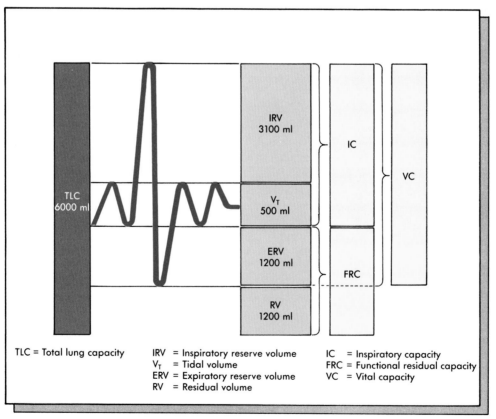

TLC = Total lung capacity	IRV = Inspiratory reserve volume	IC = Inspiratory capacity
	V$_T$ = Tidal volume	FRC = Functional residual capacity
	ERV = Expiratory reserve volume	VC = Vital capacity
	RV = Residual volume	

FIGURE 3-1
Relationship of lung volumes and capacities.

Table 3-1 ⎯⎯⎯⎯⎯⎯⎯⎯⎯⎯⎯⎯⎯⎯⎯⎯⎯⎯⎯⎯⎯⎯⎯⎯⎯⎯⎯ ∿∿

PULMONARY FUNCTION TESTS

Test	Description	Significance
LUNG VOLUME TESTS		
V_T—Tidal volume	The volume of air inspired and expired during the respiratory cycle. Normal volume is 5-8 ml/kg body weight. Measured by simple spirometer for 1 min and then divided by the number of breaths per min to determine the average V_T.	V_T should be considered only in relation to ABGs, respiratory rate, and minute volume. May be decreased in restrictive diseases.
V_E—Minute volume	The total volume of air inspired or expired in 1 minute. Measured by simple spirometer for several minutes, then divided by the number of minutes to find the average.	V_E must be considered in relation to ABGs. Most often used in exercise testing. V_E increases in hypoxia, hypercapnia, acidosis, and exercise.
V_D—Respiratory dead space	The volume of air in the lungs that is ventilated but not perfused. This includes air in anatomic dead spaces (conducting airways) and nonfunctioning alveoli. Determined approximately by the weight of the patient in pounds: $V_D = 1$ ml per 1 lb body weight.	V_D provides important information about functional lung capacity. Used primarily in exercise testing.
V_A—Alveolar ventilation	The volume of air that participates in gas exchange in the lungs. *Calculation:* $V_A = (V_T - V_D) \times$ Respiratory rate.	Used primarily in exercise testing.
ERV—Expiratory reserve volume	The maximum amount of air that can be exhaled after a resting expiratory level. Measured by simple spirometry.	ERV is about 25% of the VC. It has no diagnostic value, but ERV must be measured to calculate the RV.
IRV—Inspiratory reserve volume	The maximum amount of air that can be inspired after a normal inspiration. Measured by simple spirometry.	Abnormal IRV alone is not diagnostic of respiratory disorder. IRV decreases with normal exercise.
RV—Residual volume	The volume of air remaining in the lungs at the end of maximum expiration. *Calculation:* RV = FRC − ERV.	RV helps differentiate restrictive and obstructive diseases. Restrictive disease: usually decreased. Obstructive disease: increased.
LUNG CAPACITY TESTS		
VC—Vital capacity	The maximum amount of air that can be expired slowly and completely after a maximum inspiration. Other values that can be calculated from VC are ERV, IRV, V_T, and IC. Measured by simple spirometry. *Calculation:* VC = ERV + V_T + IRV.	Decreased in both restrictive and obstructive diseases, loss of lung tissue, and depression of the respiratory center of the brain.
FRC—Functional residual capacity	The volume of air remaining in the lungs at the end of normal expiration. It is a calculated measure of airway resistance. Performed by either gas spirometry or body plethysmography. *Calculation:* FRC = ERV + RV.	FRC is helpful in differentiating between restrictive and obstructive diseases. Restrictive disease: decreased. Obstructive disease: increased.

Continued.

Table 3-1 ─── ∿

PULMONARY FUNCTION TESTS—cont'd

Test	Description	Significance
LUNG CAPACITY TESTS—cont'd		
IC—Inspiratory capacity	The largest volume of air that can be inspired in one breath from the resting expiratory level. *Calculation:* IC = V_T + IRV.	Normal: IC = about 75% of VC. Restrictive disease: decreased. Obstructive disease: decreased or normal.
TLC—Total lung capacity	The volume of air contained in the lung at the end of a maximal inspiration. *Calculation:* TLC = FRC + IC *or* VC + RV.	TLC is helpful in differentiating between restrictive and obstructive disease. Restrictive disease: decreased. Obstructive disease: increased.
RV/TLC ratio	This ratio expresses the percent of TLC that can be defined as RV.	Values higher than 35% are seen in patients with chronic air trapping or emphysema.
PULMONARY SPIROMETRY TESTS		
FVC—Forced vital capacity	The volume of air expired forcefully and rapidly after maximal inspiration. Validity depends on patient's best effort. Measured directly.	Normal: FVC = VC Restrictive disease: FVC decreased and VC nearly normal. Obstructive disease: Both FVC and VC decreased or normal.
FEV_T—Forced expiratory volume timed	The FVC measured over a specific interval of time (T), usually 0.5, 1, or 3 seconds (written as $FEV_{0.5}$, FEV_1, and FEV_3).	Normal: FEV_T = FVC The single most common screening test for detecting obstructive disorders, in which FEV_T is always reduced.
FEV—FEV_T/FVC ratio	The ratio of FEV_T to FVC, expressed as the percent of FVC that a given FEV_T represents.	Normal: FEV_T − FVC Restrictive disease: FEV_T/FVC increased or normal. Obstructive disease: FEV_T/FVC always decreased.
$FEF_{25\%-75\%}$—Forced expiratory flow	The average flow during the middle 50% of an FEV. This value is compared with the VC. Previously called the maximum expiratory flow rate (MMEF or MMF).	$FEF_{25\%-75\%}$ is an index of the status of medium-sized airways. Restrictive disease: increased or normal. Obstructive disease: decreased.
PEFR—Peak expiratory flow rate	The maximum flow rate attainable at the beginning of forced expiration.	Decreased PEFR may indicate a mechanical problem, such as upper airway obstruction or obstructive disease.
MVV—Maximum voluntary ventilation	The largest volume of air that can be breathed per minute by voluntary effort. Actually testing period is 10 or 15 secs. Results rely on the patient's best efforts.	MVV measures the performance of the respiratory muscles, the resistance of airways and tissues, and the compliance of the lung and thorax.
GAS EXCHANGE		
DL_{CO}—Diffusing capacity of CO	A measure of gas exchange. It assesses the number of functioning pulmonary capillary beds in contact with functioning alveoli. Measured by the single-breath Krogh method.	Decreased DL_{CO} in the presence of thickened alveolar-capillary membrane indicates interstitial disease, such as pulmonary fibrosis and emphysema.
R_{AW}—Airway resistance G_{AW}—Airway conductance	R_{AW} is the pressure difference required for a unit flow change. G_{AW} is the flow generated per unit of pressure drop in the airway. G_{AW} is the reciprocal of R_{AW}. Measured at the same time as FRC with a body plethysmograph.	R_{AW} and G_{AW} increase in obstructive diseases. Calculations are most useful in evaluating patient's response to various bronchodilators.

SIMPLE SPIROMETER

The simple spirometer is a basic office tool used in routine screening, but it can also distinguish between obstructive and restrictive patterns of pulmonary disease. There are two types of spirometers, volume and flow, both of which are usually computerized and may be either water-filled or rolling-seal spirometers.

As the patient exhales or inhales into the mouthpiece (Figure 3-2), the water or air inside the spirometer is displaced, causing a pan to touch the rotating drum and record the respiratory pattern. The flow-volume loop (Figure 3-3) is a graphic display of the forced vital capacity (FVC), the basic measure of lung volume. The lung function measurements are compared with the normal values for a person of the same age, sex, and height. Race and weight also influence lung function. The spirometric standards for the American population are shown in Appendix A.

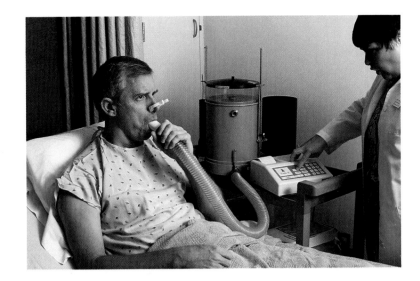

FIGURE 3-2
Simple spirometer.

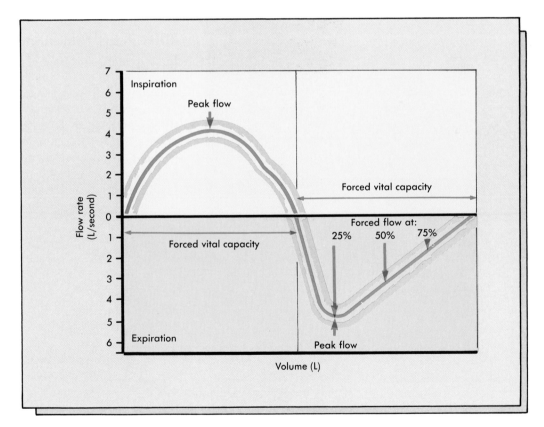

FIGURE 3-3
Flow-volume loop. *PIF,* peak inspiratory flow; *PEF,* peak expiratory flow; *FEV,* forced expiratory flow at x% FVC; *FVC,* forced vital capacity.

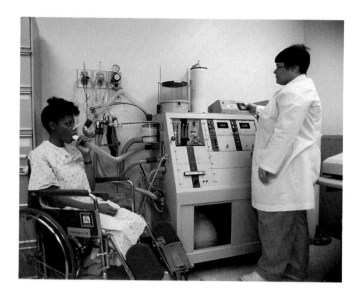

FIGURE 3-4
Spirometer with gas dilution.

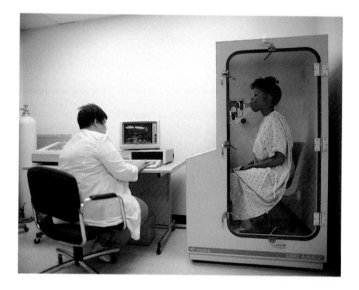

FIGURE 3-5
Body plethysmography.

SPIROMETER WITH GAS DILUTION

The spirometer with gas dilution permits calculation of the functional residual capacity (FRC) remaining in the lungs after a normal expiration. Either helium or oxygen is used to assess gas distribution throughout the lungs, diffusion across the respiratory membrane, and the efficiency of vascular perfusion in the alveoli. In the helium dilution technique, the patient rebreathes a known concentration of diluted helium through a mouthpiece (Figure 3-4) until the helium concentrations in the patient's lungs and the spirometer are equal. Because helium does not cross the alveolar-capillary membrane, the total amount of helium (that in the lungs and in the spirometer) does not change. In the nitrogen washout technique, the patient breathes 100% oxygen from one source and exhales the expired gas into the spirometer. The FRC measurements by the gas dilution method do not detect gas trapped beyond closed or narrowed airways.

The diffusing capacity of carbon dioxide (DL_{CO}) can be measured by the single-breath Krogh method: the patient deeply inhales a mixture of air containing 0.3% carbon monoxide and 10% helium, holds the breath for 10 seconds, and then exhales. Carbon monoxide levels are then measured. The DL_{CO} provides a measure of gas exchange.

BODY PLETHYSMOGRAPHY

In body plethysmography, the patient sits in an airtight chamber (also called a body box) and breathes through a mouthpiece that is connected to a transducer (Figure 3-5). Pressure is measured at both the mouthpiece and the patient's chest. To calculate thoracic gas volume the patient is instructed to pant into the mouthpiece while keeping the cheeks rigid and the glottis open. The R_{AW} and G_{AW} are calculated mathematically as the patient breathes rapidly and shallowly.

Body plethysmography has the advantage of measuring all respiratory gas, including gas trapped behind poorly communicating airways or in closed spaces (e.g., pneumothorax).

INDICATIONS

Routine screening
To evaluate: Obstructive vs. restrictive pulmonary disease
Surgical risk
Therapeutic effectiveness of bronchodilators and steroids
Need for mechanical ventilation

CONTRAINDICATIONS

Meal 4 to 6 hours before test

ABNORMAL FINDINGS

Lung disorders that cause abnormalities of ventilation are classified as either **restrictive** or **obstructive** disorders. Restrictive disorders develop in conditions that inhibit lung expansion, including muscle or neurologic disease, pulmonary infiltrates, pleural thickening, space-occupying tumors, and after lung resection. Obstructive disorders include asthma, bronchitis, emphysema, and bronchiectasis and any disease that causes narrowing of the tracheobronchial tree.

ARTERIAL BLOOD GASES (ABGS)

Blood gas analysis is an essential test in diagnosing and monitoring patients with respiratory disorders. These tests are performed on arterial blood because this provides more direct information about ventilatory function. In some cases, particularly patients undergoing hemodynamic monitoring with a pulmonary catheter, both arterial and venous blood samples are analyzed. If continuous monitoring of oxygen saturation is needed, the noninvasive technique of pulse oximetry can be used (Figure 3-6).

There are two procedures for collecting arterial blood: direct puncture of the artery (see box on page 42) and collecting a sample from an intraarterial catheter (see page 44).

Blood gas analysis determines the pH, saturation, and partial pressure of oxygen and also the partial pressure of carbon dioxide. Table 3-2 shows the normal values of blood gases and the clinical significance of abnormal values. Acid-base imbalances are outlined in Table 3-3; additional information on compensatory mechanisms can be found on page 14, Transport of Respiratory Gases.

INDICATIONS

Signs of acidosis or alkalosis
Cyanosis
Hyperventilation or hypoventilation
Respiratory distress

CONTRAINDICATIONS

None. However, direct puncture requires special precautions in patients with known clotting disorders and in those taking anticoagulants.

NURSING CARE

Treatments such as bronchodilators and intermittent positive pressure breathing may be withheld before pulmonary function testing. Patients with dentures should wear them during the test because this will help form a good seal around the mouthpiece. During testing, observe the patient for signs of tiring and dizziness. Provide a rest period after the test.

PATIENT TEACHING

Explain the procedure and its purpose. Assure the patient that the test is painless and that the accuracy of test results relies on his or her best efforts.

NURSING CARE

The radial artery is the first choice for direct puncture because it has excellent blood flow, is easily accessible, and is relatively insensitive to pain. However, the Allen test must be performed first to evaluate collateral blood flow. If the Allen test is negative, the radial artery cannot be used. The brachial artery is the second choice, and the third choice is the femoral artery. Follow procedures carefully for collecting arterial blood.

PATIENT TEACHING

Explain the reason a blood sample is needed. If direct puncture will be done, tell the patient that an anesthetic will be injected first, which will feel like a "stick" and initially cause a cold sensation, followed by tingling and numbness. The patient will feel pressure when the needle is inserted into the artery.

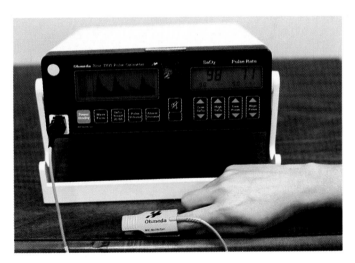

FIGURE 3-6
Monitoring arterial oxygen saturation (Sao$_2$) by pulse oximetry. A diode and photodetector are attached to a finger, earlobe, or pinna of the ear. The photodetector distinguishes between the color of oxygenated and deoxygenated hemoglobin and transmits the information to a microprocessor. The percentage of saturation is displayed on the screen.

DIRECT PUNCTURE METHOD FOR COLLECTING ARTERIAL BLOOD

1. Assemble the following equipment: 2 or 3 ml syringe with 25-gauge needle; 10 ml syringe with 20- or 21-gauge needle (21- or 28-gauge needle for children) and 1 ml heparin sodium (1:1000) or preheparinized syringe; rubber stopper or Luer-Lok cap; lidocaine or procaine: alcohol and iodophor prep; sterile gauze pads; nonsterile gloves; and basin with crushed ice and water.
2. Heparinize the 10 ml syringe by using the 20- or 21-gauge needle to draw up 0.3 ml of heparin, wetting the cylinder and plunger. Hold the syringe upright and expel the heparin and air bubbles. Recover the needle and lay the syringe aside. (Pre-heparinized syringes are also available.)
3. Position the patient in either a sitting or a supine position.
4. If the radial artery is to be used, first perform the Allen test to be sure that the collateral blood supply is adequate. If the hand flushes within 15 seconds, the test is positive and the radial artery may be used. If the test is negative, do not use that artery. The remaining description assumes the radial artery will be used.

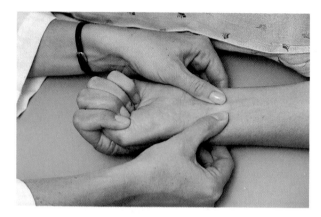

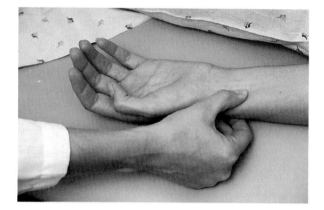

The Allen test for evaluating collateral circulation of the radial artery. Step 1: While the patient's fist is closed tightly, obliterate both the radial and ulnar arteries simultaneously. Instruct the patient to relax the hand, and watch for blanching of the palm and fingers.

Step 2: Release the obstructing pressure from only the ulnar artery. Wait 15 seconds, observing the hand for flushing caused by capillary refilling. This indicates a positive Allen test, verifying that the ulnar artery alone is capable of supplying the entire hand. If flushing does not occur within 15 seconds, the Allen test is negative and the radial artery cannot be used. The test may be performed in unconscious patients by elevating the patient's hand straight up until blanching occurs; obliterate the arteries as described, lower the hand, and release pressure over the ulnar artery while observing for flushing.

5. Wash hands thoroughly and don nonsterile gloves.
6. Palpate the radial artery to locate the area where maximum pulsation occurs.
7. Cleanse the area with iodophor prep, then wipe with alcohol swab.
8. Inject the skin with the anesthetic agent using the small syringe and 25-gauge needle.

DIRECT PUNCTURE METHOD FOR COLLECTING ARTERIAL BLOOD—CONT'D

9. With one hand, locate the radial pulse proximal to the cleansed area and keep this hand on the pulse. With the other hand, insert the heparinized needle into the radial artery distal to the palpating fingers. The angle between the needle and the artery should be about 45 degrees to make an oblique puncture, which allows the muscle fiber to seal the puncture as soon as the needle is withdrawn. Do not make more than two attempts at any one site.

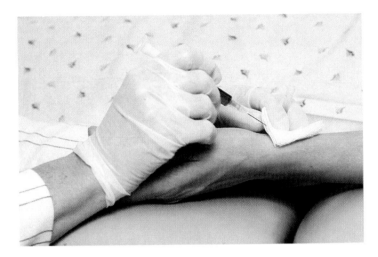

Drawing arterial blood by the direct puncture method. Note that the needle is at a 45-degree angle.

10. Once the artery is punctured, the pulsating blood will push up the hub of the syringe.
11. After 3-5 ml of blood are obtained, remove the needle and apply sterile gauze to the puncture site. Keep firm, continuous pressure over the site for at least 5 minutes. If the patient is on anticoagulants, maintain pressure for 20 minutes or longer until the bleeding stops.
12. Remove all air bubbles from the syringe so that the test results are not affected. Apply the rubber stopper or Luer-Lok cap.
13. Place the capped syringe in the basin of crushed ice and water to preserve the gas and pH levels of the specimen.
14. Record the following data: the time that blood sample was drawn, the patient's temperature, the ventilator settings, and the percentage of oxygen administered. Send the specimen and report to the laboratory immediately.

COLLECTION FROM ARTERIAL CATHETER

1. Assemble the following equipment: 3 to 6 ml sterile syringe; 6 ml sterile syringe; sterile gauze; alcohol swab; basin containing ice and cold water; nonsterile gloves; flush solution of 500 ml normal saline with 2,000 units of heparin.
2. Wash hands thoroughly and don nonsterile gloves.

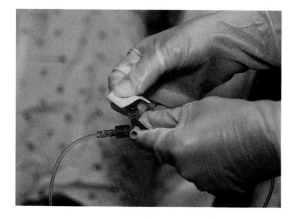

3. Clean entry port. Note stopcock is turned "off" to the flush solution.

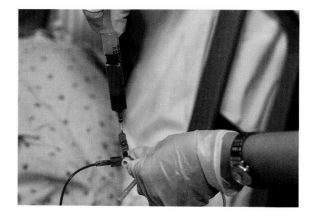

4. Attach 3 or 6 ml syringe to stopcock and turn stopcock to the pressure bag to "off" position.
5. Remove the amount of blood equal to the deadspace in the catheter and any extension tubing deadspace (about 10 ml). Discard both the blood and the syringe.

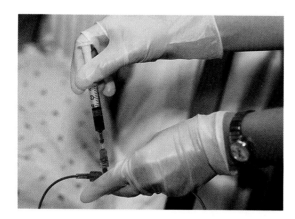

6. Attach the 6 ml syringe to the stopcock and withdraw 4.5 ml of blood. Place this immediately in the basin containing the ice and send the specimen to the laboratory.

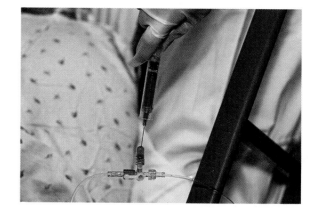

7. Flush arterial line until blood is cleared from the tubing.

8. Flush the stopcock opening into the sterile gauze. This prevents the blood from clotting in the stopcock.
9. Clean the port with alcohol swab to remove any blood and replace the stopcock cap.

Table 3-2

NORMAL AND ABNORMAL VALUES FOR BLOOD GASES

Test	Normal values	Purpose	Significance of Abnormal Values
pH: Arterial **Venous**	7.35-7.45 7.32-7.43	To assess acid-base status	See Table 3-3.
P$_{CO_2}$: Arterial **Venous**	35-45 mm Hg 35-50 mm Hg	To evaluate ventilation	*Hypocarbia* occurs in hyperventilation from rapid removal of CO_2. *Hypercarbia* occurs in hypoventilation from retention of CO_2.
P$_{O_2}$ Arterial	80-95 mm Hg	To measure amount of O_2 dissolved in plasma (not amount carried by hemoglobin)	*Hypoxemia* is caused by hypoventilation, ventilation-perfusion imbalance, or reduction in inspired O_2. *Hyperoxemia* occurs in patients breathing high O_2 concentrations (above 21%).
HCO$_3^-$: Arterial **Venous**	21-28 mEq/L 22-29 mEq/L	To evaluate metabolic component	*Alkalosis* is caused by excess renal absorption of bicarbonate or by excessive H^+ loss. *Acidosis* is caused by excessive H^+ production or by excessive loss of bicarbonate.
SaO$_2$	95-99%	To measure the percentage O_2 carried by hemoglobin in arterial blood	*Decrease* is caused by venous blood shunting to the arterial system or carbon dioxide poisoning. *No increase* is possible.

Table 3-3

ACID-BASE IMBALANCES

Type	Blood gas analysis	Causes
Respiratory acidosis	pH<7.35, Pa$_{CO_2}$ >45 mmHg, HCO$_3$ >28 mEq/L if compensating	Hypoventilation, asphyxia, central nervous system depression
Respiratory alkalosis	pH>7.45, Pa$_{CO_2}$<35 mm Hg, HCO$_3$ <21 mEq/L if compensating	Hyperventilation, respiratory stimulation
Metabolic acidosis	pH <7.35, HCO$_3$ <21 mEq/L, PaCO$_2$ <35 mm Hg if compensating	HCO$_3$ less from diarrhea, inadequate acid excretion from renal disease, excessive acid production from hepatic or endocrine disorders, shock, or drug intoxication
Metabolic alkalosis	pH >7.45, HCO$_3$ >28 mEq/L, Pa$_{CO_2}$ >45 mm Hg if compensating	Loss of hydrochloric acid from vomiting or gastric suctioning, potassium loss from diuretics or steroids, excessive alkali ingestion

COMPLETE BLOOD CELL COUNT (CBC)

The hemogram, or complete blood cell count (CBC), is a routine screening test that provides general information about overall state of health and respiratory function. The procedure is simple because venous blood is used. CBC determinations are made by automated equipment, and the results can be available quickly.

The elements of the CBC that most directly relate to the respiratory status are the red blood cell (RBC) count, hematocrit (Hct), hemoglobin (Hgb), white blood cell (WBC) count, and the differential WBC count. Table 3-4 shows the normal laboratory values for these tests. Other determinations that can be made from the CBC are the mean corpuscular volume (MCV), mean corpuscular hemoglobin (MCH), and mean corpuscular hemoglobin concentration (MCHC).

Table 3-4

COMPLETE BLOOD CELL COUNT (CBC)

Test	Normal Adult Values	Purpose	Clinical Significance
Red blood cell	Men: 5.11 ± 0.38 Women: 4.51 ± 0.36 (10^5 μL)	To determine oxygen carrying capacity of blood	*Increases:* Erythrocytosis and secondary polycythemia are attempts to compensate for chronic hypoxia; seen in chronic lung disease. *Decreases:* Anemia results from blood loss, abnormal destruction of RBCs, or bone marrow suppression.
Hemoglobin	Men: 15.5 ± 1.1 Women: 13.7 ± 1.0 (g/dl)	To determine oxygen carrying capacity of blood	*Increases:* Same as for RBC count. *Decreases:* Same as for RBC count.
Hematocrit	Men: 46.0 ± 3.1 Women: 40.9 ± 3 (%)	To determine the percentage of RBCs and hydration status	*Increases:* Severe dehydration causes loss of blood plasma, increasing percent concentration of RBCs. In patients with normal hydration, increased Hct indicates increased number of RBCs. *Decreases:* Overhydration. If hydration status is normal, indicates decreased number of RBCs. Total WBC may be increased or decreased in infections and increased in inflammation. See below.
White blood cell count	4500-110 (cells/mm$_3$)	To determine immune system response to antigens	*Increases:* Neutrophilia is seen in acute bacterial infections, chronic inflammatory diseases, carcinoma, severe trauma, Cushing's disease, diabetes mellitus, acute hemorrhage, and hemolytic anemia.
Granulocytes Neutrophils	56 (%)	Because they are involved in phagocytosis, the neutrophil count often reflects inflammatory process	*Decreases:* Neutropenia seen in acute viral infections, bone marrow depletion resulting from overwhelming infection, B_{12} or folic acid deficiency, and drug toxicity from nafcillin, penicillin, and cephalosporins. *Increases:* Eosinophilic leukocytosis seen in allergic disorders (e.g., asthma, hay fever), parasitic infections, Hodgkin's disease, colitis, eosinophilic leukemia.

Table 3-4

COMPLETE BLOOD CELL COUNT (CBC)—cont'd

Test	Normal Adult Values	Purpose	Clinical Significance
Granulocytes—cont'd			*Decreases:* Eosinophilic leukopenia is seen with increased levels of adrenal steroids.
Basophils	0-2 (%)	Basophils contain vasoactive chemicals (histamine and serotonin) and may play a role in allergic reactions.	*Increases:* Basophilic leukocytosis is seen in myeloproliferative disorders. *Decreases:* Basophilopenia is seen in anaphylactic reactions.
Monocytes	1-8 (%)	To determine phagocytic activity	*Increases:* Monocytosis is seen in acute infections such as tuberculosis, typhoid fever, malaria, and subacute bacterial endocarditis. Monocytosis can occur with no increase in total WBC count. *Decreases:* None.
Lymphocytes	15-45 (%)	To determine activity of antibody production	*Increases:* Lymphocytosis is seen in acute viral and chronic bacterial infections, thyrotoxicosis, Cushing's disease, and leukemia. *Decreases:* Lymphopenia is seen in immune deficiency states, including AIDS, and as a result of drugs that are immunosuppressive such as corticosteroids and cytotoxic agents used in cancer therapy.

CBC ELEMENTS

Red blood cell (RBC) count

A count of the number of red blood cells (erythrocytes) per cubic millimeter (mm^3) of blood.

Hematocrit (Hct, Crit)

The percentage of red blood cells in the plasma.

Hemoglobin (Hgb or Hb)

A component of the red blood cell made of pigment (heme), which carries oxygen, and protein (globin).

White blood cell (WBC) count and differential (Diff)

The number of white blood cells in a cubic millimeter (mm^3) of blood. A differential count is the determination of the proportions of each of five types of white blood cells in a sample of 100 white blood cells. The difference is reported in percentages.

INDICATIONS

For routine examination and screening
To diagnose respiratory disorders
To evaluate treatment

CONTRAINDICATIONS

None. However, precautions should be taken in patients with known clotting disorders.

NURSING CARE

Blood samples are usually obtained from one of the large superficial veins at or just below the antecubital fossa. Nonsterile gloves should be worn. Occlude the vein above the elbow and cleanse the puncture site with alcohol. Insert the needle into the vein at about a 45-degree angle. After withdrawing the needle, press a sterile gauze pad against the puncture site for about one minute and then cover it with a sterile adhesive strip.

If only a hematocrit value is needed, obtain a small blood sample by the finger stick method (heel stick in infants).

PATIENT TEACHING

Explain the procedure and the purpose of the blood test. Warn the patient that the needle will sting briefly. After withdrawing the needle, ask the patient to flex her arm tightly against the gauze pad to help stop the bleeding.

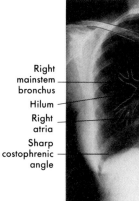

FIGURE 3-7
Patient positioned for chest x-ray.

CHEST X-RAYS

Chest x-rays (roentgenograms) are an essential diagnostic tool for evaluating disorders of the chest. They provide visualization of the lungs, ribs, clavicles, humeri, scapulae, vertebrae, heart, and major thoracic vessels. Chest x-rays are useful in identifying foreign bodies, infiltration, and abnormal shadows. They also identify whether a disorder involves the lung parenchyma or the interstitial spaces. Finally, chest x-rays are invaluable for visualizing the location of invasive lines such as endotracheal and nasogastric tubes.

The best x-rays of the chest are obtained with the patient in an upright position, the film exposed during deep inspiration, and the x-ray tube at least 6 feet away from the film (Figure 3-7). Alterations in these conditions can change the appearance of the thoracic structures and result in inaccurate interpretations. However, in many clinical situations deep sustained inspiration is not possible for unconscious patients or those on mechanical ventilators.

The standard series for chest x-rays are the posteroanterior (PA) and lateral views (Figure 3-8). In the supine patient, the anteroposterior (AP) view is used. Small pleural effusions are often best seen in the lateral decubitus view. Because abnormalities in the apex of the lung can be obscured by the clavicles and first ribs, an apical lordotic view is sometimes necessary.

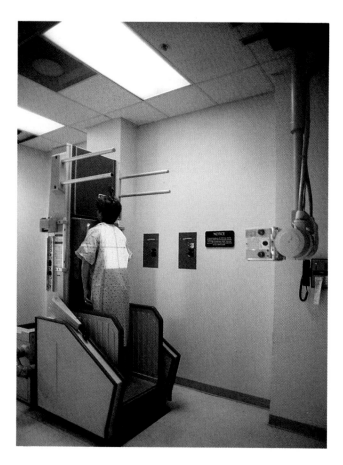

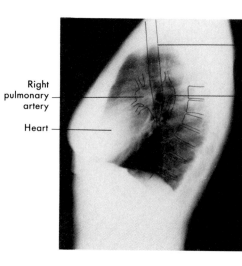

FIGURE 3-8
Normal PA and lateral chest x-rays.

INTERPRETATION OF CHEST FILMS

The white bony densities of the scapulae, clavicles, humeri, ribs, and vertebrae are inspected for fractures or deformities. Eight or nine ribs should be visible on the PA view.

The hemidiaphragms should appear round, smooth, and clearly defined, with the right hemidiaphragm slightly elevated because of the liver. An elevated hemidiaphragm indicates poor inspiration, whereas a flattened silhouette may suggest overinflation of the lungs. If no hemidiaphragm is seen, atelectasis is suspected if the patient is afebrile and pneumonia is suspected if fever is present.

The costophrenic angle (CVA) is formed by the lateral junction of the rib cage and the diaphragm. Blunting or absence of the CVA may indicate pleural effusion.

The tracheobronchial tree is elevated for tracheal deviation from midline, an angle at which the mainstem bronchi bifurcate (the carina), and the vascular markings that arise in the hilar area and extend through the lung fields. The carina normally is located one-half to one vertebral body below the aortic knob. The intrapulmonary bronchi should be visible. Infiltration of the lungs will show as grey areas (fluid) surrounding white areas (air), which makes the intrapulmonary bronchi visible.

Normal lung fields appear black with vascular markings that are seen as thin, wispy, white streaks originating from the hili. Greyness in the lung fields suggests pleural effusion. In upright patients this will be at the base of the lung. In supine patients the greyness will appear homogenous, and the x-ray should be repeated with the patient in an upright position to confirm that the fluid shifts to the lung bases.

USE IN CRITICAL CARE SITUATIONS

Chest x-rays are used in the critical care setting to check the placement of tubes and lines.

- Endotracheal (ET) tubes are placed in the trachea 5-7 cm above the carina. An ET tube positioned too high will not provide adequate ventilation, whereas an ET tube placed too low can pass into the right mainstem bronchus and block ventilation to the left lung.
- Nasogastric tubes should be checked for kinks and for correct placement below the diaphragm into the stomach.
- The effectiveness of chest tubes for either pneumothorax or fluid drainage can be assessed to determine lung reexpansion.
- Pulmonary artery catheters should be in the proximal main pulmonary artery or the descending

RADIOLOGIC TESTS

Roentgen rays are part of the spectrum of electromagnetic radiation that penetrates the body according to the thickness and density of different tissues. Tissue with little density absorbs a greater number of x-rays, producing black images on the photographic film. Conversely, the more dense the tissue, the fewer x-rays can pass through the tissue; and lighter images are produced. Thus air-filled spaces such as the lungs appear black, fluid-filled structures such as blood vessels appear grey, and metal-containing structures, such as bones, calcium deposits, surgical wires and clips, and prosthetic devices, appear white. Figure 3-8 demonstrates the different densities of roentgenographic images.

right or left pulmonary artery. Chest x-rays are also taken to detect pneumothorax or hemothorax resulting from pulmonary catheters.

- A central venous pressure (CVP) line should be checked routinely to verify placement in the superior vena cava and to identify iatrogenic damage on the side of insertion. The CVP line is often seen in the subclavian artery or right atrium.

INDICATIONS

Routine screening
To diagnose: Atelectasis
　　　　　　　Pleural effusion
　　　　　　　Hemothorax or pneumothorax
　　　　　　　Infiltrates
　　　　　　　Foreign bodies
　　　　　　　Thoracic fractures
To monitor: Endotracheal tubes
　　　　　　　Nasogastric tube
　　　　　　　Central venous or pulmonary artery catheters
　　　　　　　Cardiac pacemaker wires

CONTRAINDICATIONS

Pregnancy

NURSING CARE

Have the patient remove all neck jewelry and wear a hospital gown. After the machine is positioned and the film is inserted into the carrier, position the patient. Instruct the patient to take a deep breath and hold it.

PATIENT TEACHING

Explain the purpose of the x-ray.

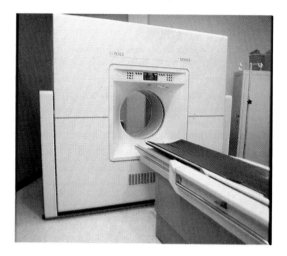

FIGURE 3-9
Clinical setting for computed tomography.

TOMOGRAPHY

Tomography consists of a series of roentgenographic images of thin cross-sections (0.8 to 1.3 cm) of the thorax. Images can be obtained in the sagittal or horizontal plane. Because tomograms provide morphologic detail, the exact characteristics and location of lesions can be determined. Tomographic images are much sharper and more detailed than those obtained by conventional x-rays. The technique shows pulmonary densities such as cavitation and calcification. Radiation exposure is very low with tomography, and the need for invasive diagnostic procedures is reduced.

LAMINAGRAM OR PLANIGRAM

This basic application of the tomogram produces three-dimensional images in a single plane with other planes blurred out. The camera moves around the patient to bring different layers of the thorax into focus.

COMPUTED TOMOGRAPHY (CT)

The CT scan produces three-dimensional images, supplying more detailed analysis than is possible in the one-dimensional images of the planigram. For a CT scan of the thorax, the patient lies on a narrow table with the upper body inside the tunnel-like scanner. The scanning camera rotates around the patient, taking pictures from different angles (Figure 3-9). This information is recorded on a computer printout, and film prints are made. Figure 3-10 shows a transverse CT scan of the chest.

INDICATIONS

To diagnose: Pulmonary densities
Space-occupying tumors
Mediastinal lymph nodes

CONTRAINDICATIONS

Pregnancy

NURSING CARE

Have the patient remove all neck jewelry and wear a hospital gown. Instruct the patient to lie very still during the procedure.

PATIENT TEACHING

Discuss the reason for the test. Explain that the patient will lie on a narrow table and that the camera will make a clicking noise. The procedure will take approximately 20-30 minutes to complete. A two-way intercom system will allow communication between the patient and the x-ray personnel. Reassure the patient that the procedure is painless.

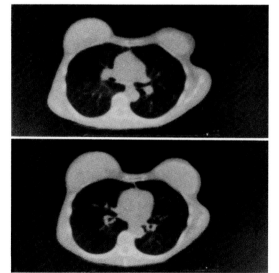

FIGURE 3-10
Transverse CT scan of female patient. Bilateral breast shadows, heart, pulmonary arteries, and main bronchi are visible.

LUNG SCANS

Radionuclide lung scans are performed to evaluate either perfusion or ventilation. After the contrast material is introduced, a scintillation camera records the radioactivity in the lungs for about 5 minutes to determine how much gas enters the lungs and how long it takes for the gas to be exhaled (Figure 3-11). If both perfusion and ventilation are to be evaluated, the perfusion scan is performed first.

PERFUSION LUNG SCANS

Perfusion is assessed after injecting technetium Tc 99m into a peripheral vein. Because the radioactive particles are retained in the pulmonary capillary beds, scanning shows the distribution of blood flow through the lungs (Figure 3-12).

VENTILATION LUNG SCANS

Ventilation lung scans are performed after the patient takes a deep breath of a mixture of radioactive gas (xenon (Xe) 133 or krypton (Kr) 85) and oxygen. Because the radioactive particles are too large to diffuse across the alveolar-capillary membrane, scanning shows the air spaces in the lung. Evaluation is performed in three stages to detect ventilation abnormalities: (1) at initial inspiration to determine TLC, (2) during normal tidal breathing (wash-in), and (3) during elimination while the patient breathes room air (wash-out). Areas of decreased ventilation show as delayed appearance of radionuclide during wash-in and prolonged retention during wash-out.

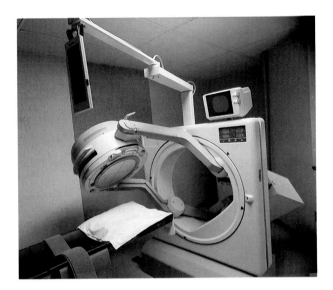

FIGURE 3-11
Clinical setting for lung scanning.

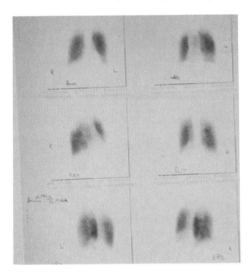

FIGURE 3-12
Lung scans.

INDICATIONS

Perfusion scan
To diagnose and evaluate pulmonary emboli
Preoperative assessment before lung resection
Ventilation scan
To detect regional differences in lung function

CONTRAINDICATIONS

Pregnancy. However, precautions should be taken for patients with a history of allergic reactions to iodine.

NURSING CARE

Determine whether the patient has had a previous reaction to diagnostic dyes or a history of allergic reactions to shellfish or iodine. Obtain informed consent. After perfusion lung scan, encourage the patient to drink fluids to flush the contrast material from the kidneys.

PATIENT TEACHING

Explain the procedure and its purpose. If a perfusion scan is to be performed, explain that the dye will be injected into a vein and may cause a flushing sensation or nausea. Assure the patient that these symptoms are brief. Inform the patient that the imaging time is 20 to 40 minutes, that he will lie under a camera, and that a mask may be placed over his nose and mouth during the test.

If a ventilation scan is to be performed, explain that the patient will inhale gas but that it does not cause symptoms. Inform the patient that scanning will take only about 5 minutes.

THORACENTESIS

Thoracentesis involves inserting a needle through the chest wall and into the pleura to remove pleural fluid. A local anesthetic is used, and the patient sits on a table, leaning slightly forward (Figure 3-13). Complications associated with thoracentesis are hemothorax, pneumothorax, air embolism, and subcutaneous emphysema.

Stains and cultures are always performed on pleural fluid, even when there is no evidence of infection. Histopathologic studies and cell profiles can help determine the cause of the effusion. Pleural effusions with blood counts greater than 100,000/ml often result from trauma, malignancy, and pulmonary thromboembolism. A lymphocytic effusion containing more than 50% lymphocytes may have a tuberculous or malignant origin.

Chemical studies are done to determine whether the fluid is an exudate or a transudate, which can help isolate the cause.

INDICATIONS

Pleural effusion
Suspected malignancy

CONTRAINDICATIONS

None

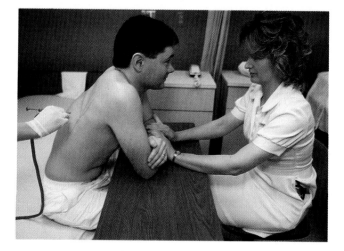

FIGURE 3-13
Patient positioned for thoracentesis.

NURSING CARE

Obtain written consent. Administer preprocedure sedative as ordered. Chest x-rays are made after thoracentesis. Assess the patient for signs of complications.

PATIENT TEACHING

Explain the procedure and its purpose. Inform the patient that a local anesthetic will be used to minimize the discomfort and that some pressure will be felt when the needle is inserted.

SKIN TESTS

Skin tests are performed to diagnose bacterial, fungal, or viral pulmonary diseases. The antigen is injected intradermally (Figure 3-14) rather than subcutaneously, which can produce a false negative reaction. The injection site is circled and later inspected to determine the result. If induration is present, the diameter is measured in millimeters. Reddened, flat areas should not be measured.

Because the exact procedure for administering and interpreting skin tests varies with the antigen used, the manufacturer's instructions must be followed carefully.

MANTOUX TEST

The Mantoux test, or tuberculin test, detects present or previous *Mycobacterium tuberculosis* infection. It is performed by injecting 0.1 ml of intermediate strength purified protein derivative (PPD) into the inner forearm. The test is read 48-72 hours after injection.

Induration of 10 mm or more is a positive reaction and indicates past or present infection. An induration of 5-9 mm is classified as a doubtful reaction and suggests

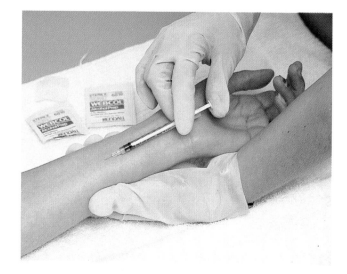

FIGURE 3-14
Intradermal injection in forearm for skin testing.

probable prior infection with other mycobacteria. In clinical practice, it usually is considered negative in patients without symptoms of tuberculosis. However, it is likely to be positive in patients who have had close contact with an infected person who has clinical signs, radiographic evidence, or positive sputum for tuberculosis. Induration of 0-4 mm is considered negative, and repeat testing is not required unless the patient has clinical signs of tuberculosis.

MULTIPLE PUNCTURE TESTS

Multiple puncture tests (Heaf, Tine, or Mono-Vac) are used in mass screenings to determine how a patient's immune system reacts to the tubercle bacillus. They are administered by pressing an applicator firmly against the inside forearm to push a drop of antigen through the skin. The area is evaluated 48-72 hours later.

These tests usually produce several separate areas of induration. Measure the diameter of the largest single reaction. A blisterlike elevation of vesiculation indicates a positive reaction. An induration of 2 mm or more is classified as doubtful, but patients with this reaction should be retested using the Mantoux test. A negative reaction is less than 2 mm. A positive finding should always be followed by the Mantoux test.

INDICATIONS

To diagnose tuberculosis

CONTRAINDICATIONS

None

NURSING CARE

Read and follow the manufacturer's instructions carefully because the proper administration and interpretation of each test varies. Inject the antigen intradermally, not subcutaneously, on the inside of the forearm. You may wish to circle the injection site with a ballpoint pen. On the patient's chart, draw a diagram of the forearm, labeling the injection site and noting whether the left or right arm was tested. In interpreting the results, measure the induration in millimeters, using a good light source to inspect the area. Reddened, flat areas should not be measured.

PATIENT TEACHING

Explain the test and its purpose. Tell the patient that the injection will feel like a "stick" or will sting slightly. Instruct the patient not to wash or otherwise remove the circle drawn on the skin until after the test is evaluated. Inform the patient when the results will be evaluated, giving date and time outpatient should return.

SWEAT TEST

The sweat test is a noninvasive test for cystic fibrosis. Iontophoresis, a technique that initiates a small electric current, is used to deliver the drug pilocarpine to stimulate sweat production in an area on the skin (Figure 3-15). The sweat is collected on filter paper and analyzed for sodium and chloride concentration. Values above 65 mEq/L for both electrolytes suggest cystic fibrosis. The degree of elevation does not necessarily correlate with the severity of disease. In a variant of cystic fibrosis (characterized by *Pseudomonas* bronchitis and normal pancreatic function), chloride concentrations are between 40 and 60 mEq/L.

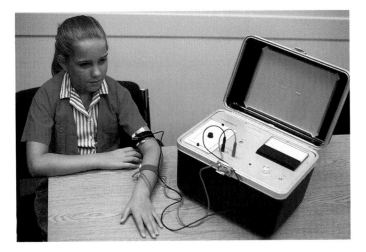

FIGURE 3-15
Child undergoing sweat test for cystic fibrosis.

The sweat test can be done as early as 24 hours after birth, but it is difficult to obtain an adequate amount of sweat for testing until the infant is 4 weeks old. The test is painless and without complication.

INDICATIONS

To screen for cystic fibrosis

CONTRAINDICATIONS

None

NURSING CARE

There is no specific nursing care.

PATIENT TEACHING

Explain the test and its purpose to the parents. Give a simple, age-appropriate explanation to children and reassure them the test will not hurt. The sweat test takes about 40 minutes.

BRONCHOSCOPY

Bronchoscopy has a multitude of uses in diagnosing and treating disorders of the tracheobronchial tree. It allows direct inspection of the larynx, trachea, and bronchi to localize bleeding or tumors. Biopsies can be obtained, and secretions can be collected for cytologic or bacteriologic examination for culturing fungi, acid-fast bacilli, *Pneumocystis carinii*, and *Legionella pneumophila*. It is used to remove foreign bodies and mucus plugs and to implant radioactive gold seeds for treating tumors.

The **flexible fiberoptic bronchoscope** is the instrument of choice in most cases because it is small and permits visualization of the segmental and subsegmental bronchi. Figure 3-16 illustrates both the instrument's structure and its application. The flexible fiberoptic bronchoscope has an external diameter between 3 and 6 mm and contains four channels: two light channels, one vision channel, and one open channel that accommodates biopsy forceps, cytology brush for obtaining samples, suction tube, lavage tube, anesthetic, or oxygen. With the aid of a fluoroscope, forceps and brushes can be advanced beyond the bronchoscope field of vision to obtain specimens. When alveolar tissue is obtained, this is termed a transbronchial biopsy.

The **rigid bronchoscope** is necessary to remove foreign bodies, excise endobronchial lesions, evaluate tracheal lesions, and control massive hemoptysis. The rigid bronchoscope is a hollow metallic tube with a light at its end.

General anesthesia is sometimes used. However, in most cases the patient is sedated and a local anesthetic is sprayed or swabbed over the mouth, tongue, and throat. An oxygen tube is inserted into one nostril and left in place throughout the procedure. Lidocaine jelly is generally used to both lubricate the bronchoscope and suppress the gag and cough reflexes. The bronchoscope is introduced through the nose or mouth, through the trachea, and into the mainstem bronchi. Evaluation of distal lesions or transbronchial biopsy requires fluoroscopic guidance.

Just before the procedure the patient is given atropine to dry respiratory secretions. A narcotic for sedation and a sedative or tranquilizer (such as Valium) for muscle relaxation are also given.

Complications of bronchoscopy include bleeding, infection, and pneumothorax.

FIGURE 3-16
Flexible fiberoptic bronchoscope. The four channels consist of two that provide a light source, one vision channel, and one open channel that accommodates instruments or allows administration of an anesthetic or oxygen.

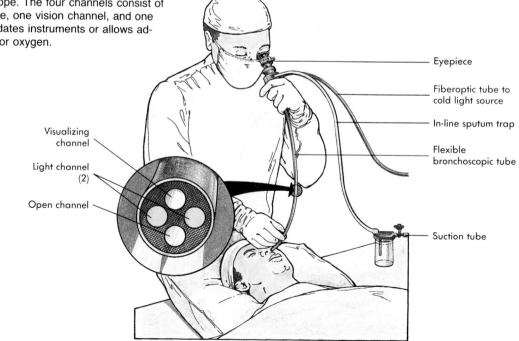

Visualizing channel

Light channel (2)

Open channel

Eyepiece

Fiberoptic tube to cold light source

In-line sputum trap

Flexible bronchoscopic tube

Suction tube

INDICATIONS

Severe or chronic lung infection
Lung tumor
Hemoptysis
Foreign body
Mucus plug
Implant radioactive seeds

CONTRAINDICATIONS

None

NURSING CARE

The patient should be kept NPO for 6-8 hours before the procedure. Remove any dental prosthesis and warn the physician about any loose teeth. Administer sedative as ordered.

After the procedure, patients should be kept in a semi-Fowler's position, although they may be turned from side to side. Talking should be discouraged; in fact, temporary loss of voice is common. Provide the patient with pencil and paper to communicate. Oxygen may be ordered.

Fluids may be given after the gag and swallow reflexes return, usually about 2 hours after the procedure. Throat discomfort is to be expected. Warm drinks, warm saline gargles, and throat lozenges will help to ease the soreness. If swallowing is painful, a soft diet can be offered.

Assess breath sounds and respiratory rhythm and be alert for signs of pneumothorax. Subcutaneous emphysema, which presents as crepitus around the patient's neck and face, indicates a leak in the pleura. Laryngeal stridor and dyspnea suggest laryngeal edema or laryngospasm. Pink-tinged secretions after bronchoscopy are normal, but hemoptysis suggests hemorrhage. Vigorous coughing after a biopsy must be discouraged because it could dislodge a clot.

PATIENT TEACHING

Before bronchoscopy is performed, explain the purpose of the procedure. Assure the patient that he will be sedated to minimize the discomfort. Explain that he must breathe through the tube, which initially may produce a feeling of suffocation, but that he should try to relax and not fight against it. He will not be able to talk while the tube is in place. Bronchoscopy takes about 45-60 minutes. Results of most tests usually are available the following day, although the acid-fast bacilli test may take up to 6 weeks. Patients who are undergoing bronchoscopy to determine whether a malignancy is operable may need extra support.

PULMONARY ANGIOGRAPHY

Pulmonary angiography provides visualization of the entire pulmonary vascular tree, making it an essential diagnostic tool in disorders involving pulmonary circulation. It is performed with pulmonary artery catheterization.

The patient is awake during the procedure. A catheter is inserted into the median basilic, cephalic, or femoral vein. Using fluoroscopy for guidance, the catheter is advanced into the right atrium, through the tricuspid valve into the right ventricle, and into the pulmonary artery. A radiopaque dye is then injected through the catheter. A series of radiographic films are made to track the dye as it flows through the pulmonary vasculature.

The standard filming techniques are cineangiography and serial angiography. Cineangiography produces a motion picture of the fluoroscopic images. Serial angiography uses a rapid film changer to produce a series of roentgenograms.

Patients are continuously monitored by electrocardiogram during cardiac catheterization to detect dysrhythmias and other adverse events. Blood gas sampling is available in the event of severe dysrhythmias or cardiac arrest.

Pulmonary angiography has a very low rate of complications and is often performed as an outpatient procedure. Complications during the procedure include adverse reactions or anaphylaxis to the contrast medium, dysrhythmias requiring cardioversion, and perforation leading to cardiac tamponade. Postprocedure complications include myocardial infarction, stroke, dysrhythmias, embolism, thrombosis, aneurysm, infection, pulmonary edema, and hematoma or hemorrhage at the insertion site.

For an illustration of the pulmonary arteries, see Figure 1-13.

INDICATIONS

To diagnose: Arteriovenous malformations in the lung
Pulmonary hypertension
Pulmonary thromboembolism
To evaluate: Abnormalities found on chest x-ray
Collapsed lung for preoperative assessment

CONTRAINDICATIONS

Severe respiratory distress
Patients with histories of allergic reactions to iodine or contrast medium require special precautions.

NURSING CARE

Before the procedure obtain written consent. Determine whether the patient is allergic to shellfish or iodine or has had a previous reaction to contrast media. Maintain the patient NPO for 4 to 6 hours. Shave and cleanse the insertion site and administer a sedative as ordered.

After the procedure, monitor vital signs every 15 minutes for the first hour or until the patient is stable. Keep a pressure dressing over the insertion site. Check the site for bleeding, hematoma, and signs of infection and monitor the area distally for pulse, circulation, numbness, and tingling. Maintain the patient on bed rest for 4 to 6 hours. Encourage fluid intake during the first 8 hours to encourage renal excretion of the contrast medium.

PATIENT TEACHING

Explain the procedure and its purpose. Reassure the patient that although no anesthetic is used, the procedure should cause very little discomfort. The patient will need to follow instructions given by the physician during the procedure, such as coughing. Explain that insertion of the catheter will cause a feeling of pressure and that injection of the dye will produce a flushing sensation or nausea, but these symptoms are temporary. Assure the patient that he will be monitored during the procedure, which usually takes about 2 hours. Explain that soreness at the insertion site and muscle cramping are common, but these after-effects disappear in a few days.

SPUTUM EXAMINATION

The microbiologic examination of sputum is essential in evaluating patients with respiratory disorders. Culture and sensitivity (C & S) and Gram stain are the two laboratory tests routinely performed on sputum specimens. The specimen is cultured to diagnose bacterial infection, and the sensitivity test determines whether the bacterial strain is resistant to certain antibiotics. Because the results of a C & S may take 24 to 48 hours, a Gram stain is performed to determine whether the organisms are gram-negative or gram-positive. The Gram stain report is available quickly (in a few hours) and is useful for selecting antibiotic therapy until the C & S report is available.

An acid-fast stain is done to detect acid-fast bacilli when tuberculosis is suspected. The result of acid-fast stain is usually available in 3-6 weeks. Specimens from 3 consecutive days are required for acid-fast stain.

Cytology is performed if a malignancy is suspected. A single sputum specimen is collected in a special container with a fixative solution.

INDICATIONS

To diagnose: Malignancy
              Tuberculosis
To evaluate: Pneumonia
To select an effective antibiotic

CONTRAINDICATIONS

None

TECHNIQUES

Sputum is collected early in the morning, at which time it is more plentiful and concentrated from pooling while the patient slept. The specimen is put directly into a sterile container and transported immediately to the lab. Collection may be by either the direct method or the indirect method or by gastric lavage.

Direct Method

The patient coughs voluntarily to produce sputum. If coughing fails to produce a specimen, breathing a heated, nebulized mist of distilled water or sodium chloride for several minutes will often liquify secretions enough to produce a specimen. The patient should expectorate directly into a wide-mouthed sterile container with a tight-fitting lid. The direct method of sputum collection has no associated complications.

Indirect Method

Sputum can be obtained from patients who are unable to cough up a specimen by either nasotracheal suctioning or transtracheal aspiration. Nasotracheal suctioning is the simpler technique because it involves passing a catheter through a nostril and into the trachea. Hypoxemia is a possible complication of nasotracheal suctioning.

Transtracheal aspiration is the preferred method, however, because better specimens are obtained. A needle puncture is made through the cricothyroid membrane and into the trachea, where sputum is aspirated. Transtracheal aspiration requires sterile technique and is uncomfortable for the patient, although a local anesthetic is used. Complications arising from this procedure include subcutaneous or mediastinal emphysema and infection at the puncture site.

Gastric Lavage

Obtaining sputum by gastric lavage is occasionally necessary in uncooperative patients, particularly very young children, and acutely ill patients suspected of having malignancy or tuberculosis. This method is based on the assumption that the patient swallows sputum while sleeping and during early morning coughing.

A nasogastric tube is inserted through the nose and into the stomach. Gastric contents are aspirated with a large syringe, placed in a sterile container, and sent immediately to the laboratory. The nasogastric tube is then removed.

NURSING CARE

Regardless of the technique used, note the color, consistency, odor, and amount of the sputum. As soon as the specimen is collected, transport it directly to the lab. When serial specimens are needed, number the specimens for each of the 3 days.

In obtaining sputum by the direct method, first have the patient brush teeth and gargle to reduce contamination with saliva and mouth bacteria. Instruct the patient to expectorate any postnasal secretions. Then have the patient take a deep breath to full capacity and exhale with an expulsive deep cough directly into the sterile container.

For nasotracheal suctioning, assist the patient into a sitting position. Administer oxygen during this procedure. The nurse or physician passes a catheter through the patient's nose. Monitor the patient's cardiovascular and respiratory status during and after the procedure.

For transtracheal aspiration, assemble the sterile equipment needed: gloves, gauze sponges, large-bore intracatheter needle, 10 cc syringe, sterile specimen cup, local anesthetic with needle and syringe, and iodophor for cleaning the skin. Administer high-flow oxygen during the procedure. Position the patient in a supine position with neck hyperextended with a pillow under the shoulders. Monitor the patient's respiratory and cardiovascular status. After the procedure, maintain light pressure over the injection site for 3-5 minutes. Assess for complications. Anaerobic culture specimens should be sent to the laboratory in the aspirating syringe after all excess air has been expelled.

For gastric lavage, the patient should be maintained NPO for 8 hours before the procedure.

PATIENT TEACHING

Explain the procedure and its purpose.

PERCUTANEOUS LUNG BIOPSY

Percutaneous lung biopsy is performed on patients who have an unexplained diffuse pulmonary process, unidentified pulmonary infection, or suspected malignancy. There are essentially two types of percutaneous techniques for lung biopsy, one performed with a narrow-gauge needle and one using a cutting needle. Because a local anesthetic is used rather than general anesthesia, percutaneous lung biopsy requires a cooperative patient. Both techniques carry the risk of pneumothorax, hemorrhage, cardiac arrest, vagal reflex stimulation, air emboli, and infection.

The tissue specimen is sent to the laboratory for microbiologic, histologic, cytologic, and immunologic studies.

PERCUTANEOUS NEEDLE BIOPSY WITH ASPIRATION

A 22- to 24-gauge needle is inserted percutaneously into the suspected lesion under the guidance of a fluoroscope. Once the needle is in place, the syringe is rotated during aspiration of fluid and cells to obtain an adequate specimen. This technique is used to remove a peripheral nodule or to identify an infectious process.

PERCUTANEOUS BIOPSY WITH A CUTTING NEEDLE

Use of a cutting needle is indicated in patients with diffuse pulmonary infiltrates because a larger tissue sample is obtained. Any one of three techniques can be used: (1) punch biopsy with a Vim-Silverman needle, (2) drill biopsy with a high-speed trephine that automatically seals off blood vessels, or (3) suction excision biopsy with an Abrams needle or a modification of an Abrams needle. Biopsy with a cutting needle carries a higher rate of complications than aspiration with a narrow-gauge needle.

INDICATIONS

Suspected malignancy
Unexplained diffuse lung disease
Unidentified infectious process

CONTRAINDICATIONS

Emphysematous bullae in the area to be biopsied
Pulmonary hypertension
Respiratory insufficiency
Uncooperative patient

NURSING CARE

Obtain written consent. Follow standard preoperative procedures. Disinfect the patient's skin and prepare a sterile field. Administer preoperative sedative as ordered. After the procedure carefully assess the patient for signs of pneumothorax, hemorrhage, and cardiac dysrhythmias.

PATIENT TEACHING

Explain the procedure and its purpose. Inform the patient that a local anesthetic will be used, which will sting when injected, and pressure will be felt when the needle is inserted. Assure the patient that discomfort during the procedure will be minimal. Instruct the patient to hold her breath for 15-30 seconds while the tissue sample is obtained.

OPEN LUNG BIOPSY

Open lung biopsy, or exploratory thoracotomy, is a surgical procedure for obtaining large specimens of lung tissue. The procedure is usually performed only when percutaneous needle biopsy has failed to establish a diagnosis. With the patient under general anesthesia, a standard thoracotomy incision is made, and the lung is inspected and biopsied. The specimen is submitted for microbiologic, histologic, cytologic, and immunologic studies.

Complications of open lung biopsy are considerable and include respiratory failure, emphysema, and bronchopleural fistula.

INDICATIONS

Suspected malignancy
Unexplained diffuse lung disease
Unidentified infectious process

CONTRAINDICATIONS

Pulmonary hypertension
Respiratory insufficiency
Uncontrolled coughing

NURSING CARE

Standard preoperative procedures should be followed. Keep the patient NPO for 8-12 hours before surgery. Shave the incision area and give preoperative medications as ordered. One or two days after surgery, use a chest tube connected to water-seal drainage to reverse the surgically induced pneumothorax. Monitor the patient closely for signs of respiratory complications. A series of chest x-rays are usually taken over several days.

PATIENT TEACHING

Explain the procedure and its purpose.

Noninfectious Respiratory Disorders

According to the National Institutes of Health (NIH), lung diseases cause one out of every eight deaths and play a role in one out of every four.

About 17 million Americans have some form of chronic lung disorder. In the United States, respiratory diseases account for approximately 21 million days of hospital care, and lung diseases account for more workdays lost (over 31 million annually) than any other category of illness.

Smoking is the single most common cause of chronic respiratory disorders and lung cancer. Approximately 10 million Americans have chronic obstructive pulmonary disease (COPD), and at least 80% of these cases result from smoking. COPD is the fifth most common cause of death in the United States, but the actual mortality rate is considerably higher. Patients with COPD have high complication rates from influenza, and deaths are often attributed directly to pneumonia.

Asthma affects about 7 million Americans and is the most common chronic disease of childhood, affecting over 3 million children under age 15. The high absenteeism from school among asthmatic children leads to learning impairments.

Environmental insults are also a leading cause of lung disorders. Although it is difficult to establish a clear picture of the impact of air pollutants on the general population, occupational lung diseases continue to rank as an important cause of chronic disability. These disorders have a range of clinical manifestations, including asthma, COPD, allergic alveolitis, and lung cancer. Despite efforts by the federal government to reduce hazardous pollutants in some industries, several occupational lung diseases continue to be a problem. Silicosis, coal worker's pneumoconiosis, and asbestos-related diseases are the major occupational lung disorders.

Dyspnea is the primary symptom that prompts most patients to seek medical attention. When severe, it is a frightening experience that can induce panic, which only increases the patient's dyspnea. Patients experiencing chest pain, particularly if it is sharp or severe, also tend to seek early medical care.

Unfortunately, other symptoms of respiratory disorders may be ignored for longer periods of time. Chronic cough develops gradually and is frequently dismissed by patients, particularly smokers, even when it is productive. Patients with hemoptysis are generally more likely to become alarmed and seek medical attention.

Adult Respiratory Distress Syndrome (ARDS)

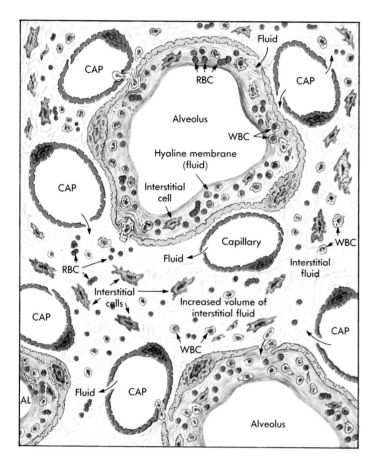

In **adult respiratory distress syndrome (ARDS),** capillary permeability is increased, precipitating a clinical condition in which lungs are wet and heavy, congested, hemorrhagic, stiff, and unable to diffuse oxygen.

ARDS results from pulmonary edema and respiratory failure secondary to increased capillary permeability. Disorders that may lead to ARDS include trauma, inhaled toxins, liquid aspiration, hematologic disorders, infections, drug overdose, and toxic metabolic disorders. During World War I ARDS was called posttraumatic pulmonary insufficiency, during World War II it was called wet lung, and during the Vietnam war it was called DaNang lung.

PATHOPHYSIOLOGY

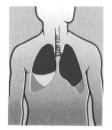

Regardless of the cause of ARDS, the tissue response of the lung and the response of the body do not vary. On biopsy examination the lung is congested and bleeding and looks like a liver. The amount of secretions in the large airways is insignificant, and there is no visible blockage of the major vessels.

There is always a time sequence in the development of ARDS. For example, it may be seen 12 to 24 hours after an injury resulting in hypovolemic shock or lung contusion, or it may appear 5 to 10 days following the development of sepsis. In either case the sequence of response and the symptoms remain the same.

Figure 4-1 outlines the physiologic process. The subsequent physiologic manifestations are stiff lungs and shunting. The lungs are stiff because the alveoli are filled with a proteinaceous exudate that has leaked out of damaged pulmonary capillaries. Stiff lungs are manifested by decreased compliance. As a result more airway pressure is required for each breath, making less air volume available for oxygen transfer. Stiff lungs also reduce the functional residual capacity (FRC). FRC is the volume of air in the lungs at the end of tidal volume. The FRC decreases because alveoli filled with fluid tend to collapse at the end of expiration. The collapsed alveoli lessen lung tissue available to exchange oxygen.

Both physiologic shunting and alveolar dead space ventilation occur in ARDS. Since the alveoli are filled with fluid, oxygen cannot diffuse from the alveoli to the pulmonary capillaries nor can carbon dioxide diffuse from the pulmonary capillaries to the alveoli. This results in a venous admixture, which accounts for profound hypoxemia. The dead space ventilation occurs in later stages of ARDS. While some alveoli are filled with fluid, others are relatively underperfused and overventilated, creating extra dead space and increasing the dead space/tidal volume ratio ($\dot{V}_D/\dot{V}_T$).[71]

As a result of this process the following major problems occur:

1. A reduction in the functional vital capacity
2. Bronchovascular edema, resulting in a decrease of the interstitial negative pressure, distal atelectasis, and decreased vital capacity
3. Decreased lung compliance caused by congestion, resulting in a decreased functional residual capacity (FRC)
4. Hypoxia caused by shunting in the lungs
5. Increased oxygen consumption, increased airway resistance, and increased venous blood return to the heart caused by the patient's attempt to increase minute breathing

One of the most important assessment rules in the care of the patient with ARDS or potential ARDS is to have good baseline data. Should the patient's condition deteriorate, subtle changes can be identified.

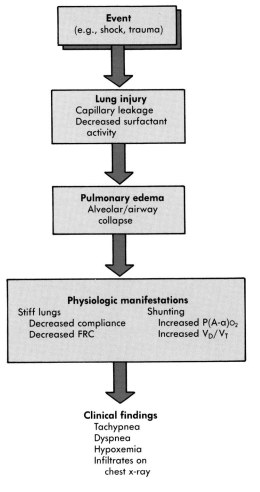

FIGURE 4-1
Pathogenesis of adult respiratory distress syndrome.

COMPLICATIONS

Dysrhythmias
Secondary infections
Sepsis
Stress ulcers
Disseminated intravascular coagulation
Barotrauma
Congestive heart failure
Renal failure

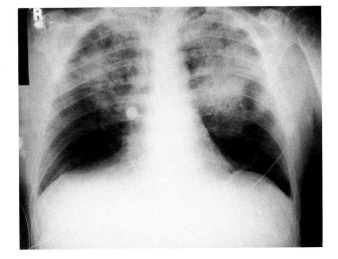

FIGURE 4-2
Chest x-ray of patient with adult respiratory distress syndrome. Heart is normal size; note diffuse infiltrates in upper and middle zones of lungs. (Courtesy R. Keith Wilson, M.D., Baylor College of Medicine, Houston, Tex; From Thompson.)[99]

Respiratory failure is a condition in which the arterial Pco_2 is above 50 mm Hg when the patient is at rest and breathing room air or in which the Pao_2 is less than 55 mm Hg.

Respiratory failure refers to the inability of the lungs to maintain normal oxygenation of the blood (hypoxic failure) and/or elimination of carbon dioxide (hypoventilatory failure).

In its most severe state, acute respiratory failure is referred to as adult respiratory distress syndrome (ARDS).

Respiratory failure is not a disease but is a disorder of ventilation that may be caused by a variety of conditions either directly or indirectly.

Respiratory failure may be divided into three types:

Type I: Causes of severe hypoxemia with an abnormally low Pao_2 include the following:
1. Increased pulmonary capillary pressure resulting from such conditions as:
   a. Left ventricular heart failure
   b. Pulmonary edema or fluid overload
2. Increased pulmonary capillary permeability from such conditions as:
   a. Pneumonia
   b. Tuberculosis
   c. Fungal infections
   d. Near drowning
   e. Chemical or smoke inhalation
   f. Liquid aspiration

Type II: In type II respiratory failure the diseased lung is unable to normally excrete CO_2. Usually this is manifested by some type of chronic breathing problem accompanying such conditions as the following:
1. Chronic bronchitis
2. Emphysema
3. Massive obesity
4. Severe kyphoscoliosis
5. Asthma

Type III: The third type of respiratory failure is due to the inability of the neuromuscular system to ventilate normal or nearly normal lungs. There are two basic causes for this:
1. Respiratory center depression due to a malfunctioning central nervous system. This can be caused by:
   a. Drug overdoses
   b. Central nervous system lesions or infections
2. Inability of a normally functioning central nervous system to generate respiratory muscle power. Examples of disorders of neuromuscular transmission include the following:
   a. Guillain-Barré syndrome
   b. Multiple sclerosis
   c. Spinal cord injury
   d. Myasthenia gravis
   e. Muscular dystrophies
   f. Poliomyelitis
   g. Tetanus

DIAGNOSTIC STUDIES AND FINDINGS

Diagnostic Test	Findings
Pulmonary function tests	Decreased vital capacity, minute volume, and functional residual capacity indicating stiff lungs due to fluid-filled alveoli
	Compliance (c): Below normal, indicating stiff lungs
Laboratory tests	
Arterial blood gases	Pao_2 <55 mm Hg indicates hypoxia
	$Paco_2$ >45 mm Hg indicates retention of CO_2
	HCO_3 <26 mEq/L indicates kidneys' attempt to compensate for respiratory acidosis; pH increased in beginning; as ARDS becomes worse, pH decreases—indicates respiratory acidosis
Alveolar-arterial oxygen gradient $P(A-a)o_2$ (also A-a Do_2)	300-500 mm Hg; reflects the difficulty with which oxygen crosses the alveolar-capillary membrane
Shunt fraction ($\dot{Q}s-\dot{Q}t$)	May be > 15% to 20%, measures the degree of intrapulmonary shunting; normal value <6%
Lactic acid levels	Increased regardless of measurement technique—reflects excess due to lack of oxygen
	Normal values:
	80-100 Wacker units
	120-340 IU/I
	150-450 Wroblewski units
Chest x-rays	There must be a large increase in lung fluid before abnormalities are observed on chest x-rays; early diagnostic radiographic changes include thickened or blurred margins of the bronchi or vessels; Figure 4-2 shows diffuse and hazy blurred appearance throughout the lung fields
	Diffuse pulmonary infiltrates

MEDICAL MANAGEMENT

The major medical plan is focused in three areas: **1. Supportive,** to provide adequate oxygenation and mechanical ventilation to reverse the hypoxemia and expand the distal gas exchange units so as to prevent further airway and alveolar collapse. **2. Therapeutic,** to treat the systemic responses caused by the alterations in pulmonary function. **3. Curative,** to locate and halt the causal insult.

GENERAL MANAGEMENT

Fluid and electrolyte therapy: Fluids are monitored carefully. Excessive intravascular fluid administration may result in cardiogenic pulmonary edema. Patients with capillary damage from ARDS are especially susceptible to fluid leakage into the alveolar spaces.

Fluid types: There is some controversy regarding the use of colloids and crystalloids. It is most generally believed that colloidal fluids should be used in hypoalbuminemic patients. All other patients should receive crystalloid fluids.

Quantity of fluids: PCWP is much more reliable than the CVP when trying to determine the quantity of fluids to be administered. In most situations, maintenance of the PCWP at 10-15 mm Hg provides adequate, but not excessive, intravascular volumes. Certainly clinical parameters such as pulse, urinary output, and peripheral vasoconstriction should also be considered as assessment variables.

Oxygenation: Oxygen support via mask may be used in the very early stages of ARDS but will not be sufficient as the syndrome becomes worse. The goal is to provide the lowest oxygen concentration to maintain the mixed venous oxygen at a level > 40 mm Hg.
If oxygen concentrations > 50% are required to maintain adequate blood gas oxygen levels, intubation and mechanical ventilation are indicated.
The purpose of mechanical ventilation for ARDS is to produce a rapid inspiratory flow rate while also exerting a continuous PEEP (See Chapter 6).

Cardiovascular monitoring: Invasive cardiovascular monitoring (e.g., with the pulmonary artery catheter) should be used whenever cardiovascular compromise is anticipated. Once the catheter is in place, the PCWP should be optimized to 10-15 mm Hg.

Electrocardiogram: Monitor cardiac response.

Alimentation: Alimentation should be undertaken from the onset. External alimentation with a small feeding tube is best, but intravenous hyperalimentation should be instituted if enteral alimentation is not possible. The use of antacids and H_2 blockers to maintain gastric pH above 4 is warranted for prophylaxis for stress ulcers.

DRUG THERAPY

There are no specific drugs used to treat the syndrome. Drugs used are primarily supportive to other therapeutic measures such as mechanical ventilation.

Morphine 3-5 mg/h IV: May be given as sedation for mechanical ventilator patients who are restless and experiencing tachypnea.

Pancuronium bromide (Pavulon): May be used as a neuroblocking agent to completely paralyze the voluntary respirations of the patient. Dosage must be carefully and individually calculated for each patient. The initial intravenous dosage range for an adult is 0.04-0.1 mg/kg.

Corticosteroids: Use is controversial. Evidence remains speculative that they are helpful in reducing pulmonary edema and stabilizing pulmonary membranes.

Heparin: Has been advocated by some sources as a drug to combat microvascular emboli. Most authorities, however, question the real benefits of heparin and warn that its risks outweigh any potential benefit for these critically ill individuals.

Diuretics: Used to keep the patient on the "dry" side. The PCWP is kept as low as possible without impairing cardiac output. Fluid therapy is discussed above.

1 ASSESS

ASSESSMENT	OBSERVATIONS
Respiratory	Respiratory distress: nasal flaring, chest wall retractions, tachypnea or bradypnea, decreased chest wall movement, dyspnea, crackles Breath sounds: crackles, sonorous wheezes (rhonchi) and sibilant wheezes, decreased, bilaterally unequal Breathing pattern: labored, irregular Increased sputum, persistent cough, wet-sounding breathing Hypercapnia: headache, dizziness, confusion, unconsciousness, twitching, hypertension, sweating, flushed face Hypoxia: restlessness, confusion, impaired motor function, hypotension, cyanosis, tachycardia
Cardiovascular	Decreased cardiac output: restlessness, lethargy, tachycardia, hypotension, decreased urinary output Pulmonary pressures: increased PCWP, increased PAP
Psychosocial	Anxiety, fear of suffocation, fear of being out of control if on ventilator, fear of unknown, inability to communicate

2 DIAGNOSE

NURSING DIAGNOSIS	SUBJECTIVE FINDINGS	OBJECTIVE FINDINGS
Impaired gas exchange related to alveolar-capillary membrane changes	Complains of SOB, expresses need for supplemental oxygen	Crackles (rales), decreased breath sounds, dyspnea, tachypnea Pa_{O_2} <70 mm Hg Pa_{CO_2} >35 mm Hg pH <7.35 Increased lactic acid Diffuse infiltrates on chest x-ray Confusion, somnolence, restlessness
Ineffective breathing pattern related to decreased compliance	Complains of fatigue, pain when breathing, and inability to breathe Expresses need for oxygen	Dyspnea, tachypnea, use of accessory muscles, nasal flaring, cyanosis of nailbeds and mucous membranes Pa_{O_2} <55 mm Hg Pa_{CO_2} >35 mm Hg pH <7.35 Decreased tidal volume, decreased minute volume
Activity intolerance related to hypoxia	Complains of being too tired to perform activities	Unable to perform usual ADL; sleeps more than usual
Ineffective airway clearance related to pulmonary and interstitial edema	Complains of difficulty breathing; expresses anxiety	Crackles (rales), rhonchi, and wheezes Tachypnea, dyspnea, cough, fever, use of accessory muscles

NURSING DIAGNOSIS	SUBJECTIVE FINDINGS	OBJECTIVE FINDINGS
Altered nutrition: less than body requirements related to inadequate intake secondary to hypoxia and fatigue	Complains of being too tired to eat; complains of being too short of breath to eat	Inadequate intake of food and fluid Weight loss Decreased albumin and lymphocytes Decreased triceps skinfold and midarm circumference measurements
Fear related to suffocation, to being on mechanical ventilator, to the uncertainty of prognosis, and to inability to verbally communicate	Expresses fears	Tachypnea, tachycardia, scared facial expression
Potential for infection related to decreased pulmonary function, possible steroid therapy, and ineffective airway clearance	Complains of fatigue and inability to breathe	Crackles (rales), decreased breath sounds, decreased albumin and lymphocytes, inadequate sleep, intubated

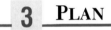 3 PLAN

Patient goals

1. Patient will have adequate oxygenation of tissues.
2. Patient will have an effective respiratory pattern.
3. Patient will be able to perform daily activities without fatigue.
4. Patient's airways will be patent with clear breath sounds.
5. Patient will maintain adequate nutritional status.
6. Patient will report decrease in fear.
7. Patient will have no infection.
8. Patient will demonstrate understanding of home care and follow-up instructions.

4 IMPLEMENT

NURSING DIAGNOSIS	NURSING INTERVENTIONS	RATIONALE
Impaired gas exchange related to alveolar-capillary membrane changes	Auscultate lungs for sonorous wheezes, crackles (rales), and sibilant wheezes.	Determines adequacy of gas exchange and detects atelectasis.
	Observe changes in awareness, orientation, and behavior.	May indicate hypoxia.
	Observe skin color and capillary refill.	Determines circulatory adequacy.
	Monitor ABGs.	Determines acid-base balance and need for oxygen.

NURSING DIAGNOSIS	NURSING INTERVENTIONS	RATIONALE
	Monitor CBC.	Detects amount of hemoglobin to carry oxygen and presence of infection.
	Assess PAP, PCWP, and jugular vein distention.	Indicates adequacy of tissue perfusion; may increase as a complication of PEEP.
	Monitor ECG and cardiac status for dysrhythmias.	Hypoxia can cause dysrhythmias. Tachycardia may occur as a complication of PEEP.
	Monitor lactic acid levels.	May increase during respiratory acidosis.
	Administer oxygen as ordered.	Improves gas exchange; decreases work of breathing.
	Administer corticosteroids as ordered.	Corticosteroids reduce edema and stabilize pulmonary membranes; also reduce inflammation.
	Administer diuretics as ordered.	Diuretics reduce pulmonary edema.
	Administer morphine as ordered.	Morphine sedates patient receiving mechanical ventilation.
	Administer heparin as ordered.	Heparin prevents formation of thrombi.
	In collaboration with physician, administer packed RBCs.	Increases hemoglobin so that more oxygen can be transported.
	Maintain PEEP.	To increase lung volumes, compliance, and mean airway pressure as well as decreasing shunting.
	Pace activities to patient's tolerance.	Decreases oxygen demand.
Ineffective breathing pattern related to decreased compliance	Observe changes in respiratory rate and depth.	Determines adequacy of breathing pattern.
	Review chest x-rays.	Identifies areas of infiltration and congestion.
	Measure tidal volume and vital capacity.	Determines lung's compliance and volume of air moving in and out of lungs.
	Supervise use of ventilator.	Maintains inhalation using mechanical assistive devices.
	Assist patient to use relaxation techniques.	Relieves anxiety and slows respiratory rate.

NURSING DIAGNOSIS	NURSING INTERVENTIONS	RATIONALE
Activity intolerance related to hypoxia	Observe response to activity.	Determines extent of activity intolerance.
	Identify factors contributing to intolerance (e.g., stress, side effects of drugs).	Guides selection of therapeutic interventions.
	Assess patient's sleep patterns.	May document a causative factor.
	Plan rest periods between activities.	To reduce fatigue.
	Perform activities for patient until he/she is able to perform them.	Meets patient's need without causing fatigue.
	Provide progressive increase in activity as tolerated.	Slowly increases the number of and endurance of activities.
	Administer oxygen as needed.	To decrease work of breathing during activity.
Ineffective airway clearance related to pulmonary and interstitial edema	Auscultate lungs for rhonchi, crackles, or wheezing.	Determines adequacy of gas exchange and extent of airway obstructed with secretions.
	Assess characteristics of secretions: quantity, color, consistency, odor.	Detects presence of infection.
	Assess patient's hydration status: skin turgor, mucous membranes, tongue, intake and output over 24 hours.	Determines need for fluids.
	Monitor chest x-rays.	Shows extent of lung involvement.
	Monitor sputum and culture and sensitivity reports.	Guides therapeutic interventions; identifies microorganisms present.
	Monitor tidal volume and vital capacity.	Indicates ventilatory sufficiency.
	Assist patient with coughing as needed.	Removes secretions.
	Perform endotracheal or tracheostomy tube suctioning as needed.	Stimulates cough reflex and removes secretions.
	Position patient in proper body alignment for optimal breathing pattern (head of bed up 45°, if tolerated up to 90°).	Secretions move by gravity as position changes. Elevating head of bed moves abdominal content away from diaphragm to enhance diaphragmatic contraction.
	Assist patient with ambulation/position changes (turning side-to-side).	Secretions move by gravity as position changes.
	Perform chest physiotherapy (e.g., postural drainage, percussion, vibration).	Facilitates loosening and mobilizing of secretions.

NURSING DIAGNOSIS	NURSING INTERVENTIONS	RATIONALE
Altered nutrition: less than body requirements related to inadequate intake secondary to hypoxia and fatigue	Weigh patient weekly.	Provides data on adequacy of nutrition.
	For patient with tracheostomy, inspect tracheal aspirate for food particles at each feeding. Stop feedings if aspiration is found.	Determines if patient is aspirating feedings.
	Auscultate bowel sounds.	Documents gastrointestinal peristalsis.
	Measure fluid intake and output.	Determines fluid balance.
	Monitor albumin and lymphocytes.	Indicates adequacy of visceral protein.
	Measure mid-arm circumference and triceps skinfold.	Indicates protein and fat stores, respectively.
	Administer TPN/tube feeding and fluids as ordered.	Provides complete nutrition and maintains fluid balance without overhydrating patient.
Fear related to suffocation, to being on mechanical ventilation, to the uncertainty of prognosis, and to inability to communicate verbally	Validate sources of fear with patient. Assess patient's perception of unmet needs/expectations.	Guides therapeutic interventions.
	Assist patient to identify coping skills used successfully in the past.	Facilitates problem solving.
	Encourage patient to ask questions and express feelings.	May relieve anxiety; helps patient put thoughts into perspective.
	Provide accurate information about ARDS.	Knowledge can decrease fears.
	Provide oxygen as ordered.	Decreases the work of breathing.
	Provide alternate forms of communication when patient is unable to speak.	Facilitates communication, may decrease fear.
Potential for infection related to decreased pulmonary function, possible steroid therapy, and ineffective airway clearance	Monitor leukocytes and albumin.	Indicates adequacy of secondary defense and immune system.
	Assess nutritional status.	Adequate nutritional status supports the immune system.
	Monitor pulmonary function studies.	Indicates extent of pulmonary disease.

NURSING DIAGNOSIS	NURSING INTERVENTIONS	RATIONALE
	Assist with nebulizer treatments and physiotherapy.	Maintains clear airways and prevents stasis of secretions.
	Administer prophylactic antibiotics as ordered.	May prevent infections.
	Use strict aseptic technique in giving care.	Prevents introduction of microorganisms.
Knowledge deficit	See Patient Teaching.	

5 EVALUATE

PATIENT OUTCOME	DATA INDICATING THAT OUTCOME IS REACHED
Breathing pattern is effective.	Vital capacity measurements including tidal volume and minute volumes are optimal for patient. ABGs are within normal limits (Pa_{O_2} = 80-100 mm Hg, Pa_{CO_2} = 35-45 mm Hg, pH = 7.35-7.45); patient is breathing without difficulty.
Gas exchange is improved.	ABGs are within normal limits (see above).
Able to perform activities without fatigue.	Completes activities of daily living without dyspnea.
Airway is patent.	Breath sounds are clear; cough has subsided.
Nutritional status has improved.	Patient is eating a balanced diet and is gaining weight. Albumin = 3.2-4.5 g/dl Lymphocytes = 2100 or 35-40% per ml^3 blood Triceps skinfold = 12.0 mm (men) 23.0 mm (women) Midarm circumference = 32.7 cm (men) 29.2 cm (women)
Fear is decreased.	Patient states he is less fearful.
There is no infection.	Patient is afebrile. WBCs are within normal limits. Cultures are negative.
Knowledge deficit is resolved.	Patient demonstrates knowledge of disease process and home care management.

→ > >

PATIENT TEACHING

1. Teach the patient adaptive breathing techniques. Emphasize importance of periodic turning, coughing, and deep breathing.
2. Teach the importance of not fighting the ventilator and relaxing instead to permit maximum ventilation. Assure the patient that oxygen is being supplied.
3. Teach adaptive exercise and rest techniques.
4. Teach eating and food choice modifications.
5. Provide the patient and family with information regarding all medications the patient is taking: name, dosage, time of administration, and side effects.

Asthma

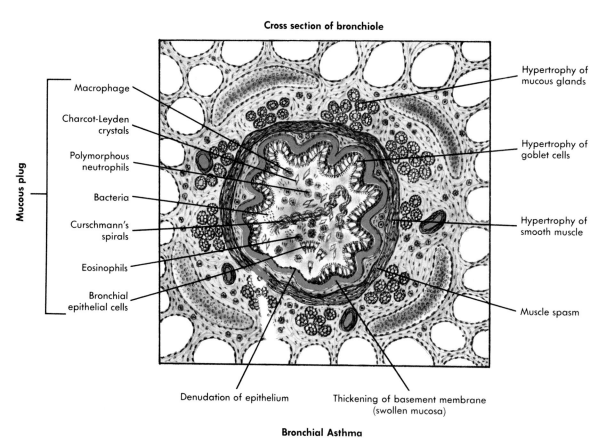

Cross section of bronchiole

Macrophage

Charcot-Leyden crystals

Polymorphous neutrophils

Bacteria

Curschmann's spirals

Eosinophils

Bronchial epithelial cells

Mucous plug

Hypertrophy of mucous glands

Hypertrophy of goblet cells

Hypertrophy of smooth muscle

Muscle spasm

Denudation of epithelium

Thickening of basement membrane (swollen mucosa)

Bronchial Asthma

Asthma, a disease marked by increased responsiveness of the trachea and bronchi to various stimuli, results in widespread narrowing of the airways that improves either spontaneously or with therapy. Status asthmaticus is an intense, unrelenting bronchospasm that does not respond to the usual modes of therapy.

Bronchial asthma is a broad clinical syndrome rather than a specific disease. There is bronchial hypersensitivity marked by reversible airway bronchospasm. The bronchospasm causes increased mucosal edema; constriction of the bronchial muscles; production of viscous mucus, which eventually leads to increased mucus plugs; bronchial airway obstruction; and overdistention of the lungs.

Asthma affects about 2% to 3% of the U.S. population and has a death rate of 1 per 100,000 persons.[100] In about 50% of patients the disease begins before 10 years of age, and in another 30% it occurs before age 40. During childhood there is a 2:1 male/female prevalence. This ratio equalizes during adolescence and thereafter.[45]

Asthma is the most common chronic disease for children and adults. It is responsible for about 150,000 hospital admissions and 1,275,000 hospital days a year. Asthma accounts for at least 85 million days of restricted work and 5 million days of work lost each year.[45]

Asthma may be divided into two types: extrinsic (atopic) asthma and intrinsic (nonatopic) asthma (Table 4-1).

Extrinsic asthma is caused by external agents such as dust, lint, insecticides, mold spores, foods, pollen, danders, or feathers. This type is best understood as an allergic reaction to specific allergens. Exposure to an allergen can cause an attack.

Intrinsic asthma indicates that the specific causes cannot be identified. It may be precipitated by many situations, such as a common cold, upper respiratory infection, or even exercise. This type usually begins in persons over 35 years of age and develops into a life-long condition, becoming worse and occurring more often.

Status asthmaticus has been defined as a severe asthmatic attack that does not respond to pharmacologic treatment within a few hours. Status asthmaticus is an acute progressive and life-threatening event that leads to respiratory failure if not properly treated.

PATHOPHYSIOLOGY

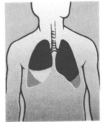

Whereas the trigger mechanism and physiologic response for intrinsic and extrinsic asthma differ, the clinical response appears the same. Figure 4-3 summarizes the proposed pathogenesis for the two causes of an asthmatic response.

Extrinsic (atopic or allergic) asthma is an example of a Type I hypersensitivity reaction termed *anaphylactic reaction*. Upon exposure to an allergen, the β lymphocytes are stimulated and differentiated into plasma cells that produce immunoglobulin E (IgE) antibodies. The IgE antibodies attach to mast cells and basophils in the bronchial walls. The mast cells in turn release chemical mediators—histamine, prostaglandins, bradykinin, and SRS (slow-reacting substance of anaphylaxis). Locally the histamine stimulates bronchial smooth muscle contraction and increases vascular permeability, causing leakage of protein and fluids into bronchial mucosa. (See Figure 4-4.)

Both parasympathetic and sympathetic nerves affect bronchi. Bronchial muscle tone is regulated by vagal nerves via the parasympathetic nervous system. In intrinsic asthma, when afferent (sensory) nerves endings are stimulated by mechanical or chemical stimuli (e.g., pollen, dust, or air pollution), the release of acetylcholine increases, causing reflex bronchoconstriction and production of chemical mediators (histamine, bradykinin, prostaglandins, and SRS), which also cause bronchoconstriction. One possible explanation for asthma is that asthmatics have a low threshold for parasympathetic responses.[81]

Both alpha and beta adrenergic receptors of the sympathetic nervous system are found in bronchi. Stimulation of alpha adrenergic receptors causes bronchoconstriction, while stimulation of beta receptors causes bronchodilation. Alpha and beta receptors are balanced by cyclic adenosine monophosphates (c-AMP). Alpha adrenergic stimulation results in decreased levels of c-AMP, causing increased mast cell release of chemical mediators and causing bronchoconstriction. Conversely, beta adrenergic stimulation increases levels of

Table 4-1

INTRINSIC VERSUS EXTRINSIC ASTHMA

Characteristic	Extrinsic	Intrinsic
Allergens as precipitants	Yes	No
Immediate skin test	Positive	Negative
Elevated IgE	Common	Uncommon
Eosinophilia	Yes	Yes
Childhood onset	Common	Uncommon
Other allergies	Common	Uncommon
Family history of multiple allergies	Common	Uncommon
Hyposensitization therapy	Helpful	Equivocal
Typical attack	Acute and self-limiting	Often fulminant and severe
Relationship of attack to infection	May be present	Common

Data from Miller and Kazemi[75] and Weiss.[110]

c-AMP, which inhibits release of chemical mediators and causes bronchodilation. One proposed explanation for asthma is that there is a block of beta adrenergic stimulation.[81]

A major difficulty in diagnosing asthma in adults who are not experiencing an acute attack is the lack of signs or symptoms. Patients may complain of cough, dyspnea on exertion, or weakness, but have normal arterial blood gases and chest x-rays. Pulmonary function tests, however, are performed before and after the inhalation of a bronchodilator.

Table 4-2 summarizes this assessment of the severity of asthma.

COMPLICATIONS

Mediastinal or subcutaneous emphysema
Bronchitis
Pulmonary hypertension
Cor pulmonale
Respiratory failure following status asthmaticus

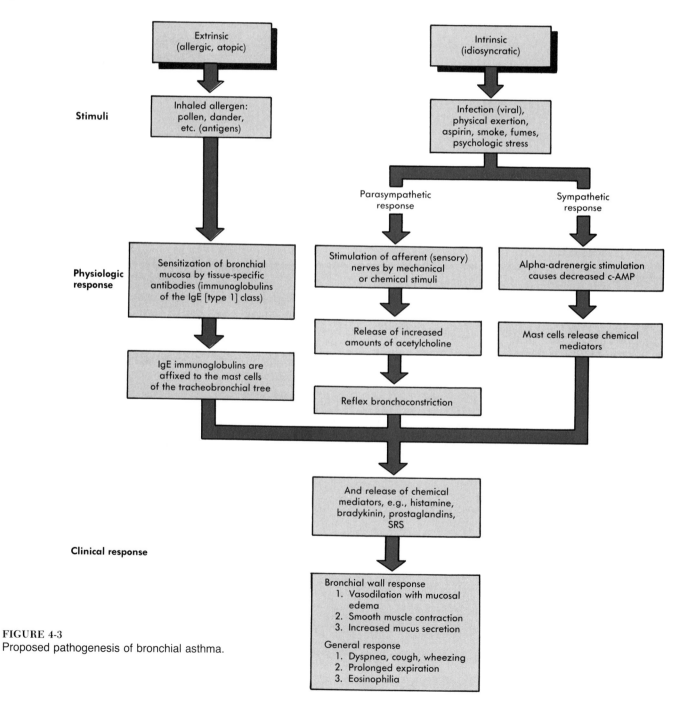

FIGURE 4-3
Proposed pathogenesis of bronchial asthma.

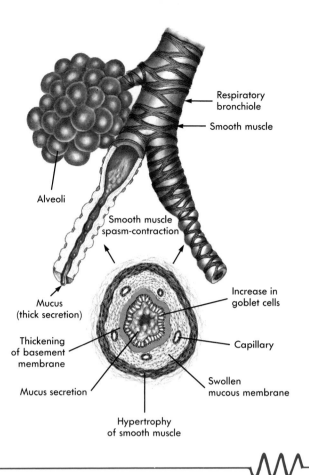

FIGURE 4-4
With bronchial asthma, the bronchiole is obstructed on expiration, particularly by muscle spasm, edema of the mucosa, and thick secretions.

Table 4-2 ⎯⎯⎯⎯⎯⎯⎯⎯⎯⎯⎯⎯⎯⎯⎯⎯⎯⎯⎯⎯⎯⎯⎯⎯ -\/\/\/-

ASSESSMENT OF SEVERITY OF ASTHMA

	Mild	Moderate	Severe
Episode of Severity Analysis*			
Acute phase	Mild dyspnea	Respiratory distress at rest	Marked respiratory distress
	Diffuse wheezes	Hyperpnea	Marked wheezes or absent breath sounds
	Adequate air exchange	Marked wheezes	
		Air exchange normal or $\downarrow$	Pulsus paradoxus >10 mm
			Chest wall retractions
	FEV_1 = 80% normal	FEV_1 = 50% normal	FEV_1 = 25% normal
	pH = Normal or $\uparrow$	pH = Generally $\uparrow$	pH = Normal or $\downarrow$
	Pao_2 = Normal or $\downarrow$	Pao = $\downarrow$	Pao_2 = $\downarrow$
	$Paco_2$ = Normal of $\downarrow$	$Paco_2$ = Generally $\downarrow$	$Paco_2$ = normal or $\uparrow$
Disease Severity Analysis†			
General assessment	Attacks no more than once per week	Cough and wheeze episodes more than once per week	Daily wheezing
	Responds to bronchodilators in 24 h	Cough and low-grade wheeze between acute episodes	Frequent severe episodes
	No signs of asthma between episodes	Exercise tolerance diminished	Hospitalization frequently required to break cycle
	No sleep interruption due to asthma	May be up at night because of cough and wheeze	Poor exercise tolerance
	No hyperventilation	Hyperinflation seen on chest roentgenogram	Much sleep interruption
	Normal chest roentgenogram	Lung volumes increased	Chest deformity due to chronic hyperinflation
	Minimal evidence of airway obstruction		Airway obstruction not completely reversible by bronchodilators
	No to minimal degree of increase in lung volume		Lung volumes markedly increased

*Modified from Berkow[11]
†From Ellis[30]

DIAGNOSTIC STUDIES AND FINDINGS

Diagnostic Test	Findings
Pulmonary function	FEV_1 (young healthy adult individual)
	Asthma before treatment, abnormally low after treatment, at least 2 L
	Peak expiratory flow rate (PEFR) (young healthy adult individual)
	Asthma before treatment, as low as 100 L/min
	After treatment, at least 300 L/min
	TLC: increases during acute episode because of air trapping
	RV: increases during acute episode
	VC: < 1 L
Laboratory	
ABGs	Pao_2 normal or slightly decreased secondary to decreases in $\dot{V}/\dot{Q}$; has direct linear relationship with FEV_1 (as FEV_1 decreases, so does Pao_2 [<60 mm Hg])
	$Paco_2$: increases only when FEV_1 is decreased by at least 20% ($\geq$ 40 mm Hg); pH: normal or decreased
	HCO_3^-: normal or decreased
CBC	Eosinophilia usually seen, which indicates allergic response
Theophylline level	Any asthmatic patient taking theophylline should have baseline monitoring of theophylline levels; therapeutic level of theophylline in the blood is 10-20 µg/ml
Chest x-ray	Usually clear; hyperinflation secondary to air trapping may be seen in persistent and long-standing cases; transient migratory pulmonary infiltrations may also be seen
ECG	Sinus tachycardia may be seen in acute episodes; prominent P waves occur in chronic asthma

MEDICAL MANAGEMENT

The intent of the immediate medical plan for the patient with asthma is to decrease the amount of bronchospasm and to increase pulmonary ventilation.

After the acute event is passed, the medical plan is to identify precipitating stimuli and to promote maximum health with this potentially degenerative chronic disease.

GENERAL MANAGEMENT

Oxygenation: Humidified oxygen should be administered by nasal cannula or mask to counteract clinical and laboratory signs of hypoxemia. Oxygen is administered to keep Pao_2 in range of 60-70 mm Hg to result in oxygen saturation greater than 90%.

Volume-cycled ventilator: Should the patient's condition continue to deteriorate despite aggressive therapy (1% to 3% of hospitalized asthma patients), endotracheal intubation and mechanical ventilation may become necessary.

The goal of ventilation by this method is to ensure adequate alveolar ventilation without hypercapnia or hypocapnia. To do this the practitioner should (1) decrease tidal volume as tolerated to allow lower cycling pressures, (2) decrease respiratory rate as tolerated to allow adequate duration of expiration, (3) supply heated, humidified oxygen to maintain Pao_2, (4) sedate patient as required and ordered, (5) continue to administer medications as listed under the drug section, and (6) administer chest physiotherapy and continue to encourage coughing.[75]

Chest physiotherapy: Postural drainage with chest percussion should be administered at least 2-4 h as long as the patient has congestion. See pp. 235-239 for techniques.

Environment: Provide an atmosphere void of known allergens.

DRUG THERAPY

Drug therapy for asthma can be divided into three categories: (1) acute phase therapy; (2) status asthmaticus therapy; and (3) interim therapy. For each of these treatment categories, two types of pharmacologic agents are used. Bronchodilators are used to increase the airway diameter, and corticosteroids are used to reduce the inflammatory response.

MEDICAL MANAGEMENT—cont'd

Category I: Acute phase
Bronchodilators
Parenteral
Epinephrine 1:1000: 0.3-0.8 ml subcutaneously q 15-30 min
Theophylline (Quibron, Theo-Dur): loading dose 5-6 mg/kg in normal saline over 20 min; lower dose for patients over 40 years of age; obtain theophylline levels in 12-24 h and maintain level at 10-20 μg/ml
Terbutaline (Brethine, Bricanyl): 0.2-0.3 ml subcutaneously q 30 min for 3 doses
Aminophylline: 250 mg in 20-30 ml normal saline (or 5.6-6 mg/kg in 100 ml normal saline); maximum rate 25 mg/min
Aerosols: 1 or 2 inhalations from hand nebulizer q 3-4 h or 0.5 ml in 2.5 or 3 ml normal saline by nebulization
Isoproterenol (Isuprel) 1:200
Isoetharine (Bronkosol) 1:200
Corticosteroids
Parenteral
Hydrocortisone sodium succinate (Solu-Cortef): 100-250 mg
Oral
Prednisone (Deltasone, others): 40-60 mg/d in divided doses; tapered rapidly over 3 wk if possible

Category II: Status asthmaticus
Bronchodilators
Epinephrine: same as for category I
Aminophylline (loading dose): 5.6-6 mg/kg in 100 ml normal saline for 20-30 min; maximum rate 25 mg/min
Continued therapy dose
    Young adult smokers: 1 mg/kg/h for 12 h, then reduce to 0.8 mg/kg/h
    Healthy, nonsmoking adults: 0.7-0.9 mg/kg/h for 12 h; then reduce to 0.5 mg/kg/h
    Older adults with cor pulmonale: 0.6 mg/kg/h for 12 h; then reduce to 0.3 mg/kg/h
    Adults with congestive heart failure and liver failure: 0.5 mg/kg/h for 12 h; then reduce to 0.1-0.2 mg/kg/h
    Subsequent doses should be determined by therapeutic serum level of aminophylline of 10-20 μg/ml
Corticosteroids
Parenteral
Hydrocortisone sodium succinate (Solu-Cortef), 4 mg/kg IV q 4 h
Methylprednisolone sodium succinate (Solu-Medrol), 2 mg/kg IV q 4 h
Oral (may also start on oral medications then reduce IV medications)
Hydrocortisone sodium succinate (Solu-Cortef): 300 mg/d divided into 4 doses
Prednisone (Deltasone, others): 20 mg/d divided into 4 doses
Methylprednisolone (Medrol): 16 mg/d divided into 4 doses

Category III: Interim phase
Bronchodilator: Maintenance doses to keep serum level at 10-20 μg/ml
Oral
Theophylline (Aerolate, Elixophyllin, Quibron, Tedral, Theo-Dur, Theolair): 16 mg/kg/d in single dose or divided doses
Aminophylline (Aminodur, Aminophyl, Somophyllin), 3.5-5 mg/kg/q 6 h
Aerosol
Albuterol (Proventil Inhaler, Ventolin Inhaler): 1-2 inhalations q 4-6 h
Corticosteroids
Aerosol
Beclomethasone dipropionate (Vanceril inhaler, others) 2 inhalations qid; long-acting and not systemically absorbed

Fluid and electrolyte therapy
    The purpose of fluid therapy is to liquefy secretions and to have a method by which to administer intravenous drugs. Providing that the patient has no cardiovascular dysfunction, fluid therapy should be aggressive. Dextrose 5% in water or 5% dextrose in 0.02 normal saline are adequate intravenous solutions.

1 ASSESS

ASSESSMENT	OBSERVATIONS
History	Known family or personal history of allergy, infantile eczema, or previous episodes of asthma; previous recent severe attack; prolonged attack (24-36 h); previous hospitalization for asthma
Current medications	Careful and complete history of current respiratory-related medications, as well as most recent dose and time before hospital arrival
Physical assessment Respiratory status	Airway obstruction: with severe airway obstruction, breath sounds diminished in certain lung regions Respiratory distress: dyspnea, tachypnea, cough, prolonged expiration, use of accessory muscles, retractions Breath sounds: inspiratory and expiratory wheeze, coarse rhonchi; in severe cases only coarse bronchial sounds heard; bilateral sounds heard throughout chest
Circulatory status	Cardiovascular findings result from hypoxia and include tachycardia often >130/min, pulsus paradoxus >15/min, premature ventricular contractions, right bundle-branch block with severe hypoxia
Skin	Increased diaphoresis as respiratory distress increases
Hydration	Intake and output to monitor hydration
Psychosocial	Fear of suffocation

2 DIAGNOSE

NURSING DIAGNOSIS	SUBJECTIVE FINDINGS	OBJECTIVE FINDINGS
Ineffective breathing pattern related to anxiety and decreased lung expansion	Complains of SOB	Dyspnea, tachypnea, short inspiratory period, use of accessory muscles, tachycardia, chest wall retraction with a severe attack
Ineffective airway clearance related to tenacious secretions and bronchospasm	Complains of SOB	Inspiratory/expiratory wheezing, coarse rhonchi, cough (often ineffective), dyspnea $Pa_{O2} <60$ mm Hg, $Pa_{CO2} \geq 40$ mm Hg, pH normal to <7.35
Activity intolerance related to fatigue and imbalance between oxygen supply and demand	Complains of fatigue; complains of SOB on exertion	Tachypnea on exertion, tachycardia on exertion, inability to perform activity
Potential for infection related to steroid therapy and ineffective airway clearance	Complains of difficulty breathing	Thick purulent sputum, taking corticosteroids

NURSING DIAGNOSIS	SUBJECTIVE FINDINGS	OBJECTIVE FINDINGS
Anxiety related to threat of death from suffocation	Increased tension, apprehension, short of breath	Decreased lung expansion, diaphoretic, pupil dilation, tachypnea

3 PLAN

Patient goals

1. Patient's breathing pattern will be effective without fatigue or dyspnea.
2. Patient's airways will be patent.
3. Patient will be able to perform usual activities without fatigue or dyspnea.
4. Patient will show no signs of pulmonary infection.
5. Patient's anxiety will be relieved.
6. Patient will demonstrate understanding of home care and follow-up instructions.

4 IMPLEMENT

NURSING DIAGNOSIS	NURSING INTERVENTIONS	RATIONALE
Ineffective breathing pattern related to anxiety and decreased lung expansion	Observe changes in respiratory rate and depth.	Determines adequacy of breathing pattern.
	Observe breathing pattern for SOB, nasal flaring, pursed-lip breathing, or prolonged expiratory phase and use of accessory muscles and intercostal retractions.	Identifies increased work of breathing.
	Observe for changes in awareness, orientation, and behavior.	May indicate hypoxia.
	Monitor ABGs.	Determines acid-base balance and need for oxygen.
	Review chest x-rays.	Indicates severity of lung involvement.
	Measure tidal volume and vital capacity.	Indicates volume of air moving in and out of lungs.
	Monitor ECG.	Detects tachycardia.
	Assess emotional response.	Detects use of hyperventilation as a contributing factor.
	Administer oxygen as ordered.	Improves gas exchange and decreases work of breathing.
	Position patient in optimal body alignment in high Fowler's position for breathing.	Optimizes diaphragmatic contraction.

→ > >

NURSING DIAGNOSIS	NURSING INTERVENTIONS	RATIONALE
	Administer bronchodilators as ordered.	Increases airway diameter to decrease the work of breathing.
	Encourage use of blow bottles or incentive spirometry.	Facilitates deep breathing.
	Assist patient to use relaxation techniques.	Relieves anxiety and reduces work of breathing.
Ineffective airway clearance related to tenacious secretions and bronchospasm	Auscultate lungs for rhonchi, crackles, or wheezes.	Determines adequacy of gas exchange and extent of airway obstructed with secretions.
	Assess sputum for color, tenacity, and amount.	Detects presence of infection and need for fluids.
	Assess patient's hydration status: skin turgor, mucous membranes, tongue, intake and output over 24 h, Hct.	Determines need for fluids.
	Monitor theopylline levels if appropriate.	Determines blood level of theophylline. Normally between 10-20 mEq/L.
	Assist patient with coughing as needed.	Removes secretions to improve airway patency.
	Perform endotracheal or tracheostomy tube suctioning as needed.	Stimulates cough reflex and removes secretions.
	Position patient in proper body alignment for optimal breathing pattern (head of bed up 45°, if tolerated up to 90° or leaning on over bed table).	Secretions move by gravity as position changes. Elevating head of bed moves abdominal content away from diaphragm to enhance diaphragmatic contraction.
	Keep environment allergen-free (e.g., dust, feathers, smoke) according to individual needs.	To prevent allergic reactions, e.g., bronchial irritation.
	Assist patient with ambulation/position changes (turning side to side).	Secretions move by gravity as position changes.
	Increase room humidification.	Humidifies secretions to facilitate their elimination.
	Administer corticosteroids as ordered.	Reduces inflammation.
	Administer bronchodilators as ordered.	Facilitates mobilization of secretions.
	Perform chest physiotherapy (e.g., postural drainage, percussion, vibration).	Facilitates loosening and mobilizing of secretions.

NURSING DIAGNOSIS	NURSING INTERVENTIONS	RATIONALE
	Avoid suppressing cough reflex unless cough is frequent and nonproductive.	Cough reflex needed to mobilize secretions.
	Encourage increased fluid intake to 1½ to 2 L/day unless contraindicated.	Liquifies secretions.
	Assist patient with oral hygiene as needed.	Removes taste of secretions.
Activity intolerance related to fatigue and imbalance between oxygen supply and demand	Observe response to activity.	Determines extent of tolerance.
	Identify factors contributing to intolerance, e.g., stress, side effects of drugs, dyspnea.	Guides selection of therapeutic interventions.
	Assess patient's sleep patterns.	May document a causative factor.
	Plan rest periods between activities.	Reduces fatigue.
	Encourage use of adaptive breathing techniques during activity.	Decreases work of breathing.
	Perform activities for patient until he/she is able to perform them.	Meets patient's needs without causing fatigue.
	Provide progressive increase in activity as tolerated.	Slowly increases the number of and endurance of activities.
	Keep frequently used objects within reach.	Provides convenient use for patient; decreases oxygen demand.
	Problem solve with patient to determine methods of conserving energy while performing tasks, e.g., sit on stool while shaving; dry skin after bath by wrapping in terry cloth robe instead of drying skin with a towel.	Identifies ways to conserve energy, thereby using less oxygen and producing less carbon dioxide.
Potential for infection related to steroid therapy and ineffective airway clearance	Monitor leukocytes and albumin.	Indicates adequacy of secondary defense and immune system.
	Assess nutritional status.	Adequate nutritional status supports the immune system.
	Monitor pulmonary function studies.	Indicates extent of pulmonary disease.
	Monitor temperature.	Detects fever indicating actual infection.
	Assess mouth and oral mucosa for irritation.	Detects secondary infection from aerated corticosteroids.

→ > >

NURSING DIAGNOSIS	NURSING INTERVENTIONS	RATIONALE
	Encourage effective coughing and deep breathing.	Maintains clear airway, prevents atelectasis.
	Encourage an increase in fluid intake unless contraindicated.	Liquifies secretions so they can be coughed more easily.
	Assist with nebulizer treatments and physiotherapy.	Maintains clear airways and prevents stasis of secretions.
	Administer antibiotics as ordered.	Prevents or reduces growth of microorganisms.
	Encourage oral hygiene after using aerated corticosteroids.	Prevents mouth irritation.
	Encourage optimum nutrition.	Supports the immune system function.
Anxiety related to threat of death from suffocation	Assess patient's level of anxiety (mild, moderate, severe, panic).	Guides therapeutic interventions.
	Assist patient to identify coping skills used successfully in the past.	Facilitates problem solving.
	Encourage patient to ask questions and express feelings.	May relieve anxiety; helps patient put thoughts into perspective.
	Provide accurate information about asthma and all procedures.	Knowledge can decrease anxiety.
	Provide comfort measures, e.g., back rub.	Facilitates relaxation; may decrease respiratory rate.
	Stay with patient during acute asthma attack.	Reduces anxiety/fear.
	Maintain rest periods.	Facilitates recovery.
	Limit visitors as necessary.	May help to reduce anxiety.
Knowledge deficit	See Patient Teaching.	

5 EVALUATE

PATIENT OUTCOME	DATA INDICATING THAT OUTCOME IS REACHED
Respiratory pattern is effective.	Vital capacity measurements are optimum for patient's status, including FEV_1, TLC, and RV. Clear breath sounds. Serum level for IgE is normal for patient.
Airways are patent.	Clear breath sounds. Breathing occurs without obstruction. Blood gas values are within normal limits.
Usual activities are performed without dyspnea and fatigue.	Patient demonstrates ability to perform ADL without dyspnea or fatigue.
There is no pulmonary infection.	Patient is afebrile. WBCs are within normal limits.
Anxiety is relieved.	Patient reports lessened anxiety with the return of adequate breathing pattern and with knowledge about how to lessen the frequency of asthma attacks.
Knowledge deficit is resolved.	Patient demonstrates knowledge of disease process and home care management.

PATIENT TEACHING

1. Teach about prescribed medications such as bronchodilators and corticosteroids: name, dosage, purpose, time of administration, and side effects.
2. Provide the patient and family with information about asthma as a disease, how to assess an asthmatic response, what to do during the process of care, and criteria for requesting professional assistance and acute emergency care.
3. Assist the patient and family to examine secondary factors that may precipitate asthmatic episodes, such as emotional stress, fatigue, or environmental changes or specific allergen contacts such as dust, animal dander, feathers, and pollen.
4. Teach the patient adaptive breathing techniques and breathing exercises such as pursed-lip breathing and positioning.
5. Teach the patient and family effective coughing techniques.
6. Teach the importance of consuming large quantities of fluid to liquefy secretions.
7. Teach relaxation techniques.
8. Provide the patient and family with information regarding the care, cleaning, and maintenance of inhalation equipment being used in the hospital or to be used at home.
9. Provide the patient and family with respiratory-related health information such as pollution indexes, secondary infection exposure, and community support groups.
10. Teach the patient to obtain vaccine for influenza and pneumococcal pneumonia.
11. Teach the patient the signs and symptoms to report to the physician, e.g., changes in sputum characteristics, excessive fatigue, increased cough, increased SOB, fever, chills, chest discomfort, and wheezing.
12. Teach the patient to avoid contact with people who have respiratory infections.

Chronic Obstructive Pulmonary Disease (COPD)

Chronic obstructive pulmonary disease (COPD) is a group of diseases that includes asthma, bronchitis, emphysema, and bronchiectasis.[47]

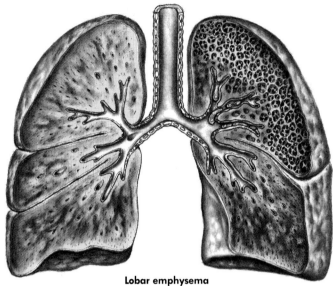

Lobar emphysema

Chronic bronchitis

Recurrent obstruction of airflow is common to each of these diseases. At one end of the spectrum are periodic asthmatic attacks, and at the other end is pure emphysema. Chronic bronchitis and emphysema are discussed here. Asthma is discussed on pages 70-81. Bronchiectasis is discussed on pages 186-194.

COPD is a major cause of death and disability in the United States. About 15% of the older population have some degree of COPD. The estimated economic costs for treatment are greater than $1 billion per year.[43] The actual incidence of COPD is difficult to determine be-

cause of the lack of agreement regarding diagnosis and because two or more obstructive diseases may be present at the same time. In most patients with COPD, two or more histopathologic elements aggravate the breathing process.[18]

Figure 4-5 illustrates the interrelatedness of these diseases and the many host and environmental factors that tend to affect them. The degree of involvement and the response to therapy are individual.

CHRONIC BRONCHITIS AND EMPHYSEMA

Obstructive airway disease refers to a continuum of pulmonary responses to various noxious stimuli. At one end of the spectrum is pure chronic bronchitis and at the other end is pure emphysema. Because of this complexity, these two pure disease states are discussed in combination. Where possible, their differences are pointed out.

Chronic bronchitis refers to excessive mucus secretion in the bronchial tree. This mucus causes chronic productive coughing.

Emphysema refers to anatomic alterations of the air spaces distal to the conducting airways. There is an abnormal enlargement of the air spaces. This causes physiologic destruction of the alveolar walls, which in turn causes increased lung compliance, decreased diffusing capacity, and increased airway size on inspiration, with collapse of airways on expiration.

Chronic bronchitis and emphysema represent a variety of respiratory disorders that all lead to a slowly progressive airway-obstructive disease. The airway obstruction is persistent and irreversible.

The development of chronic bronchitis or emphysema is determined by evaluating the interrelatedness of the individual's genetic vulnerability and environmental factors.[47] The incidence of the diseases has increased dramatically in recent years. The American Lung Association attributes this increase to smoking and airborne irritants and to a better understanding of

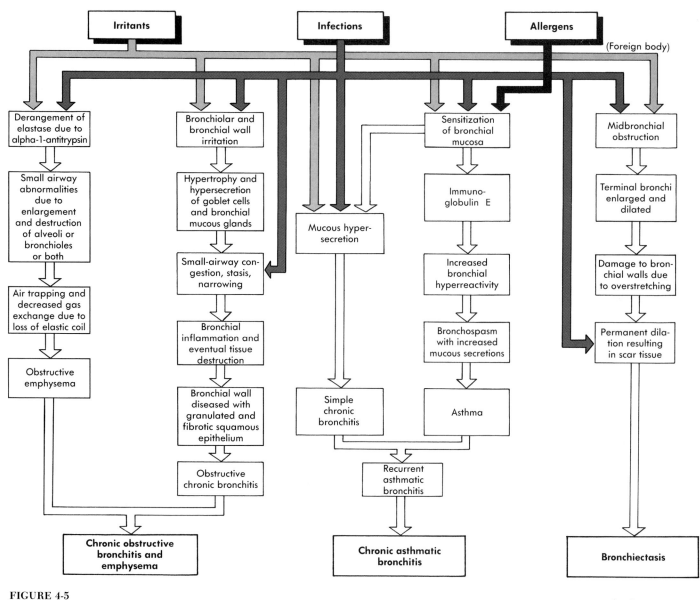

FIGURE 4-5
Overview of obstructive lung disease.

the physiologic processes and diagnostic criteria.[2] The incidence of chronic bronchitis and emphysema remains greater in men than in women, possibly because of smoking history and choice of occupation.

The course of the diseases before the symptoms develop is unclear. Probably the forced expiratory volume in 1 second (FEV_1) decreases before the signs of illness appear. Once signs are evident, the FEV_1 measurement (after bronchodilator administration) may be the best indicator of the prognosis. In addition to predicting outcome, the FEV_1 may be a useful guide for evaluating death rates. Table 4-3 summarizes the relationship between the FEV_1 and activities of daily living.

Table 4-3

RELATIONSHIP BETWEEN FEV_1 AND ACTIVITIES OF DAILY LIVING

FEV_1 (L)	Activity Response
3.7-4	Normal value for adult
2-1.5	Complaints of dyspnea on exertion such as carrying packages or climbing stairs
about 1	Breathlessness when trying to perform activities of daily living such as cooking, cleaning, bathing, dressing, walking Subject to complications of carbon dioxide retention and cor pulmonale
<0.75	Individual unable to work, usually housebound

Data from Fries and Ehrlich[45]

PATHOPHYSIOLOGY

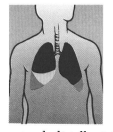

Chronic bronchitis. One of the earliest changes in chronic bronchitis appears in the secretory glands. Hypertrophy and hypersecretion occur in the goblet cells and bronchial mucous glands. The goblet cells and the mucous gland cells increase in size and number. The goblet cells extend distally into the terminal bronchioles, where they are not normally found. The net result is increased amounts of sputum, bronchial congestion, and narrowing of bronchioles and small bronchi. With time the normally sterile lower respiratory tract becomes colonized by bacteria, and an increased number of polymorphonuclear neutrophil (PMN) leukocytes is found in the secretions.[47] These leukocytes probably stimulate further bronchial swelling and eventual tissue destruction.[93] As the bronchial wall becomes diseased, granulated and fibrotic squamous epithelium replaces the normal ciliated epithelium. This scarring leads to stenosis and airway obstruction.

Emphysema. The main defect underlying emphysema is the derangement of lung elastin by the neutral proteases, the most important of which is elastase. Elastase is made and released by PMN leukocytes and alveolar macrophages. Under normal conditions, proteases become fused with bacteria that find their way to the alveolar level. A fraction of the total protease produced is liberated in the lung in response to inhaling particles and following cell death. Normally there is a counterbalancing supply of the protease inhibitor alpha-1-antitrypsin. Recurrent infections, environmental irritants, and cigarette smoking, along with an alpha-1-antitrypsin deficiency, probably cause a situation in which elastin in the distal airways and alveoli is degraded.[47] There is also evidence that cigarette smoking alone depresses the activity of alpha-1-antitrypsin.[85] The imbalance in this elastase-antielastase system allows for the destruction of the basic elastin structure of the distal airways and alveoli. As septal walls are lost, blood vessel density also is reduced and emphysema results.[47] (**Note:** Alpha-1-antitrypsin deficiency is probably responsible for less than 10% of the identified cases of emphysema.[47])

The lungs of a patient with emphysema appear large, overinflated, and pale. The walls of the bronchioles undergo destructive changes, and large bullae may form. There are two types of emphysema: centriacinar (centrilobular) and panacinar (panlobular). The anatomic changes of each of these are shown in Figure 4-6. Centriacinar emphysema is the more common type and is characterized by dilation of the respiratory bronchioles. Chronic bronchitis often is associated with centrilobular emphysema. Panacinar emphysema is characterized by dilation and destruction of alveolar walls throughout the acinus. This latter type often is found in elderly persons with no evidence of chronic bronchitis. Individuals with true alpha-1-antitrypsin deficiency are more likely to have panlobular emphysema.[81]

Two important consequences of emphysema are air trapping and decreased gas exchange. The air trapping is caused by a loss of elastic recoil. Ventilation is regionally decreased, not only because of the elastic recoil but also because of poor support of terminal airways. This increases collapsibility of the noncartilaginous peripheral bronchioles. The decreased gas exchange causes both pulmonary diffusion and perfusion abnormalities. Pulmonary diffusion is reduced because of a loss of alveolar surface area and pulmonary vasoconstriction. The resulting hypoxemia causes a more generalized pulmonary artery constriction, shunting blood away from even the normal areas of the lung.[67] The measurable result of these two processes is an increase in the functional residual capacity (FRC), increased compliance, and hypoxia.

Chronic bronchitis and emphysema are typically "silent" for years before the patient has even minimal symptoms. When symptoms appear, diagnostic studies evaluating the shortness of breath and cough are generally performed.

COMPLICATIONS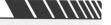

Cor pulmonale
Acute respiratory failure
Peptic and esophageal reflux
Pneumonia
Polycythemia
Dysrhythmias

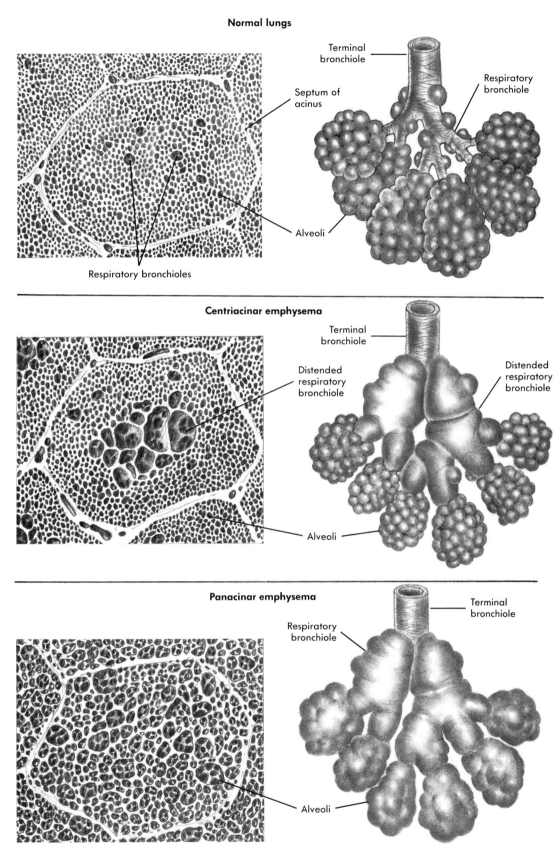

FIGURE 4-6
Types of emphysema. (From McCance.)[73]

AIR TRAPPING

Mechanisms of air trapping in COPD. Mucus plugs and narrowed airways cause air trapping and hyperinflation on expiration. During inspiration the airways enlarge, allowing gas to flow past the obstruction. During expiration the airways narrow and prevent gas flow. This mechanism of air trapping, known as "ball valving," occurs in asthma and chronic bronchitis.

Mechanisms of air trapping in emphysema. Damage or destroyed alveolar walls no longer support and hold open the airways, and alveoli lose their property of passive elastic recoil. Both of these factors contribute to collapse during expiration.[73]

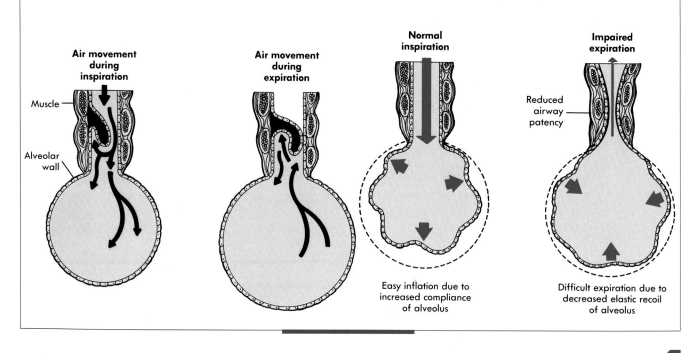

DIAGNOSTIC STUDIES AND FINDINGS

Diagnostic Test	Findings
Laboratory studies	
ABGs	Alveolar-arterial (A-a) oxygen gradient: widened
	Pao_2: decreased; $Paco_2$: increased; patients with pure chronic bronchitis are more prone to CO_2 retention than are those patients with emphysema of comparable severity
Serum electrolytes	Chloride: decreased from salt depletion and diuretics; Potassium: decreased from diuretics
Pulmonary function tests	FEV_1: decreased, may fall as much as 50-75 ml per year; FVC: decreased; FEV_1/FVC ratio: decreased; TLC: increased in emphysema because of decreased elastic recoil; RV: increased in emphysema because of decreased elastic recoil and in chronic bronchitis because of air trapping; FRC: increased in emphysema because of decreased elastic recoil; may be normal in pure chronic bronchitis; C: increased in emphysema; R_{aw}: increased in both chronic bronchitis and emphysema
Chest x-ray	May have flattened diaphragm and increased anterior-posterior diameter
	In emphysema, vascular markings may be decreased and intercostal spaces widened, and bullae may be present
	Abnormalities such as hyperinflation and increased lung markings are usually due to concomitant emphysema or other complicating causes
	In chronic bronchitis, cardiac enlargement, evidence of chronic inflammation and congested lung fields are seen

MEDICAL MANAGEMENT

The goal of medical management for patients with emphysema and chronic bronchitis is to stop the progress of the disease and to maximize breathing by reducing airway secretions and inflammation and halting bronchospasms.

GENERAL MANAGEMENT

Acute exacerbations

Oxygenation: Administered at rates sufficient to maintain a Pa_{O_2} between 50-60 mm Hg, usually by nasal cannula at a flow rate of 1-3 L/min. Because patients with chronic bronchitis and emphysema may have chronic hypercapnia, CO_2 ceases to be a stimulus for breathing; instead low O_2 levels become the stimulus. This means that their borderline or diminished ventilatory drive may be further suppressed by increasing the Pa_{O_2}. Care must be taken to closely monitor oxygen administration and to increase the flow slowly and carefully. Use of the Venturi mask allows more precise oxygen administration.

Mechanical ventilation: Intubation and mechanical ventilation may be necessary if supplemental O_2 cannot maintain the Pa_{O_2} above 40 mm Hg with a pH greater than 7.25. If mechanical ventilation becomes necessary, the intermittent mandatory ventilation (IMV) technique becomes useful.

Long-term management

Oxygenation: Intermittent (at least 18 h/day) oxygen therapy via nasal prongs may be indicated for patients who are unable to maintain a Pa_{O_2} of at least 50 to 55 mm Hg while at rest and breathing room air. The flow rate should be adjusted to maintain a resting Pa_{O_2} close to 60 mm Hg.

Chest physiotherapy: Percussion and postural drainage may be administered at regular intervals for patients with large amounts of sputum production. See pp. 235 to 239 for techniques.

Physical training program: Physical training programs are based on the premise that improved ventilatory and cardiac muscle function might compensate for nonreversible lung disease. Bicycle and treadmill training appear to lead to decreased oxygen consumption with exercise and increased work capacity. These physical training techniques are currently used as methods of rehabilitation.[75]

DRUG THERAPY

Acute exacerbation management
  Antibiotics
Ampicillin(Amcill, Omnipen, others), 250-500 mg po q 6 h for 10 days
Tetracycline (Achromycin, others), 250-500 mg po q 6 h for 10 days
Long-term management
Bronchodilators: Therapeutic theophylline levels should be maintained between 10 and 20 mEq/ml
Corticosteroids: If pulmonary function tests are improved after 3-4 wk by corticosteroids, they may be continued at low doses; the goal is discontinuation of the medication
Influenza and pneumococcal vaccines

1 ASSESS

ASSESSMENT	OBSERVATIONS
History	
Smoking and irritants	Smoking history and history of known respiratory irritants, including duration of exposure to each; history of previous respiratory diseases, infections, allergies; history of chronic cough and characteristics; family history of respiratory diseases; description of activity tolerance, including fatigue and dyspnea precipitation
Medications	Careful and complete history of respiratory-related medications, as well as use of over-the-counter medication and inhalers
Use of oxygen	History of use of oxygen, IPPB, or other related respiratory assistive devices; history to include amount, frequency, duration, and therapeutic response

→ › ›

ASSESSMENT	OBSERVATIONS
Physical assessment	
Respiratory	Respiratory distress as evidenced by dyspnea, cough, prolonged expiration; audible expiratory wheeze; diminished breath sounds over diseased area; anxiety; bronchospasm; sputum-producing cough; hyperresonance owing to overinflation of lungs; barrel chest; cyanosis of nail beds and mucous membranes; posturing and use of accessory muscles during breathing; respiratory failure signs
Cardiovascular	Cardiovascular findings result from hypoxia and include tachycardia, hypotension, and pulsus paradoxus; ECG changes may show atrial dysrhythmias; tall, symmetric P waves in leads II, III, and aV_F; vertical QRS axis; and signs of right ventricular hypertrophy late in the disease
Neurologic	Neurologic changes result from hypoxia and include restlessness and confusion
Gastrointestinal	Anorexia owing to chronic hypoxic state, weight loss, and constipation
Psychosocial	Depression, anxiety, fear
Vital signs	Increased temperature, increased pulse, decreased BP, increased respiratory rate

2 DIAGNOSE

NURSING DIAGNOSIS	SUBJECTIVE FINDINGS	OBJECTIVE FINDINGS
Ineffective airway clearance related to tenacious bronchial secretions	Complains of SOB	Productive cough of tenacious sputum Dyspnea Rhonchi crackles (rales), and wheezes heard on auscultation Tachypnea Changes in depth of respiration
Ineffective breathing pattern related to fatigue, decreased lung expansion, and tracheobronchial obstruction	Complains of SOB	Dyspnea Increased anterior-posterior diameter Productive cough Pursed-lip breathing Reduced vital capacity Pa_{O2} <60 mm Hg Pa_{CO2} >normal for patient pH <7.35 Tachypnea
Impaired gas exchange related to alveolar-capillary membrane changes	Complains of SOB	Inability to move secretions Restlessness, irritability Hypoxia (Pa_{O2} <60 mm Hg) Hypercapnia (Pa_{CO2} >normal for patient) Tachycardia Dyspnea Use of accessory muscles
Altered nutrition: less than body requirements related to dyspnea and fatigue	Complains of fatigue and/or SOB, leading to inability to eat	Weight loss Anorexia Poor muscle mass Albumin <3.5 g/dl Lymphocytes <2100 or 30% of leukocyte Triceps skinfold <16.5 mm (men)

NURSING DIAGNOSIS	SUBJECTIVE FINDINGS	OBJECTIVE FINDINGS
		<12.5 mm (women) Mid-arm circumference <29.3 cm (men) <25.8 cm (women)
Activity intolerance related to fatigue	Complains of weakness, inability to perform usual activities, and SOB on exertion; also reports decreased food intake and sleep pattern disturbances	DOE Pallor Decreased independent activity
Sleep pattern disturbance related to dyspnea and/or coughing	Reports coughing and/or SOB disturbing sleep	Irritability Listlessness Expressionless face Dark circles under eyes Frequent yawning
Potential for infection related to decreased pulmonary function, possible steroid therapy, and ineffective airway clearance	Reports increase in coughing	Change in sputum to thick and purulent Fever Leukocytosis
Sexual dysfunction related to dyspnea and/or fatigue	Reports difficulties with sexual function and/or no interest in resuming sexual activity; fatigue and SOB on exertion; coughing, sputum production Decreased desire for intimacy	
Anxiety related to changes in health	Reports dyspnea and fear of suffocation	Worried, facial tension, restlessness, insomnia

3 PLAN

Patient goals

1. Patient's airways will be patent.
2. Patient's respiratory pattern will be effective without causing fatigue.
3. Patient's gas exchange will improve.
4. Patient's nutritional status will improve.
5. Patient will be able to perform usual activities without dyspnea or fatigue.
6. Patient's sleeping pattern will improve.
7. Patient will have no signs of infection.
8. Patient's sexual needs will be met.
9. Patient's anxiety/fear will be reduced.
10. Patient will demonstrate understanding of home care and follow-up instructions.

4 IMPLEMENT

NURSING DIAGNOSIS	NURSING INTERVENTIONS	RATIONALE
Ineffective airway clearance related to tenacious bronchial secretions	Auscultate lungs for rhonchi, crackles, or wheezing.	Determines adequacy of gas exchange and extent of airway obstructed with secretions.

NURSING DIAGNOSIS	NURSING INTERVENTIONS	RATIONALE
	Assess characteristics of secretions: quantity, color, consistency, odor.	Detects presence of infection.
	Assess patient's hydration status: skin turgor, mucous membrances, tongue, intake and output over 24 hours, Hct.	Determines needs for fluids.
	Monitor sputum culture and sensitivity reports.	Guides therapeutic interventions. Identifies microorganisms present.
	Monitor theophylline levels if appropriate.	Determines blood level of theophylline (normally between 10-20 mEq/L).
	Assist patient with coughing as needed.	Removes secretions.
	Teach patient and family effective coughing techniques.	Ineffective coughing can tire patient.
	Perform endotracheal or tracheostomy tube suctioning as needed.	Stimulates cough reflex and removes secretions.
	Position patient in proper body alignment for optimal breathing pattern (head of bed up 45°, if tolerated up to 90°).	Secretions move by gravity as position changes. Elevating head of bed moves abdominal content away from diaphragm to enhance diaphragmatic contraction.
	Assist patient with ambulation/position changes (turning side to side).	Secretions move by gravity as position changes.
	Increase room humidification.	Humidifies secretions to facilitate their elimination.
	Administer expectorants/bronchodilators as ordered.	Facilitates mobilization of secretions.
	Perform chest physiotherapy (e.g., postural drainage, percussion, vibration).	Facilitates loosening and mobilizing of secretions.
	Assist patient in using blow bottles, incentive spirometry.	Requires deep breathing.
	Avoid suppressing cough reflex unless cough is frequent and nonproductive.	Cough reflex needed to mobilize secretions.
	Encourage increased fluid intake to 1½-2 L/day unless contraindicated.	Liquifies secretions.
	Assist patient with oral hygiene as needed.	Removes taste of secretions.
	Administer corticosteroids as ordered.	Decreases bronchial inflammation.
	Administer antibiotics as ordered.	Inhibits and/or reduces growth of microorganisms.

NURSING DIAGNOSIS	NURSING INTERVENTIONS	RATIONALE
Ineffective breathing pattern related to fatigue, decreased lung expansion, and tracheobronchial obstruction	Inspect thorax for symmetry of respiratory movement.	Determines adequacy of breathing pattern.
	Observe breathing pattern for SOB, nasal flaring, pursed-lip breathing, or prolonged expiratory phase and use of accessory muscles.	Identifies increased work or breathing.
	Review chest x-rays.	Indicates severity of skeletal and lung involvement.
	Measure tidal volume and vital capacity.	Indicates volume of air moving in and out of lungs.
	Assess emotional response.	Detects use of hyperventilation as a causative factor.
	Position patient in optimal body alignment in semi-Fowler's position for breathing.	Optimizes diaphragmatic contraction.
	Assist patient to use relaxation techniques.	Reduces muscle tension, decreases work of breathing.
	Encourage use of blow bottles or incentive spirometry.	Facilitates deep breathing.
	Teach use of abdominal breathing exercises.	Decreases the work of breathing.
Impaired gas exchange related to alveolar-capillary membrane changes	Auscultate lungs for rhonchi, crackles, and wheezes.	Determines adequacy of gas exchange and detects atelectasis.
	Assess level of consciousness, listlessness, and irritability.	Decreased level of consciousness may indicate hypoxia.
	Observe skin color and capillary refill.	Determines circulatory adequacy.
	Monitor ABGs.	Determines acid-base balance and need for oxygen.
	Monitor CBC.	Detects amount of hemoglobin to carry oxygen and presence of infection.
	Monitor side effects and blood levels of bronchodilators.	Guides medication use.
	Monitor changes in activity tolerance.	Activity may induce breathlessness.
	Administer low flow oxygen as ordered.	Improves gas exchange; decreases work of breathing.
	Administer bronchodilators, antibiotics, and corticosteroids as ordered.	Facilitates gas flow to and from alveoli.

→ > >

NURSING DIAGNOSIS	NURSING INTERVENTIONS	RATIONALE
	Pace activities to patient's tolerance.	Decreases oxygen demand.
	Assist patient to Fowler's position.	Optimizes diaphragmatic contraction.
	Use sedation cautiously.	Avoids depressant effects on respiratory function.
	Assist the patient with pursed-lip breathing.	Decreases work of breathing. Facilitates exhalation of carbon dioxide.
	Review risk factors (e.g., smoking, pollutants).	Helps prevent recurrence.
	Teach relaxation and stress reduction techniques.	Decreases work of breathing.
Altered nutrition: less than body requirements related to dyspnea and fatigue	Assess dietary habits and needs.	Helps to individualize the diet.
	Weight patient weekly.	Provides data on adequacy of nutrition.
	For patient with tracheostomy, inspect tracheal aspirate for food particles at each feeding. Stop feedings if aspiration found.	Determines if patient is aspirating feedings.
	Auscultate bowel sounds.	Documents gastrointestinal peristalsis.
	Assess psychologic factors (e.g., depression) that might decrease food and fluid intake.	Identifies effect of psychologic factors on food intake.
	Monitor albumin and lymphocytes.	Indicates adequate visceral protein.
	Measure mid-arm circumference and triceps skinfold.	Indicates protein and fat stores, respectively.
	Provide oxygen while eating as ordered.	Reduces dyspnea.
	Encourage rest periods before meals.	Lessens fatigue during meals.
	Encourage oral care before meals.	Removes taste of sputum that may reduce appetite.
	Provide frequent small feedings.	Lessens fatigue.
	Provide high-protein diet.	Supports immune system.
	Provide a low carbohydrate diet.	Metabolism of carbohydrates yields more carbon dioxide than metabolism of proteins.
	Avoid gas-forming foods and carbonated drinks.	These foods limit movement of diaphragm and hamper abdominal breathing.

NURSING DIAGNOSIS	NURSING INTERVENTIONS	RATIONALE
	Avoid very hot and very cold foods.	May induce cough spasms.
Activity intolerance related to fatigue	Observe response to activity. Monitor pulse and respiratory rate during activity.	Determines extent of tolerance.
	Identify factors contributing to intolerance (e.g., stress, side effects of drugs).	Guides selection of therapeutic interventions.
	Assess patient's sleep patterns.	May document a causative factor.
	Plan rest periods between activities.	Reduces fatigue.
	Encourage use of adaptive breathing techniques during activity (e.g., pursed-lip breathing).	Decreases work of breathing.
	Perform activities for patient until he/she is able to perform them.	Meets patient's need without causing fatigue.
	Provide progressive increase in activity as tolerated.	Allows patient to perform only those activities he/she can do without becoming dyspneic or fatigued and progressively adds more activities as tolerated.
	Provide oxygen as needed.	Decreases work of breathing during activity.
	Problem-solve with patient to determine methods of conserving energy, while performing tasks, e.g., sit on stool while shaving; dry skin after bath by wrapping in terry cloth robe instead of drying skin with a towel.	Identifies ways to conserve energy, thereby using less oxygen and producing less carbon dioxide.
Sleep pattern disturbance related to dyspnea and/or coughing	Identify causative factors. Determine patient's usual sleep patterns and routines.	Guides therapeutic interventions.
	Alleviate causative factors as much as possible.	Facilitates sleep.
	Provide oxygen as ordered.	Decreases work of breathing.
	Position patient for optimal breathing (e.g., semi-Fowler or high Fowler).	Facilitates diaphragmatic contraction to reduce dyspnea that may contribute to sleeplessness.
	Administer cough suppressant and bronchodilators as ordered.	Reduces cough that may contribute to sleeplessness.
	Administer pain medications as ordered.	Reduces pain as cause of sleeplessness.
	Arrange care for uninterrupted periods of rest.	Decreases sleep disturbances.

NURSING DIAGNOSIS	NURSING INTERVENTIONS	RATIONALE
	Provide comfort measures before sleep such as a back rub.	Facilitates relaxation.
	Suggest limiting chocolate and caffeine prior to bedtime.	Reduces intake of stimulants.
	Increase daytime mental and physical activity.	Activity increases relaxation and aids in sleep.
Potential for infection related to decreased pulmonary function, possible steroid therapy, and ineffective airway clearance	Auscultate lungs.	Indicates airway clearance.
	Monitor leukocytes and albumin.	Indicates adequacy of secondary defense and immune system.
	Assess nutritional status.	Adequate nutritional status supports the immune system.
	Monitor pulmonary function studies.	Indicates extent of pulmonary disease.
	Measure temperature.	Detects fever, indicating actual infection.
	Encourage effective coughing and deep breathing.	Maintains clear airway, prevents atelectasis.
	Encourage an increase in fluid intake unless contraindicated.	Liquifies secretions so they can be coughed more easily.
	Assist with nebulizer treatments and physiotherapy.	Maintains clear airways and prevents stasis of secretions.
Sexual dysfunction related to dyspnea and/or fatigue	Obtain description of problem in patient's own words.	Clarifies patient perception, guides therapeutic interventions.
	Assess stress factors in patient's environment that might cause anxiety or psychologic reactions.	Guides selection of therapeutic intervention.
	Determine knowledge of effects of illness and/or medical treatment on sexual functioning.	Determines patient's knowledge base.
	Provide atmosphere in which discussion of sexual problems is encouraged/permitted.	Facilitates problem solving.
	Provide information about resources available, human or equipment (e.g., oxygen).	Facilitates problem solving.
	Discuss importance of maintaining open communication with significant other regarding individual sexual needs, desires, and concerns.	Clarifies needs, desires, and concerns between the two and facilitates problem solving.

NURSING DIAGNOSIS	NURSING INTERVENTIONS	RATIONALE
	Discuss how patient can prepare physiologically by performing airway clearance therapies (e.g., aerosol bronchodilator drug use), diaphragmatic breathing, and oxygen therapy about 1 h before sexual activity.	Prevents airway obstruction from interfering with sexual activity.
	Emphasize importance of planning sexual activity at an optimal time for the patient.	Allows time for patient to use respiratory therapies.
	Advise patient to avoid sexual intercourse after a big meal and consumption of alcohol.	A full stomach restricts diaphragmatic movement. Alcohol decreases sexual functioning.
	Encourage patient and significant other to try positions that are least stressful for the patient, e.g., sitting or elevating head and thorax with the patient on the bottom and the partner on top.	Allows patient to exert less energy in a less dominant position.
	Frequent rests during the activity will minimize pulmonary compromise of the patient and increase partner satisfaction by prolonging stimulation.	Prevents fatigue and decreases dyspnea.
	Remind patient that increased heart and respiratory rates are normal during sexual intercourse.	May relieve anxiety.
Anxiety related to changes in health status	Assess patient's level of anxiety (mild, moderate, severe, panic). Assess patient's perception of unmet needs/expectations.	Guides therapeutic interventions.
	Assist patient to identify coping skills used successfully in the past.	Facilitates problem solving.
	Encourage patient to ask questions and express feelings.	May relieve anxiety; helps patient put thoughts into perspective.
	Provide accurate information about COPD.	Knowledge can decrease anxiety.
	Provide low flow oxygen as ordered.	Decreases the work of breathing.
	Remain with patient during anxious periods.	Offers immediate support.
	Limit visitors as necessary.	Visitors may increase anxiety.
	Introduce support groups available to patient and family, e.g., Better Breathing Clubs of American Lung Association.	Offers long-term, community-based support and education.
Knowledge deficit	See Patient Teaching.	

5 EVALUATE

PATIENT OUTCOME	DATA INDICATING THAT OUTCOME IS REACHED
Airways are patent.	Clear breath sounds, fewer and less tenacious secretions, dyspnea decreased.
Respiratory pattern is effective without tiring patient.	Dyspnea decreased. Pa_{O_2} >60 mm Hg Pa_{CO_2} returns to normal for patient. Clear breath sounds. Patient demonstrates modified breathing ventilation, e.g., pursed lip breathing. Vital capacity measurements are optimal for patient's status, e.g., FEV_1, FVC, TLC, RV, and FRC.
Gas exchange is improved.	Pa_{O_2} >60 mm Hg Pa_{CO_2} returns to normal for patient. Clear breath sounds.

Nutritional status has improved.	Food and fluid intake increased.
	Weight gain.
	Albumin = 3.2-4.5 g/dl
	Lymphocytes = 2100 or 35-40% per ml^3 blood
	Triceps skinfold normal:
	    12.0 mm (men), 16.0 mm (women)
	Midarm circumference normal:
	    32.7 cm (men), 29.2 cm (women)

Usual activities are performed without dyspnea and fatigue.	Patient demonstrates ability to perform usual ADL without dyspnea or fatigue with or without the use of supplemental oxygen.
Sleep pattern is improved.	Patient sleeps at least 6 h/night with one 1½ h morning nap. Patient appears rested.
There is no infection.	Patient is afebrile. WBCs are within normal limits. Sputum cultures are negative.
Sexual needs are met.	Patient reports plans for improved sexual activity with significant other.
Anxiety is reduced.	Dyspnea reduced. Acknowledges fear/anxiety and identifies actions to cope with it.
Knowledge deficit is resolved.	Demonstrates knowledge of disease process and home care management.

PATIENT TEACHING

1. Teach patient adaptive breathing techniques, e.g., pursed-lip breathing and abdominal breathing, and work with family to teach postural drainage techniques.
2. Teach patient and family effective coughing techniques.
3. Teach patient relaxation and stress reduction techniques.
4. Teach importance of avoiding contact with persons who have upper respiratory infections and influenza.

5. Teach importance of prescribed medications, such as bronchodilators and corticosteroids: name, dosage, purpose, time of administration, and side effects.
6. Provide patient and family with information regarding chronic lung diseases, how to assess individual capabilities and responses, and what to do during an acute episode of difficult breathing.
7. Teach change in health status that must be reported to the patient's health care providers; indicators of change may include change in sputum characteristics or color, decreased activity tolerance, increased use of IPPB or oxygen, decreased appetite, and fever.
8. Instruct patient to obtain vaccine for influenza and pneumococcal pneumonia.
9. Teach importance of consuming large quantities of fluid.
10. Teach importance of not smoking and of avoiding dust-producing articles (feathers, animal dander, cleaning equipment) and strong cooking odors, which may irritate the respiratory tract.
11. Teach eating and food choice modifications, e.g., high protein and low carbohydrates.
12 Provide patient and family with information regarding care, cleaning, and maintenance of inhalation or oxygen equipment being used in the hospital or to be used at home, as well as signs of oxygen toxicity.
13. Provide patient and family with respiratory-related health information such as pollution indexes, secondary infection exposure, and community support groups.
14. Advise patient to avoid using powders and aerosol products, which may cause bronchospasm.

Cystic Fibrosis

Cystic fibrosis (CF) is an autosomal recessive disorder of the exocrine glands that causes those glands to produce abnormally thick secretions of mucus. The glands most affected are the respiratory, pancreatic, and sweat glands.

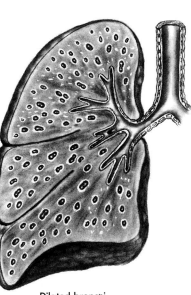

Increased goblet cells in airway epithelium
Increased submucosal size glands

Mucus plug

Mucus plug

Obstruction of small airway by mucus

Dilated bronchi filled with pus

Table 4-4

CLINICAL PRESENTATION OF CYSTIC FIBROSIS

Age	Clinical features
Infancy	Meconium ileus, protracted neonatal jaundice, hyponatremic dehydration
Childhood	Recurrent or chronic chest infection, malnutrition, intussusception, volvulus, meconium ileus equivalent, fat-soluble vitamin deficiency, pancreatitis, recurrent nasal polyps, chronic sinusitis
Adolescence	Recurrent or chronic chest infection, cor pulmonale, diabetes mellitus, male infertility

From Cherniack.[25]

CF was formerly called *mucoviscidosis,* a term no longer used. In the United States CF is the most common cause of life-threatening pulmonary disease of whites during childhood and adolescence. The disease incidence is 1 in 2000 live births. About 5% of the white population carries the disease. CF is less prevalent among blacks, Native Americans, and Asian Americans. Boys and girls are equally affected.

CF is the primary cause of pancreatic deficiency and chronic malabsorption in children. It is also responsible for many cases of intestinal obstruction in newborns. Although CF is a widespread multisystem disease, the progressive pulmonary infections are the most important clinical problem and are responsible for most of the morbidity and mortality.[77]

Although the basic defect in CF has not been determined, the CF gene has been localized on the long arm of human chromosome 7.[77] Without knowledge of the underlying biochemical defect, treatment focuses on the effects of the disease. Despite marked improvement in prognosis since CF was first described in the 1930s, the disease remains uniformly fatal, the median age of death being approximately 22 years for females and 28 years for males. Death is most commonly caused by cardiac and respiratory insufficiency.

CF can be an extremely expensive disease. Average costs just for drugs, laboratory tests, and clinic visits are estimated to be at least $2000 annually. The costs are much higher for patients requiring hospitalization, home oxygenation, or home nursing care.[45]

PATHOPHYSIOLOGY

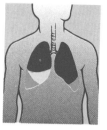

CF results from dysfunction of the exocrine glands. The goblet cells of the mucus-producing (exocrine) glands of the body produce abnormal secretions. These secretions, instead of being thin and free flowing, are thick mucoproteins that coagulate to form eosinophilic concentrations in the glands or ducts. The glands and ducts clog and widen, causing pathologic changes and thus symptoms. The pathologic changes are thought to be caused by the obstruction, not the abnormal condition of the secretions. Abnormalities of the non-mucus-producing glands are seen in saliva and sweat.

CF has a significant and predictable impact throughout the body, as shown in Figure 4-7.

Pancreas. Thick secretions block the pancreatic ducts, causing cystic widenings of the small lobes of the acini. Degenerative and fibrotic changes in the pancreas result, and the essential pancreatic enzymes (trypsin, amylase, and lipase) are unable to participate in food absorption and digestion. Thus digestion of fats, proteins, and carbohydrates is disturbed, as evidenced by increased stool fat and protein. Generalized pancreatic dysfunction places patients with CF at higher risk for diabetes mellitus.

Pulmonary system. Mucopurulent exudates are present in the upper respiratory tract. Nasal polyps occur frequently and often are associated with sinus infections. The thick mucus causes bronchial and bronchiolar obstruction, resulting in bronchiectasis in the terminal bronchioles. This leads at first to areas of atelectasis and hyperinflation. As lung involvement progresses, reduction of oxygen and retention of carbon dioxide result in hypoxia, hypercapnia, and acidosis. The heavy mucus secretions also decrease ciliary activity and thus contribute to mucus obstruction. Mucous stasis encour-

COMPLICATIONS

Pneumothorax	Intestinal obstruction
Lobar atelectasis	Esophageal varices
Pulmonary insufficiency	Portal hypertension
Lung abscess	Cirrhosis
Cor pulmonale	Arthralgia of distal long bones and associated joints (e.g., knees, ankles, wrists)
Pulmonary hypertension	
Sterility	

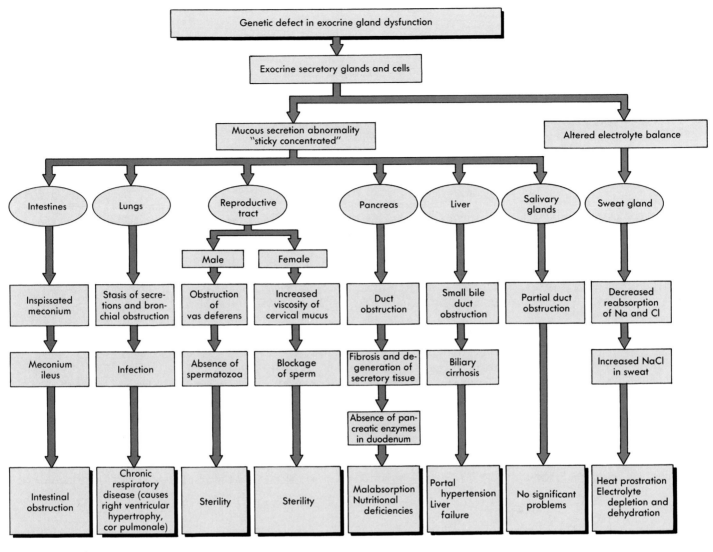

FIGURE 4-7
Pathogenesis of cystic fibrosis. (Adapted from Bullock and Rosendahl.)[17]

ages bacterial growth and resulting infection. With severe lung involvement, compression of pulmonary blood vessels and progressive lung dysfunction frequently lead to pulmonary hypertension and cor pulmonale.

Biliary system. Foci of biliary blockage and fibrosis are common and become progressively worse, resulting in a type of multilobular biliary cirrhosis. If liver involvement is extensive, portal hypertension and an enlarged spleen may also occur. Jaundice may be evidence of gallbladder obstruction.

Reproductive organs. The reproductive system of women with CF is anatomically normal. These women, however, have decreased fertility because of chronic ill-

ness, relative malnutrition, and anovulatory cycle. In girls the cervical mucous glands block the entry of sperm. Also, cervical polyps frequently develop. Boys may have atresia or obstruction of the epididymis, vas deferens, and seminal vesicles as a result of abnormal secretions during fetal development. Spermatogenesis is decreased or absent. Approximately 2% to 3% of men with CF have normal fertility, and some have fathered children.[77] As adults with CF have children, genetic risks must be considered. Affected individuals transmit the gene to every child, but the child cannot develop the disease unless both parents are carriers.[17]

Non-mucus-producing glands. Sweat and salivary gland secretions have abnormally high levels of sodium and chloride. There are no histologic abnormalities.

MEDICAL MANAGEMENT

Treatment is aimed at minimizing the bronchial plugging and attempting to inhibit the bacterial colonization.

GENERAL MANAGEMENT

Oxygenation: May be indicated for persons unable to maintain adequate oxygen levels; oxygen concentrations should be as low as possible while maintaining adequate Pao_2 level; oxygen concentration should not exceed 24%-40%; therapy may be initiated during times of infection or disease exacerbation.

Aerosol therapy: May be used intermittently in conjunction with physiotherapy.

Diet: Sufficient calories to promote normal growth (exceeding daily requirements by at least 25%); high protein (at least 1.5 to 2 g/lb/day for infants and 1.25 g/lb/day for adults); low fat (no more than 50% of normal); multivitamins with addition of vitamins A, D, and E; vitamin K if hypoprothrombinemia present; supplemental salt in hot weather.

Physiotherapy: Time-honored part of the treatment of CF; standard techniques of chest percussion and postural drainage are used to help patient expectorate mucus from various pulmonary segments; recommended treatment plan is physiotherapy for 20 min bid or tid, depending on amount of sputum produced; see pp. 235-239 for techniques.

DRUG THERAPY

Mucolytic agents: Acetylcysteine (Mucomyst), nebulization q 8-12 h with 10% solution (2-3 ml)
Antiinfective agents: May be prescribed only at time of infection or prophylactically; if prescribed for infection, antibiotic of choice depends on organism.

Expectorants: Iodinated glycerol (Organidin), 60 mg q 6 h taken with liquid; Potassium iodide (Ki-N, Pima), 300-600 mg q 4-6 h.

Bronchodilators: Salbutamol, metered aerosol 1-2 puffs q 4-6 h; Inhalation solution, inhalation 0.01-0.03 mg/kg/day; Theophylline PO or IV 18-24 mg/kg/day; Fenoterol, metered aerosol, inhalation, 1-2 puffs q 4-6 h.

Steroids: Prednisone is given daily for adults and every other day for children.

Digestive agents
Rationale: Provide enzymatic activity necessary to assist in digestion of carbohydrates, fats, and proteins.
Pancreatin (Elzyme, Viokase), 325-1000 mg with meals or snacks; Pancrelipase (Cotazym, Ilozyme, Ku-Zyme HP, Pancrease), 1-3 tablets or capsules, 0.43-1.29 g powder, or 1-2 powder packets before or with meals or snacks—has 12 times the lipase and 4 times the amylase and protease activity of pancreatin.
Contraindications: Hypersensitivity to pork or beef.
Common side effects: Nausea, diarrhea, vomiting, anorexia.

Immunizations: Routine immunization against diphtheria, tetanus, pertussis, poliomyelitis, measles, mumps, and influenza recommended as preventive measures.

SURGERY

Pulmonary lavage or bronchial washing: May be used for seriously ill patients whose bronchial airways cannot be cleared by other means.

Resection of blebs and pleural scars: May be attempted if pulmonary disease is localized; purpose is resection of blebs and pleural scars by pleural stripping.

Diagnostic Test	Findings
Laboratory Tests Sweat electrolytes	Normal mean value approximately 18 mEq/L (varies with age); sweat chloride 50-60 mEq/L suggestive of CF; sweat chloride over 60 mEq/L diagnostic of CF. Sweat test has a 2% false positive and false negative rate
Pancreatic enzymes	Examination of duodenal secretions or stool for presence of trypsin and chymotrypsin; absence of enzymes suggestive of CF
Stool examination for fat	Fat absorption tests conducted for 5 days to calculate ratio of fat in oral intake to fat in stool; impaired fat absorption in intestine, resulting in large volumes excreted in the stool (steatorrhea), suggestive of CF
Chest x-ray	Evidence of cystic bronchiectatic changes and honeycombing, particularly in the upper lung fields; upper lobes are more often affected than lower lobes and the right lung more often than the left
Bacteriology	Chronic bacterial bronchitis is a common finding in CF; children are most commonly affected with *Staphylococcus aureus*, while older patients are found to have *Pseudomonas aeruginosa*
Pulmonary function tests	Early in the disease standard spirometry indicates a restrictive pattern; as the disease progresses, an obstructive ventilatory defect develops, eventually a mixed restrictive-obstructive pattern is found; a low FEV_1 is strongly correlated with a poor prognosis.

1 ASSESS

ASSESSMENT	OBSERVATIONS
Family history	History of siblings or other family members with CF
Respiratory	Respiratory distress: cough; congestion; tachypnea; retractions; decreased chest wall movement; labored breathing; dyspnea Examination: barrel chest; tympanic percussion tone over consolidation or areas of atelectasis; clubbing of fingers and toes Breath sounds: moist crackles and rhonchi; decreased or unequal breath sounds Sputum: productive cough with thick sputum; hemoptysis Pulmonary function: decreased vital capacity; decreased FEV_1; decreased tidal volume; increased airway resistance
Cardiovascular	Decreased cardiac output: restlessness; lethargy; tachycardia
Gastrointestinal	Insufficient digestion producing bulky, foul-smelling, pale, watery stools; evidence of intestinal obstruction, fecal impaction, or rectal prolapse; evidence of gastrointestinal bleeding; tarry stools, positive guaiac findings
Hepatic and biliary	Jaundice; enlarged liver; ascites; abnormal liver function findings
Nutritional	Decreased appetite; altered percentages of carbohydrate, fat, and protein in diet; salt supplementation; evidence of malnutrition
Musculoskeletal	Pulmonary osteoarthropathy (digital clubbing) is nearly a universal clinical finding in CF
Psychosocial	Support systems; networking with cystic fibrosis resource groups; activities of daily living; self-esteem; interaction with peers; sexuality

2 DIAGNOSE

NURSING DIAGNOSIS	SUBJECTIVE FINDINGS	OBJECTIVE FINDINGS
Ineffective airway clearance related to bronchial obstruction	Complains of difficulty breathing	Rhonchi, crackles (rales), wheezes; tachypnea; productive cough; fever; dyspnea; cyanosis
Ineffective breathing pattern related to tracheobronchial obstruction	Complains of SOB	SOB; tachypnea; abnormal fremitus; hypoxia (Pa_{O_2} <60 mm Hg); hypercapnia (Pa_{CO_2} >45 mm Hg); productive cough; respiratory depth changes; nasal flaring; cyanosis
Impaired gas exchange related to alveolar-capillary membrane changes	Complains of SOB	Hypoxia (Pa_{O_2} <60 mm Hg) Irritability, restlessness
Altered nutrition: less than body requirements related to impaired pancreatic enzyme release and fatigue	Complains of decreased appetite and fatigue	Decrease in food and fluid intake Increased fat in stools, foul-smelling stools, constipation
Potential for infection related to mucopurulent sputum in the tracheobronchial tree	Complains of decreased appetite and difficulty breathing	Rhonchi, crackles, wheezes, productive cough, decreased food and fluid intake
Activity intolerance related to fatigue and dyspnea	Reports decrease in activity and energy	Decreased activity SOB during activity Remains in bed more hours than usual
Constipation related to exocrine dysfunction	Reports bowel movements occurring less often than usual Increased fat in stool Blood in stool	Bowel sounds present No recorded stool in 3 days Hard stools evacuated
Family coping: potential for growth related to having a chronically ill child and deciding whether to have additional children	Reports crisis with caring for child with chronic illness	Ineffective coping strategies Ineffective decision making

3 PLAN

Patient goals

1. Patient's airways will be patent.
2. Patient's breathing pattern will be effective without failure or dyspnea.
3. Patient's gas exchange will improve.
4. Patient's nutritional status will improve.
5. Patient will have no pulmonary infection.
6. Patient will be able to perform usual activities without fatigue or dyspnea.
7. Patient's bowel elimination will be regulated.
8. Family will be able to identify useful coping strategies.
9. Patient and family will demonstrate understanding of home care and follow-up instructions.

4 IMPLEMENT

NURSING DIAGNOSIS	NURSING INTERVENTIONS	RATIONALE
Ineffective airway clearance related to bronchial obstruction	Auscultate lungs for rhonchi, crackles, or wheezing.	Determines adequacy of gas exchange and extent of airway obstructed with secretions.
	Assess characteristics of secretions: quantity, color, consistency, odor.	Detects presence of infection.
	Assess patient's hydration status: skin turgor, mucous membranes, tongue, intake and output over 24 h, Hct.	Determines needs for fluids.
	Monitor sputum culture and sensitivity reports.	Guides therapeutic interventions; identifies microorganisms present.
	Monitor theophylline levels if appropriate.	Determines blood level of theophylline. Normally between 10-20 mEq/L.
	Assist patient with coughing as needed.	Removes secretions.
	Perform endotracheal or tracheostomy tube suctioning as needed.	Stimulates cough reflex and removes secretions.
	Perform chest physiotherapy (e.g., percussion and vibration) and postural drainage.	Facilitates loosening and mobilizing of secretions.
	Assist patient in using blow bottles, incentive spirometry.	Requires deep breathing.
	Avoid suppressing cough reflex unless cough is frequent and nonproductive.	Cough reflex needed to mobilize secretions.
	Encourage increased fluid intake to 1½ to 2 L/day unless contraindicated.	Liquifies secretions.
	Assist patient with oral hygiene as needed.	Removes taste of secretions.
	Position patient in proper body alignment for optimal breathing pattern (head of bed up 45°, if tolerated up to 90°).	Secretions move by gravity as position changes. Elevating head of bed moves abdominal content away from diaphragm to enhance diaphragmatic contraction.

→ > >

NURSING DIAGNOSIS	NURSING INTERVENTIONS	RATIONALE
	Keep environment allergan free (e.g., dust, feathers, smoke) according to individual needs.	Prevents allergic reactions, e.g., bronchial irritation.
	Encourage patient to ambulate and to turn when in bed.	Secretions move by gravity as position changes.
	Increase room humidification.	Humidifies secretions to facilitate their elimination.
	Administer mucolytic agents as ordered, e.g., Mucomyst, SSKI (saturated solution of potassium iodide).	Facilitates liquifying of secretions.
	Administer expectorants/bronchodilators as ordered.	Facilitates mobilization of secretions.
Ineffective breathing patterns related to tracheobronchial obstruction	Inspect thorax for symmetry of respiratory movement.	Determines adequacy of breathing pattern.
	Observe breathing pattern for shortness of breath, nasal flaring, pursed-lip breathing, or prolonged expiratory phase and use of accessory muscles and intercostal retractions.	Identifies increased work of breathing.
	Review chest x-rays.	Indicates severity of skeletal and lung involvement.
	Measure tidal volume and vital capacity.	Indicates volume of air moving in and out of lungs.
	Assist patient to use relaxation techniques.	Relieves anxiety.
	Encourage use of blow bottles or incentive spirometry.	Facilitates deep breathing.
	Encourage use of adaptive breathing techniques.	Decreases work of breathing.
Impaired gas exchange related to alveolar-capillary membrane changes	Auscultate lungs for rhonchi, crackles, and wheezes.	Determines adequacy of gas exchange and detects atelectasis.
	Assess level of consciousness, listlessness, and irritability.	Decreased level of consciousness may indicate hypoxia.
	Observe skin color and capillary refill.	Determines circulatory adequacy.
	Monitor ABGs.	Determines acid-base balance and need for oxygen.
	Monitor CBC.	Detects amount of hemoglobin to carry oxygen and presence of infection.

NURSING DIAGNOSIS	NURSING INTERVENTIONS	RATIONALE
	Monitor side effects and blood levels of bronchodilators.	Guides medication use.
	Administer oxygen as ordered.	Improves gas exchange; decreases work of breathing.
	Administer bronchodilators as ordered.	Facilitates gas flow to and from alveoli.
	Assist patient to Fowler's position.	Optimizes diaphragmatic contraction.
	Use sedation cautiously.	Avoids depressant effects on respiratory function.
	Teach the patient pursed-lip breathing.	Decreases work of breathing. Facilitates exhalation of carbon dioxide.
Altered nutrition: less than body requirements, related to impaired pancreatic enzyme release and fatigue	Assess dietary habits and needs.	Helps to individualize the diet.
	Weigh patient weekly.	Provides data on adequacy of nutrition.
	Auscultate bowel sounds.	Documents gastrointestinal peristalsis.
	Assess psychologic factors, e.g., depression, that might decrease food and fluid intake.	Identifies effect of psychologic factors on food intake.
	Monitor albumin and lymphocytes.	Indicates adequate visceral protein.
	Measure mid-arm circumference.	Indicates protein stores.
	Measure triceps skin fold.	Indicates fat stores.
	Provide oxygen while eating as ordered.	Reduces dyspnea.
	Encourage oral care before meals.	Removes taste of sputum that may reduce appetite.
	Provide frequent small feedings.	Lessens fatigue.
	Provide foods in appropriate consistency for eating.	Requires less energy to eat soft foods and liquids thereby reducing oxygen requirement.
	Provide high-protein diet.	Supports immune system and promotes normal growth.
	Provide a low-carbohydrate diet.	Metabolism of carbohydrates yields more carbon dioxide than metabolism of proteins.
	Provide low-fat diet.	Fat not tolerated due to inadequate pancreatic lipase.

→ › ›

NURSING DIAGNOSIS	NURSING INTERVENTIONS	RATIONALE
	Administer vitamins A, D, E, as ordered.	Supplements diet.
	Administer pancreatic enzymes as ordered.	Facilitates metabolism of foods.
Potential for infection related to mucopurulent sputum in the tracheobronchial tree	Auscultate lungs.	Indicates airway clearance.
	Monitor leukocytes and albumin.	Indicates adequacy of secondary defense and immune system.
	Assess nutritional status.	Adequate nutritional status supports the immune system.
	Monitor pulmonary function studies.	Indicates extent of pulmonary disease.
	Measure temperature.	Detects fever indicating actual infection.
	Obtain sputum for culture and sensitivity.	Guides selection of medications.
	Encourage effective coughing and deep breathing.	Maintains clear airway, prevents atelectasis.
	Encourage an increase in fluid intake unless contraindicated.	Liquifies secretions so they can be coughed easier.
	Assist with nebulizer treatments and physiotherapy.	Maintains clear airways and prevents stasis of secretions.
	Teach patient to avoid contact with people who have respiratory infections.	Prevents exposure to a contagious person.
	Encourage patient to obtain vaccine for influenza and pneumococcal pneumonia.	Increases immunity to these diseases.
	Teach patient the signs and symptoms he needs to inform the physician about, e.g., changes in sputum characteristics, excessive fatigue, increased cough, increased shortness of breath, fever, chills, diaphoresis, chest discomfort, and wheezing.	Informs patient so that he will know when to contact physician for early treatment of infection.
Activity intolerance related to fatigue and dyspnea	Observe response to activity.	Determines extent of tolerance.
	Identify factors contributing to intolerance, e.g., stress, side effects of drugs.	Guides selection of therapeutic interventions.
	Assess patient's sleep patterns.	May document a causative factor.
	Plan rest periods between activities.	Reduces fatigue.
	Encourage use of adaptive breathing techniques during activity.	Decreases work of breathing.

NURSING DIAGNOSIS	NURSING INTERVENTIONS	RATIONALE
	Perform activities for patient until he/she is able to perform them.	Meets patient's need without causing fatigue.
	Provide progressive increase in activity as tolerated.	Slowly increases the number of and duration of activities.
	Provide positive feedback about progress.	Motivates patient to continue activity.
	Provide oxygen as needed.	Decreases work of breathing during activity.
	Keep frequently used objects within reach.	Provides convenient use for patient; decreases oxygen demand.
	Problem-solve with patient to determine methods of conserving energy while performing tasks, e.g., sit on stool while shaving; dry skin after bath by wrapping in terry cloth robe instead of drying skin with a towel.	Identifies ways to conserve energy thereby using less oxygen and producing less carbon dioxide.
Constipation related to exocrine dysfunction	Auscultate bowel sounds.	Indicates presence of peristalsis needed for defecation.
	Assess stool; note odor, color, amount, consistency, and frequency.	Helps to confirm problem of constipation.
	Observe for blood in the stool.	Indicates rectal bleeding.
	Measure intake.	Determines adequacy of fluid intake.
	Increase fluid intake to 2500 ml daily, unless contraindicated.	Increases water for absorption by feces; stimulates peristalsis.
	Increase fiber in the diet.	Increases the bulk of feces to stimulate peristalsis.
	Encourage ambulation.	Stimulates peristalsis.
	Administer stool softeners as ordered.	Softens stool for easier evacuation.
	Administer laxative as ordered.	Stimulates peristalsis.
	Administer enema as ordered.	Distends colon to stimulate peristalsis.
Family coping: potential for growth related to having a chronically ill child and deciding whether to have additonal children	Assess family's psychologic status, e.g., fearful, anxious, angry, depressed.	Guides selection of therapeutic interventions.
	Identify significant others from whom family derives support.	Gives information about which persons to involve in patient's plan of care.

→ › ›

NURSING DIAGNOSIS	NURSING INTERVENTIONS	RATIONALE
	Assess ability to understand events, provide realistic appraisal of situation, e.g., understanding of diagnostic tests, disease process, prognosis, and therapies.	Guides selection of therapeutic interventions.
	Assess impact of illness on decision to have additional children.	Guides selection of therapeutic interventions.
	Explain relationship of disease processes for therapies, diet, and medications.	Promotes understanding of disease.
	Encourage family members to communicate their feelings.	May diminish fears, begins problem solving process.
	Explain genetic probability of having another child with cystic fibrosis.	Assists in decision making.
	Assist family to use problem-solving methods of coping.	Guides patients through a process that can assist coping.
	Have parents and child talk with another family who has a child with CF.	Provides a resource for family; teaches them how another family adjusted.
	Encourage parents to promote normal growth and development in their child with CF.	Discourages overprotection of child.
	Discuss financial burden with parents.	Encourages family to assess financial resources needed.
	Make appropriate referral for counseling and financial assistance if necessary.	Provides resources to help the family cope.
Knowledge deficit	See Patient Teaching.	

5 EVALUATE

PATIENT OUTCOME	DATA INDICATING THAT OUTCOME IS REACHED
Airway is patent.	Airways are clear and breathing occurs without obstruction.
Breathing pattern is effective without fatigue or dyspnea.	Patient's behavior is modified to conserve energy. Patient/family demonstrates breathing techniques. Vital capacity measurements are optimal for patient.
Gas exchange is within normal limits for patient.	$Pa_{O_2} > 80$ mm Hg $Pa_{CO_2} < 45$ mm Hg Arterial pH $= 7.35 - 7.45$ Breath sounds are clear.
Nutritional status is improved.	Weight gain. Food and fluid intake have improved. Pancreatic enzymes are normal. Stool fat content is within normal levels.

PATIENT OUTCOME	DATA INDICATING THAT OUTCOME IS REACHED
There is no infection.	Temperature within normal limits. WBC within normal limits. Cough subsided. Sputum evaluation shows no evidence of secondary respiratory infection.
Performs usual activities without fatigue or dyspnea.	Patient performs self activities, attends school/job, participates in recreation without experiencing dyspnea.
Bowel elimination is regulated.	Patient has bowel movement according to frequency usual for patient without constipation.
Family identifies useful coping strategies.	Family plans who will be responsible for household duties, for assisting patient with treatments, etc. Family identifies coping strategies they will use when needed. Family identifies support groups in the area they may attend.
Knowledge deficit is resolved.	Patient demonstrates knowledge of disease process and home care management.

PATIENT TEACHING

1. Teach the patient adaptive breathing techniques and work with the family to teach postural drainage techniques.
2. Teach the importance of avoiding contact with persons who have respiratory infections.
3. Teach the importance of obtaining appropriate immunizations and vaccinations to prevent as many childhood and communicable diseases as possible.
4. Teach the importance of prescribed medications and diet modifications. For medications, family members need to know name, dosage, time of administration, and side effects.
5. Provide the patient and family with information regarding CF, assessment of individual capabilities and responses, and actions to take during an acute episode of difficult breathing.
6. Inform the patient and family that a change in health status must be reported to the patient's health care providers. Indicators of change include change in sputum characteristics or color, decreased activity tolerance, nutritional or gastrointestinal changes, weight loss, fever, or stress symptoms indicating an inability to tolerate the disease state.
7. Teach adaptive exercise and rest techniques.
8. Provide the patient and family with information regarding the care, cleaning, and maintenance of inhalation or oxygen equipment used in the hospital or at home, as well as signs of oxygen toxicity.
9. Provide the patient and family with information related to respiratory health, such as pollution indexes, secondary infection exposure, and community support groups.

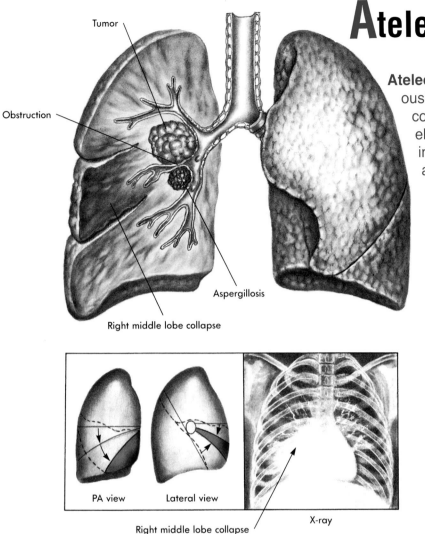

Tumor

Obstruction

Aspergillosis

Right middle lobe collapse

Atelectasis

Atelectasis is the collapse of previously expanded lung tissue or incomplete expansion at birth. Atelectasis is an acquired condition in which all or part of the normally aerated lung collapses.

PA view   Lateral view

Right middle lobe collapse   X-ray

Atelectasis is a common complication of thoracic or upper abdominal surgery. The problem is caused mostly by hypoventilation, which commonly leads to a bronchial obstruction with mucus. It may also be caused by compression of the lung tissue from hemothorax, pneumothorax, emphysema, or tumor.

PATHOPHYSIOLOGY

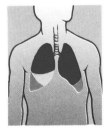

Atelectasis may occur suddenly and be extensive, or it may occur slowly and cause minor pulmonary problems. The extent of the atelectasis depends on the site and rapidity of the blockage. If the mainstem bronchus to one lung is blocked, the entire lung becomes atelectatic and respiratory compromise is great. If only a small bronchiole becomes slowly blocked because of a buildup of

secretions, symptoms may be minor and the respiratory system is able to compensate. In both cases, infection and lung tissue damage are possible.

Surfactant levels are important in atelectasis, since it must be replenished continually to keep the alveoli from collapsing. When airflow to the alveoli decreases, the alveoli collapse, and inadequate surfactant is produced. During the early stages of collapse the pores of Kohn try to maintain open alveoli by providing collateral ventilation through an interconnection between alveoli. The amount of communication, however, depends on the overall degree of inflation of the lungs (Figure 4-8). There are two types of atelectasis: compression and absorption. Compression atelectasis results from compression of lung tissue from a source outside the alveoli, such as a pneumothorax, hemothorax, pleural effusion, or tumor within the lung. Absorption atelectasis occurs when secretions in the bronchi and bronchioles obstruct these airways and prevent movement of air into the alveoli. Air trapped in the alveoli is absorbed and the alveolar sac collapses, as occurs in emphysema and pneumonia.[17]

COMPLICATIONS

Pneumonia
Pneumothorax

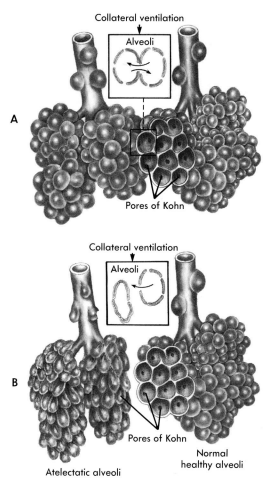

FIGURE 4-8
A, Pores of Kohn maintaining collateral ventilation. **B,** Atelectasis on the left without collateral ventilation.

DIAGNOSTIC STUDIES AND FINDINGS

Diagnostic Test	Findings
Laboratory tests	
ABGs	Pao_2 <80 mm Hg initially, often improving during first 24 h; $Paco_2$ often normal or low owing to hyperventilation
	When significant atelectasis develops, Pao_2 <60 mm Hg; when atelectasis progresses to respiratory failure, $Paco_2$ increases to 45 mm Hg
	pH decreases to <7.35
Culture and sensitivity	Sputum specimens for culture and sensitivity to identify pathogens
Serial chest x-rays	Airless area over region of atelectasis; trachea, heart, and mediastinum deviated toward atelectatic area; diaphragm elevated on affected side; rib spaces narrowed

MEDICAL MANAGEMENT

The ultimate treatment plan for atelectasis is removal of the underlying cause.

GENERAL MANAGEMENT

High tidal volumes and/or positive end-expiratory pressure (PEEP): Used to maintain open alveoli if patient is intubated; **IPPB:** Inspiratory volumes are increased by over 500 ml; **Positioning:** Patient placed with uninvolved side in dependent position to promote drainage of affected area; patient repositioned at least q 1 h; **Chest physiotherapy** with coughing and deep breathing; **Ambulation** as quickly as possible.

DRUG THERAPY

Bronchodilators: Isoetharine (Bronkosol), 2-4 ml or 0.125%-0.25% solution q 4 h; Metaproterenol sulfate (Alupent), 2-3 inhalations q 3-4 h.
Anti-infective agents (use is controversial)
Broad-spectrum antibiotic (e.g., pencillin or ampicillin) given as soon as symptoms are noted; drug may be modified appropriately if specific pathogen is isolated from bronchial secretions.
(mm2) N-acetylcysteine, can be given by IPPB or nebulizer.

SURGERY

Surgical excision or insertion of drainage tube: Performed to relieve atelectasis caused by compression component such as tumor, hemothorax, or pneumothorax.
Bronchoscopy: May be performed when atelectasis is not relieved by suction, coughing and deep breathing, or postural drainage.

_1_ ASSESS

ASSESSMENT	OBSERVATIONS
Respiratory	Tachypnea; labored breathing; dyspnea; nasal flaring; retractions; crackles, bilaterally unequal, diminished over affected area; labored or irregular breathing; hyperventilation; percussion tones dull or flat over affected area
Vital signs	Fever, tachypnea; late sign—tachycardia
Psychosocial	Fear of suffocation; fear of death

_2_ DIAGNOSE

NURSING DIAGNOSIS	SUBJECTIVE FINDINGS	OBJECTIVE FINDINGS
Ineffective airway clearance related to bronchial obstruction	Complains of difficulty breathing	Rhonchi, crackles (rales); decreased breath sounds; tachypnea; fever; dyspnea; labored or irregular breathing
Ineffective breathing pattern related to bronchial obstruction	Complains of SOB	SOB; tachypnea; hypoxia (Pa_{O_2} <60 mm Hg); hypercapnea (Pa_{CO_2} >45 mm Hg); irritability; restlessness

NURSING DIAGNOSIS	SUBJECTIVE FINDINGS	OBJECTIVE FINDINGS
Impaired gas exchange related to alveolar collapse	Complains of SOB	Hypoxia (pao_2 <60 mm Hg); hypercapnia ($Paco_2$ >45 mm Hg); irritability; restlessness
Potential for infection related to bronchial obstruction and collapse of alveoli	Reports productive sputum	Fear; thick, purulent sputum Leukocytosis
Fear related to suffocation and dying	Reports fears of suffocation and of dying	Fearful facial expression

3 PLAN

Patient goals

1. Patient's airways will be patent.
2. Patient's breathing pattern will be effective without fatigue or dyspnea.
3. Patient's gas exchange will improve.
4. Patient will show no signs of pulmonary infection.
5. Patient's fears will be reduced.
6. Patient will demonstrate an understanding of home care and follow-up instructions.

4 IMPLEMENT

NURSING DIAGNOSIS	NURSING INTERVENTIONS	RATIONALE
Ineffective airway clearance related to bronchial obstruction	Auscultate lungs for rhonchi, crackles, or wheezing.	Determines adequacy of gas exchange and extent of airway obstructed with secretions.
	Assess characteristics of secretions: quantity, color, consistency, odor.	Detects presence of infection.
	Assess patient's hydration status: skin turgor, mucous membranes, tongue, intake and output over 24 h, Hct.	Determines needs for fluids.
	Monitor sputum culture and sensitivity reports.	Guides therapeutic interventions; identifies microorganisms present.
	Assist patient with deep breathing and coughing as needed.	Removes secretions.
	Administer analgesics as ordered before coughing.	Reduces pain caused by coughing.
	Teach patient and family effective coughing techniques.	Ineffective coughing can tire patient.
	Perform nasotracheal or tracheostomy tube suctioning as needed.	Stimulates cough reflex and removes secretions.

NURSING DIAGNOSIS	NURSING INTERVENTIONS	RATIONALE
	Position patient in proper body alignment for optimal breathing pattern (head of bed up 45°, if tolerated up to 90°).	Secretions move by gravity as position changes. Elevating head of bed moves abdominal content away from diaphragm to enhance diaphragmatic contraction.
	Assist patient with ambulation/position changes (turning side to side).	Secretions move by gravity as position changes.
	Administer bronchodilators as ordered.	Facilitates mobilization of secretions.
	Perform chest physiotherapy (e.g., percussion and vibration) and postural drainage.	Facilitates loosening and mobilizing of secretions.
	Encourage increased fluid intake to 1½ to 2 L/day unless contraindicated.	Liquifies secretions.
	Administer antiinfectives as ordered.	Prevents or interrupts growth of microorganisms.
	Administer aerosol or IPPB as ordered.	Humidifies inspired air.
Ineffective breathing pattern related to bronchial obstruction and/or decreased lung expansion	Observe changes in respiratory rate and depth.	Determines adequacy of breathing pattern.
	Observe breathing pattern for SOB and use of accessory muscles.	Identifies increased work of breathing.
	Review chest x-rays.	Indicates severity of skeletal and lung involvement.
	Measure tidal volume and vital capacity.	Indicates volume of air moving in and out of lungs.
	Position patient in optimal body alignment in semi-Fowler's position for breathing or leaning forward on over bed table.	Optimizes diaphragmatic contraction.
	Assist patient to use relaxation techniques.	Relieves anxiety. Decreases work of breathing.
	Medicate with analgesic without depressing respirations.	Reduces pain that may be interfering with breathing.
	Encourage use of blow bottles or incentive spirometry.	Facilitates deep breathing.
Impaired gas exchange related to alveolar collapse	Auscultate lungs for rhonchi, crackles, and wheezes.	Determines adequacy of gas exchange and detects atelectasis.
	Assess level of consciousness, listlessness, and irritability.	Decreased level of consciousness may indicate hypoxia.
	Observe skin color and capillary refill.	Determines circulatory adequacy.

NURSING DIAGNOSIS	NURSING INTERVENTIONS	RATIONALE
	Monitor ABGs.	Determines acid-base balance and need for oxygen.
	Monitor CBC.	Detects amount of hemoglobin present to carry oxygen and presence of infection.
	Monitor side effects and blood levels of bronchodilators.	Guides medication use.
	Monitor changes in activity tolerance.	Activity may induce breathlessness.
	Administer oxygen as ordered.	Improves gas exchange; decreases work of breathing.
	Administer bronchodilators as ordered.	Facilitates gas flow to and from alveoli.
	Pace activities to patient's tolerance.	Decreases oxygen demand.
	Assist patient to Fowler's position. Use sedation cautiously.	Optimizes diaphragmatic contraction. Avoids depressant effects on respiratory function.
Potential for infection related to bronchial obstruction and collapse of alveoli	Auscultate lungs.	Indicates airway clearance.
	Monitor leukocytes and albumin.	Indicates adequacy of secondary defense and immune system.
	Assess nutritional status.	Adequate nutritional status supports the immune system.
	Monitor pulmonary function studies.	Indicates extent of pulmonary disease.
	Measure temperature.	Detects fever, indicating actual infection.
	Encourage effective coughing and deep breathing.	Maintains clear airway, prevents atelectasis.
	Encourage an increase in fluid intake unless contraindicated.	Liquifies secretions so they can be coughed more easily.
	Assist with nebulizer treatments and physiotherapy.	Maintains clear airways and prevents stasis of secretions.
	Encourage nutritional intake via oral intake, tube feeding, or parenteral nutrition.	Maintains nutritional status, which supports immune system.
	Administer antiinfective agents as ordered.	Prevents and/or inhibits growth of microorganisms.
	Administer antipyretics as ordered.	Reduces fever, relieves pain.
Fear related to suffocation and dying	Validate sources of fear with patient.	Guides therapeutic interventions.

→ › ›

NURSING DIAGNOSIS	NURSING INTERVENTIONS	RATIONALE
	Assist patient to identify coping skills used successfully in the past.	Facilitates problem solving.
	Encourage patient to ask questions and express feelings.	May relieve anxiety; helps patient put thoughts into perspective.
	Provide accurate information about atelectasis.	Knowledge can decrease fears.
	Provide alternate forms of communication when patient is unable to speak.	Reduces frustration and anxiety.
	Make referral to chaplain.	Provides resources for patient to discuss fear of death.
Knowledge deficit	See Patient Teaching.	

5 EVALUATE

PATIENT OUTCOME	DATA INDICATING THAT OUTCOME IS REACHED
Airway is patent.	Airways are clear and breathing occurs without obstruction. Breath sounds are clear.
Breathing pattern is effective without fatigue or dyspnea.	ABGs are within normal limits: Pa_{O2} = 80-100 mm Hg; Pa_{CO2} = 35-45 mm Hg; pH = 7.35-7.45. Vital capacity measurements are optimal for patient.
Gas exchange is within normal limits for patient.	Pa_{O2} = 80-100 mm Hg; Pa_{CO2} = 35-45 mm Hg; arterial pH = 7.35-7.45; breath sounds are clear.
There is no pulmonary infection.	Temperature is within normal limits. WBC within normal limits. Cough has subsided. Sputum evaluation shows no evidence of secondary respiratory infection.
Fears have been reduced.	Patient acknowledges fears of suffocation and dying. The patient's concerns are refocused to getting well and being discharged.
Knowledge deficit is resolved.	Patient demonstrates knowledge of disease process and home care management.

PATIENT TEACHING

1. Teach the patient deep breathing and coughing techniques, as well as increased movement and splinting when coughing.
2. Teach the patient about prescribed medications such as bronchodilators and antiinfectives: name, dosage, time of administration, purpose, and side effects.
3. If the patient has undergone surgery and does not have atelectasis, provide the patient and family with information about techniques to prevent its occurrence such as movement, deep breathing, and coughing, and use of an incentive spirometer to facilitate aeration of the lungs.
4. Discuss symptoms to report to physician: upper respiratory infection, influenza, difficulty breathing, persistent cough, and elevated temperature.

Pleural Effusion

A pleural effusion (pleurisy with effusion) develops when excess nonpurulent fluid accumulates in the pleural space between the visceral and parietal pleurae.

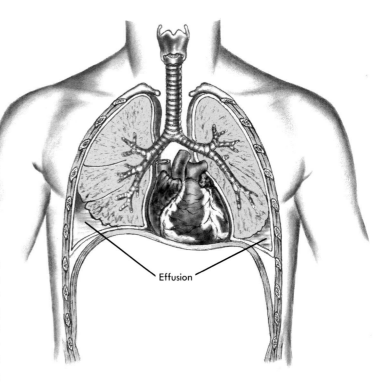

PATHOPHYSIOLOGY

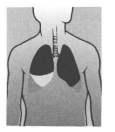

The visceral and parietal pleurae form a continuous sac between the lung and the chest wall. Normally only a potential space containing less than 10 ml of fluid separates these surfaces. The fluid is continuously moving in and out of this space because of a balance between hydrostatic pressures, colloidal osmotic pressures, and the surface characteristics of capillaries and the pleurae. Pleural effusion is rarely a disease by itself. It generally occurs as a secondary problem when one of the following physiologic processes occurs:

Increase in hydrostatic pressure, as in congestive failure

Increase in oncotic pressure, as in severe hypoproteinemia

Increase in capillary permeability, as in inflammatory and neoplastic effusion

Increase in intrapleural negative pressure, as in major atelectasis

Decrease in lymphatic drainage, as in malignancy

Movement of fluid from the peritoneal space, as in cirrhosis with ascites[77]

Pleural effusions may be divided into two categories, transudates and exudates.

The distinction between transudate and exudate is based on protein content. Transudates (hydrothorax) are produced when the flow of protein-free fluid into the pleural space is disturbed. Aspirated fluid is clear or pale yellow, has a specific gravity of 1.015 or less, and has a protein content that is either normal or less than 3 g/dl. Exudates result from a disease of the pleural surface or an obstruction in the lymphatic system that inhibits the drainage of proteins. The fluid is often dark yellow or amber and has a specific gravity greater than 1.016 and a protein content greater than 3 g/dl. An analysis of pleural fluid is provided in Table 4-5.

Following are the common causes of pleural effusions:

Exudates
  Viral infections
  Tuberculosis
  Empyema pneumonia
  Chest trauma
  Pancreatitis
  Rheumatic fever
  Collagen-vascular diseases
  Metastatic diseases
  Uremia
  Subphrenic abscess
  Pulmonary embolism
Transudates
  Peritoneal dialysis
  Pericarditis
  Cirrhosis
  Congestive heart failure
  Myxedema
  Sarcoidosis
  Hypoproteinemia
  Nephrotic syndrome
  Atelectasis

The accumulation of pleural fluid in association with pneumonia is called pneumonic effusion. Pleural empyema refers to pus in the pleural cavity; however, pleural fluid with a large number of polymorphonuclear leukocytes in the presence of pyogenic organisms can be an empyema. The accumulation of blood in the pleural cavity is called hemothorax; the presence of chyle (a milky intestinal lymph) is known as chylothorax. Air and fluid together result in hydropneumothorax; if the fluid is pus or blood, it is a pyopneumothorax or hemopneumothorax.[42]

COMPLICATIONS

Pneumothorax
Pneumonia
Empyema

Table 4-5

PLEURAL FLUID ANALYSIS

Measurement	Transudate	Exudate
Color	Pale yellow	Dark amber, blood or pus
Red blood cells (RBCs)	May increase	> 5000 RBCs/mm^3, may increase
Protein	<3 g/dl	> 3 g/dl
Specific gravity	<1.016	>1.016
Lactic dehydrogenase (LDH)	<200 U/dl	>200 U/dl
Pleural LDH/serum LDH	<0.6	>0.6
White blood cells (WBCs)	Increase indicates empyema or infected effusion	
Amylase	Exceeds serum amylase level	
	Less than serum glucose level	
Glucose	Less than serum glucose level	
Triglyceride	May be increased	
pH	<7.3	>7.3

Modified from Miller and Kazem.[75]

DIAGNOSTIC STUDIES AND FINDINGS

Diagnostic Test	Findings
Chest x-ray	Effusions typically located at base of pleural space; moderate amount of fluid (250-300 ml) must accumulate to be seen on upright PA, decubitus, or lateral chest x-ray; effusion seen as dense opacity (Figure 4-9); large effusions may obliterate hemothorax, simulating lung collapse; distinction between effusion and collapse based on shift of mediastinum away from effusion but toward lung collapse
Thoracentesis	For pleural fluid analysis; submit several hundred milliliters if possible (Table 4-5)
Laboratory tests	
Stain, culture, and sensitivity of pleural fluid	Identification of causative agent (bacterial, fungal, or viral)
Cytologic examination of pleural fluid	Evaluation of potential neoplastic involvement
	Bloody effusion without history of chest trauma suggestive of malignancy or pulmonary embolism
Pleural biopsy with tissue analysis	Indicated when fluid analysis fails to establish cause

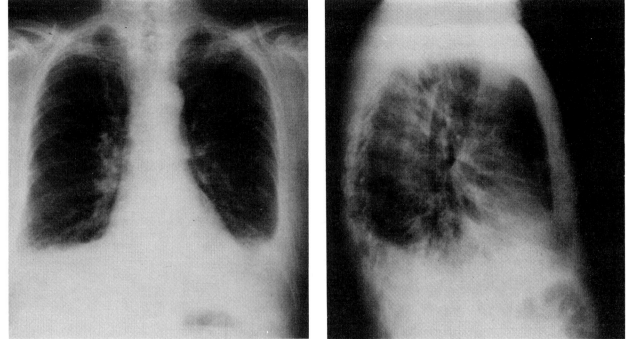

FIGURE 4-9
Chest x-ray of patient with pleural effusion. **A,** PA view: note obliteration of costophrenic angles bilaterally; pulmonary vasculature appears normal. **B,** Lateral view: note lack of costophrenic angles. (Courtesy R. Keith Wilson, M.D., Baylor College of Medicine, Houston, Tex; From Thompson.)[99]

MEDICAL MANAGEMENT

The treatment of pleural effusion depends on the etiology and clinical consequences. The following discussion refers to the general treatment of effusion.

GENERAL MANAGEMENT

Thoracentesis: To drain excess fluid from pleural space and relieve dyspnea or hypoxemia (see p. 264 for procedure and nursing care); because of potential cardiovascular response to rapid removal of pleural fluids, removal limited to 1200-1500 ml at any one time; another complication of thoracentesis is pneumothorax (see pp. 124-131)

Insertion of small chest tube
Tube may be connected to underwater seal drainage system and left in place if accumulation of fluids is large and compromising respiratory function.
If pleural effusion is caused by malignancy, tube may be inserted to drain fluid and left in place to provide insertion point for medications and therapeutic techniques.
Treatment of underlying disease or problem
Deep breathing and coughing to encourage maximal ventilation; incentive spirometer may be used; **bed rest,** which causes most effusions to absorb spontaneously.

DRUG THERAPY

Antibiotics: Specific to cause; administered if effusion is thought to be caused by infectious process.

1 ASSESS

ASSESSMENT	OBSERVATIONS
Respiratory	Dullness to percussion, which shifts with change in position; decreased or absent breath sounds over affected area; egophony above effusion site; dyspnea if effusion has occurred rapidly; if effusion is large, intercostal bulging or decreased chest wall movement during breathing
	Physical signs differ depending on the amount of fluid in the pleural space—these physical signs are summarized below:

Amount of fluid (ml)	Expansion	Fremitus	Percussion	Breath sounds	Contralateral mediastinal shift
<250	Normal	Equal, bilateral	Resonant	v	0
750	↓	↓	dull	↓ v	0
1500	↓ ↓	↓ ↓	flat	↓ ↓ bv	+
>2500	↓ ↓ ↓	absent	flat	absent	+ +

KEY: ↓, decreased; *v*, vesicular; *bv*, bronchovesicular; *0*, absent; +, present.
From Mitchell.[77]

Vital signs	Fever, tachypnea, tachycardia, hypotension
Psychosocial	Fear of dyspnea or not being able to get enough air; potential fear of unknown cause of pleural effusion

2 DIAGNOSE

NURSING DIAGNOSIS	SUBJECTIVE FINDINGS	OBJECTIVE FINDINGS
Ineffective breathing pattern related to decreased lung expansion	Complains of SOB, localized pain during a deep breath	SOB, dyspnea at rest, tachypnea, decreased chest movement Hypoxia (Pa$_{O2}$ <70 mm Hg) Labored or irregular breathing, pleural friction rub, shallow respirations
Impaired gas exchange related to alveolar-capillary membrane changes	Complains of SOB	Hypoxia (Pa$_{O2}$ <70 mm Hg) Irritability, restlessness Absent breath sounds over effusion, dullness percussed over effusion
Fear related to suffocation and dying	Reports fears of suffocation and dying	Worried facial expression
Potential for infection related to decreased pulmonary function and stasis of fluid in pleural space	Decreased lung expansion	Absent breath sounds over effusion

3 PLAN

Patient goals

1. Patient's breathing pattern will be effective without fatigue or dyspnea.
2. Patient's gas exchange will improve.
3. Patient's fear will be relieved.
4. Patient will show no signs of pulmonary infection.
5. Patient will demonstrate understanding of home care and follow-up instructions.

4 IMPLEMENT

NURSING DIAGNOSIS	NURSING INTERVENTIONS	RATIONALE
Ineffective breathing pattern related to decreased lung expansion	Observe changes in respiratory rate and depth.	Determines adequacy of breathing pattern.
	Inspect thorax for symmetry of respiratory movement.	Determines adequacy of breathing pattern.
	Observe breathing pattern for SOB, nasal flaring, and use of accessory muscles and intercostal retractions.	Identifies increased work of breathing.
	Review chest x-rays.	Indicates location of effusion.
	Assess emotional response.	Detects use of hyperventilation as a causative factor.
	Assess for pain.	Pain on inhalation or exhalation may cause an ineffective breathing pattern.
	Maintain bed rest; position patient in optimal body alignment in semi-Fowler's position for breathing.	Optimizes diaphragmatic contraction.
	Assist patient to use relaxation techniques.	Relieves anxiety and decreases work of breathing.
	Assist patient to turn, cough, and deep breathe.	Facilitates lung expansion, prevents atelectasis.
	Splint chest when coughing.	Reduces pain of coughing.
	Medicate with analgesic without depressing respirations.	Reduces pain that may be interfering with breathing.
	Encourage use of blow bottles or incentive spirometry.	Facilitates deep breathing.
	Prepare patient for thoracentesis and/or chest tube insertion.	Removes fluid from pleural space.

→ › ›

NURSING DIAGNOSIS	NURSING INTERVENTIONS	RATIONALE
Impaired gas exchange related to alveolar-capillary membrane changes	Auscultate lungs.	Determines adequacy of gas exchange and detects atelectasis.
	Assess level of consciousness, listlessness, and irritability.	Decreased level of consciousness may indicate hypoxia.
	Observe skin color and capillary refill.	Determines circulatory adequacy.
	Monitor ABGs.	Determines acid-base balance and need for oxygen.
	Monitor CBC.	Detects amount of hemoglobin present to carry oxygen and presence of infection.
	Monitor changes in activity tolerance.	Activity may induce breathlessness.
	Administer oxygen as ordered.	Improves gas exchange; decreases work of breathing.
	Maintain airway patency by assisting the patient to cough or by suctioning.	Facilitates gas flow to and from alveoli.
	Pace activities to patient's tolerance.	Decreases oxygen demand.
	Assist patient to Fowler's position.	Optimizes diaphragmatic contraction.
Fear related to suffocation and dying	Validate sources of fear with patient.	Guides therapeutic interventions.
	Assist patient to identify coping skills used successfully in the past.	Facilitates problem solving.
	Encourage patient to ask questions and express feelings.	May relieve anxiety; helps patient put thoughts into perspective.
	Provide accurate information about pleural effusion.	Knowledge can decrease fears.
	Provide oxygen as ordered.	Decreases the work of breathing.
Potential for infection related to decreased pulmonary function and stasis of fluid in the pleural space	Auscultate lungs.	Indicates airway clearance.
	Monitor leukocytes and albumin.	Indicates adequacy of secondary defense and immune system.
	Assess nutritional status.	Adequate nutritional status supports the immune system.
	Measure temperature.	Detects fever, indicating actual infection.
	Encourage effective coughing and deep breathing.	Maintains clear airway, prevents atelectasis.

NURSING DIAGNOSIS	NURSING INTERVENTIONS	RATIONALE
	Encourage an increase in fluid intake unless contraindicated.	Liquifies secretions so they can be coughed easier.
	Administer antibiotics as ordered.	Prevents or reduces microorganism growth.
	Administer antipyretics as ordered.	Reduces fever.
Knowledge deficit related to promoting recovery and preventing recurrence	See Patient Teaching.	

5 EVALUATE

PATIENT OUTCOME	DATA INDICATING THAT OUTCOME IS REACHED
Breathing pattern is effective without fatigue or dyspnea.	Chest x-rays show no evidence of fluid accumulation. Breath sounds are clear. (Pa_{O2} = 80-100 mm Hg, Pa_{CO2} = 35-45 mm Hg, pH = 7.35-7.45)
Gas exchange is within normal limits for patient.	Breath sounds are clear.
Fears have been resolved.	Patient acknowledges fears of suffocation and dying. Patient's concerns are refocused to getting well and being discharged.
There is no pulmonary infection.	Patient is afebrile, WBCs are within normal limits.
Knowledge deficit is resolved.	Patient demonstrates knowledge of disease process and home care management.

PATIENT TEACHING

1. Teach the patient the importance of positioning to facilitate ventilatory effort.
2. Teach the patient the importance of deep breathing and coughing to keep the lungs aerated and to prevent complications.
3. If pleural effusion is a recurrent problem, ensure that the patient is able to identify signs of accumulating fluid so care can be sought early.
4. Discuss symptoms to report to physician: difficulty breathing, chest pain, elevated temperature, persistent cough.
5. Discuss medication: name, dosage, time of administration, purpose, and side effects.
6. Explain need to exercise to tolerance with planned rest periods to avoid fatigue.

Pneumothorax and Hemothorax

The presence of air in the pleural space between the parietal and visceral pleurae is a **pneumothorax.** The presence of blood in the pleural space is a **hemothorax.**

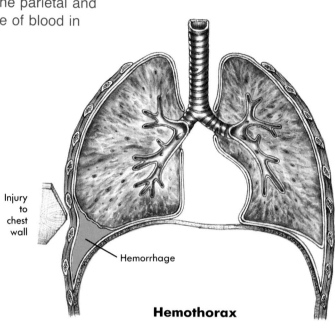

Hemothorax

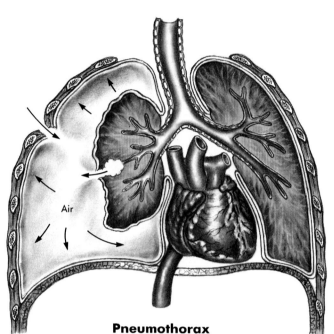

Pneumothorax

Many times, especially with trauma, victims have both pneumothorax and hemothorax. In these cases the term **hemopneumothorax** is used.

A pneumothorax may be classified as closed, open, or tension. A closed, or noncommunicating, pneumothorax develops when the air enters pleural space from within the lung without penetration of the chest wall (see Figure 4-10). A closed pneumothorax may be spontaneous, traumatic, or iatrogenic. A *spontaneous pneumothorax* may occur in apparently healthy persons, usually between 20 and 40 years of age. Often these persons are males who are tall and thin and have long, narrow chests.[42] For these persons there may be a rupture of a small air cyst (bleb) or a large air cyst (bulla) after a hard cough or sneeze, which causes the pneumothorax.[114] Pulmonary disease such as emphysema, pneumonia, and neoplasm may result in weak lung tissue where a spontaneous pneumothorax may occur due to a rupture of the bronchus or alveolus. A *traumatic closed pneumothorax* occurs following some injury to the chest when air from the lung enters the pleura, but the chest wall remains intact. A fractured rib may produce such an injury. An *iatrogenic pneumothorax* can occur after medical treatment, such as a thoracentesis, pleural biopsy, or subclavian vein or pulmonary artery catheter insertion, or after certain kinds of chest surgery, such as a thoracotomy. Patients on mechanical

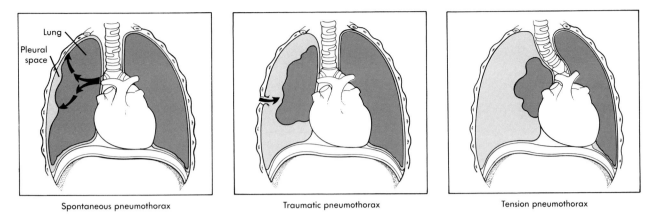

FIGURE 4-10
Spontaneous, traumatic, and tension pneumothorax.

ventilators may develop a closed iatrogenic pneumothorax. Approximately 3 to 4% of patients on ventilators have a pneumothorax; the incidence rises to 23% when PEEP is used.[84]

An open, or communicating, pneumothorax allows air to enter the pleural space through the chest wall. This is a traumatic pneumothorax which also may be called a sucking chest wound. The air enters the pleura from a penetrating injury through the chest wall such as a gun shot wound or a knife stab wound.

A tension pneumothorax develops when air leaks into the pleura and cannot escape. The tear in the pleura acts as a one-way valve. This is a life-threatening complication requiring immediate intervention.

PATHOPHYSIOLOGY

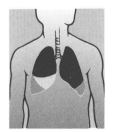 The pleural space normally maintains a negative pressure between −10 and −12 mm Hg. This negative pressure facilitates lung expansion during ventilation. When there is penetration into the pleural space by an object external to the chest wall (such as a knife or needle) or when there is penetration into the pleural space by an internal mechanism (such as a broken rib or bleb rupture of the lung), air enters the pleural space, and the negative pressure is decreased. With each inspiration air moves into the pleural space and some air moves out with each exhalation, except that in a tension pneumothorax the air cannot escape. Depending on the amount of air that enters initially and the amount that continues to enter, the lung is no longer able to remain fully inflated.

As the pleural space pressure increases and the lung collapses, there is a mediastinal shift toward the unaffected side. This shift causes pressure on the great vessels returning to the heart and thus a decreased venous return. If pneumothorax is left untreated, cardiac output is compromised and a multisystem failure may occur. The same mechanisms occur with hemothorax; however, blood is entering the pleural space rather than air.

The types of pneumothorax and hemothorax have both similarities and differences. The following diagnostic studies discuss the differences where they exist.

COMPLICATIONS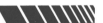

Atelectasis	Pulmonary embolus
ARDS	Pleural effusion
Infection	Empyema
Pulmonary edema	

DIAGNOSTIC STUDIES AND FINDINGS

Diagnostic Test	Findings
Spontaneous, closed or non-communicating pneumothorax Chest x-ray	The characteristic finding shows air in the pleural cavity without the lateral markings of the lungs; instead there is a sharp pleural margin seen medially, indicating that the lung has collapsed; if the lung is not entirely collapsed, this margin may not be as obvious; it is therefore desirable to take an expiratory film with the patient sitting upright—because intrapleural air first collects in the apex, partial pneumothorax identification may be made; Figure 4-11 shows a classic picture of a pneumothorax
Open, communicating, or penetrating-trauma pneumothorax Chest x-ray	See "Spontaneous, closed, or noncommunicating pneumothorax" above
Tension pneumothorax Chest x-ray	The characteristic film of an individual with a tension pneumothorax shows complete lung collapse and a shift of mediastinal structures toward the unaffected side
Hemothorax Chest x-ray	A minimum of 250 ml of intrapleural fluid is required to show a blunting of the costophrenic angle on an upright chest x-ray; it is therefore desirable to obtain an upright chest x-ray if possible
Laboratory tests ABGs	Decreased pH and Pao_2; increased $Paco_2$ regardless of the type of pneumothorax or hemothorax

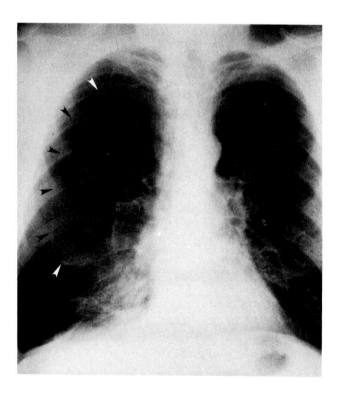

FIGURE 4-11
Chest x-ray of patient with pneumothorax. Note narrowing of pleural edge at narrow point and lack of lung markings beyond pleural line. (Courtesy R. Keith Wilson, M.D., Baylor College of Medicine, Houston, Tex; From Thompson.)[99]

MEDICAL MANAGEMENT

GENERAL MANAGEMENT

Closed-tube thoracostomy (chest tube):

This technique is used to treat most types of pneumothorax. The exception is a small, spontaneous pneumothorax in an otherwise healthy individual. For a small, spontaneous pneumothorax a one-way flutter valve (e.g., Heimlich valve) may be attached to the chest tube to allow air to escape without allowing additional air in the pleural space.[69] The indications for closed-tube thoracostomy include the following[88]: traumatic causes, pneumothorax with respiratory distress, recurrent pneumothorax, necessity for ventilatory support, moderate to large pneumothorax, pneumothorax that continues to grow despite treatment, associated hemothorax, tension pneumothorax.

Indications for this procedure for hemothorax include initial thoracostomy tube drainage greater than 1500 ml of blood; persistent bleeding rate greater than 500 ml/h; increasing hemothorax seen on chest roentgenogram; and patient in an unstable and hypotensive state despite adequate blood replacement.[88]

The chest tube should be inserted in the fifth or sixth intercostal space at the midaxillary line. If the tube is positioned posteriorly and toward the apex of the lung, it can effectively remove air and fluid. The lateral placement is preferred not only because it is most efficient but also because it does not produce a cosmetic defect, as does the anterior site of the second intercostal space at the midclavicular line.[105] See pp. 264-268 for discussion of chest tubes and their care.

Tension pneumothorax requires immediate and specific medical intervention. The building pressure in the pleural space must be reversed. A mechanism must be provided to release the pressure. The most effective way to release the pressure is to insert a large-bore needle (16 to 18 gauge) either anteriorly at the midclavicle line between the second and third intercostal space or at the midlateral line between the fifth and sixth intercostal space. Once the needle is inserted, the patient's condition should improve remarkably.

Airway maintenance: Done by positioning, a simple airway, or endotracheal intubation, depending on patient's condition.

Oxygenation: Provide oxygen to maintain adequate blood gas levels.

Mechanical ventilation with PEEP: If patient shows evidence of respiratory failure, may be initiated after chest tubes have been inserted and determined to be functioning adequately; see pp. 258-263 for discussion of technique. If the patient has communicating pneumothorax, entrance wound into the chest wall should be immediately covered by petrolatum jelly gauze; three sides of the gauze pad should be taped; the fourth is left open to permit exhale ventilation; if gauze is placed on too tightly, tension pneumothorax may result.

DRUG THERAPY

Hemothorax requires aggressive intravenous therapy to restore the circulating blood volume.

Narcotic analgesics: Analgesics such as meperidine (Demerol) may be given for pain if respirations are adequate; drugs such as morphine and barbiturates are generally contraindicated because they may cause respiratory depression.

Adrenergic agents: Antihypotensives such as dopamine may be indicated. Dopamine (Intropin): Dilute 1 ampule (200 mg) in 250 ml D5W; use with microdrip administration set; usual dose is 2-5 mg/kg/min initially; then titrate to desired response.

1 ASSESS

ASSESSMENT	OBSERVATION

Spontaneous, closed, or noncommunicating pneumothorax

History
Patient generally is male between the ages of 20 and 40 years and is in good health
Patient is older and has a COPD, pneumonia, or neoplasm
Patient usually awakens to note SOB and chest pain

Respiratory
SOB and chest pain in only 50% of all cases; patient may appear acutely ill with cyanosis, dyspnea, and tachypnea or may appear to be healthy; the difference in the clinical signs is dependent on the size of the pneumothorax; breath sounds are generally diminished; percussion tones are hyperresonant over involved area; approximately 25% of patients have subcutaneous emphysema[105]

Cardiovascular
Patient demonstrates syncope and Hamman's sign (a crunching sound with each heartbeat owing to mediastinal air accumulation)

Open, communicating, or penetrating-trauma pneumothorax

History
Some event that has caused a penetration of the chest wall

Respiratory
Penetration of the chest wall, a sucking sound on inspiration as the chest wall rises, and varying signs of respiratory distress depending on the size of the pneumothorax, dyspnea, cyanosis, tachypnea

Tension pneumothorax

History
Blunt trauma to chest that may have resulted in fractured ribs or penetrating injury to chest that permits air to enter chest wall but then seals off as air tries to escape

Respiratory
As the positive pressure on the affected side increases, the clinical signs will become more severe; dyspnea, paradoxic movement of the chest, deviated trachea toward the unaffected side, cyanosis, absence of breath sounds on the affected side, and hyperresonance on percussion of the affected side

Cardiovascular
Distant heart sounds, tachycardia, hypotension from cardiogenic shock because of lack of oxygenated blood, and neck vein enlargement due to pressure on superior vena cava

Hemothorax

History
Same as for open pneumothorax or tension pneumothorax

Respiratory
Same as above with the addition of dullness on chest percussion

Cardiovascular
Same as for tension pneumothorax with the addition of signs of hypovolemic shock, such as pallor and anxiety; the severity of the hemothorax may be determined by the amount of blood accumulation: less than 300 ml is considered minor and may not cause significant clinical signs; 300 to 1400 ml is moderate; and over 1400 ml is severe, indicating that most clinical signs will also be present

Psychologic
Fear, pain, confusion

2 DIAGNOSE

NURSING DIAGNOSIS	SUBJECTIVE FINDINGS	OBJECTIVE FINDINGS
Ineffective breathing pattern related to decreased lung expansion	Complains of SOB and stabbing pain on the affected side that may radiate to the shoulder	SOB, dyspnea, tachypnea, air hunger, labored or irregular breathing, shallow respirations, cough with or without hemoptysis

NURSING DIAGNOSIS	NURSING INTERVENTIONS	RATIONALE
Impaired gas exchange related to alveolar-capillary membrane changes	Complains of SOB and need for supplemental oxygen	Crackles (rales) Absent or decreased breath sounds on involved side Dyspnea Tachypnea Pa_{O_2} <70 mm Hg Pa_{CO_2} <35 mm Hg pH >7.45 Cyanosis Tachycardia Confusion, somnolence Restlessness Hyperresonant over involved areas Decreased tactile fremitus on affected side
Fear related to suffocation and uncertainty of prognosis	Expresses fears	Tachypnea, tachycardia, scared facial expression

3 PLAN

Patient goals

1. Patient's breathing pattern will be effective.
2. Patient's gas exchange will be improved.
3. Patient's fear will subside.

4. Patient will demonstrate an understanding of home care and follow-up instructions.

4 IMPLEMENT

NURSING DIAGNOSIS	NURSING INTERVENTIONS	RATIONALE
Ineffective breathing pattern related to decreased lung expansion	Observe changes in respiratory rate and depth, pulse, and blood pressure.	Determines adequacy of breathing pattern and status of cardiovascular system.
	Inspect thorax for symmetry of respiratory movement.	Determines adequacy of breathing pattern.
	Observe breathing pattern for SOB, nasal flaring, and use of accessory muscles and intercostal retractions.	Identifies increased work of breathing.
	Review chest x-rays.	Indicates severity of skeletal and lung involvement.
	Assess emotional response.	Detects use of hyperventilation as a complicating factor.
	Assess for pain.	May be a contributing factor.
	Position patient in optimal body alignment in semi-Fowler's position for breathing.	Optimizes diaphragmatic contraction.

NURSING DIAGNOSIS	NURSING INTERVENTIONS	RATIONALE
	Encourage patient to suppress cough during the acute symptoms but encourage coughing and deep breathing after acute episode to help reexpand the lung.	Decreases air/blood moving into pleural space.
	Assist with chest tube insertion as ordered.	Helps to reexpand lung.
	Provide chest tube care consistent with guidelines on pp. 264-268.	Maintains airtight drainage system.
	Medicate with analgesic without depressing respirations.	Reduces pain that may be interfering with breathing.
	Assist patient to use relaxation techniques.	Relieves anxiety and decreases the work of breathing.
	Should mechanical ventilation become necessary, provide care and monitoring consistent with the guidelines on pp. 258-263.	Maintains ventilation.
Impaired gas exchange related to alveolar-capillary membrane changes	Auscultate lungs.	Determines adequacy of gas exchange and detects atelectasis.
	Assess level of consciousness, listlessness, and irritability.	Decreased level of consciousness may indicate hypoxia.
	Monitor electrocardiogram.	Detects dysrhythmias secondary to altered blood gases.
	Observe skin color and capillary refill.	Determines circulatory adequacy.
	Monitor ABGs.	Determines acid-base balance and need for oxygen.
	Monitor CBC.	Detects amount of hemoglobin to carry oxygen and presence of infection.
	Remain with patient.	To allow close observation.
	Maintain patent airway.	To decrease work of breathing.
	Administer oxygen as ordered.	Improves gas exchange; decreases work of breathing.
	Pace activities to patient's tolerance.	Decreases oxygen demand.
	Have emergency equipment available: emergency cart and intubation tray.	Prepares for tension pneumothorax or intubation.
Fear related to suffocation, and to uncertainty of prognosis	Validate sources of fear with patient.	Determines the fears perceived so that appropriate interventions can be implemented.

NURSING DIAGNOSIS	NURSING INTERVENTIONS	RATIONALE
	Remain with patient; ask another person to notify physician.	Provides support and allows close observation.
	Reassure and try to calm patient.	Provides support.
	Encourage patient to ask questions and express feelings.	May relieve anxiety; helps patient put thoughts into perspective.
	Provide accurate information about pneumothorax.	Knowledge can decrease fears.
	Provide oxygen as ordered.	Decreases the work of breathing.
Knowledge deficit	See Patient Teaching.	

5 EVALUATE

PATIENT OUTCOME	DATA INDICATING THAT OUTCOME IS REACHED
Respiratory pattern is effective.	Chest x-rays show full lung expansion with no evidence of pneumothorax or hemothorax. Vital capacity measurements are optimum for patient's status, including FEV_1, TLC, and RV. Clear breath sounds. Blood gas values are within normal limits (see below).
Gas exchange is within normal limits.	Pa_{O_2} = 80-100 mm Hg Pa_{CO_2} = 35-45 mm Hg Arterial pH = 7.35-7.45 Breath sounds are clear.
Fear has been reduced.	Reports fear has lessened. Appears relaxed.
Knowledge deficit is resolved.	Demonstrates knowledge of disease process and home care management.

PATIENT TEACHING

1. Teach the patient and family about the chest tubes: their purpose, function, and care that must be taken during their use.
2. Teach the patient adaptive breathing techniques to maximize lung reexpansion and prevent complications.
3. Teach importance of avoiding contact with persons who have upper respiratory infections and influenza.
4. Teach importance of regular medical reevaluations for an extended period following the pneumothorax.
5. Discuss symptoms to report to the physician: cold, sore throat; flu; elevated temperature; cough; sudden, sharp chest pain; difficulty breathing; any redness, pain, swelling, or tenderness at puncture site of chest tube.
6. Explain importance of avoiding strenuous activity or exercise.
7. Discuss medications: name, dosage, time of administration, purpose, and side effects.
8. If patient had a spontaneous pneumothorax, discuss possibility of recurrence (10% to 60% possibility). Recurrences usually occur within 2 to 3 years, but may be as long as 20 years. The recurrence rate for a third spontaneous pneumothorax is 50% to 80%.

Pulmonary Embolism

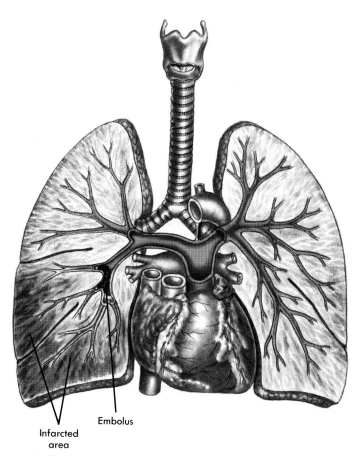

Infarcted
area

Embolus

Pulmonary embolism is the blockage of a pulmonary artery by foreign matter, such as a thrombus, that usually arises from a peripheral vein, fat, air, or tumor tissue. The blockage obstructs blood supply to the lung tissue.

The incidence of pulmonary embolism in the United States is estimated to be 6500 cases annually. Of this number approximately 38% of the patients die from the emboli. The mortality is five to six times greater in those patients in whom the diagnosis is missed. Ten percent die in the first hour after blockage of the pulmonary artery. Of the 90% who survive the first hour, only 27% are diagnosed. Of the diagnosed cases, 8% die and 92% are successfully treated. Of those not diagnosed, 32% die and 68% survive without treatment.[115] Resolution of the embolus occurs within 7 to 10 days.[99]

PATHOPHYSIOLOGY

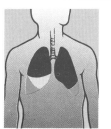

Three factors (Virchow's triad) are related to the development of a venous thrombus: venous stasis, injury to the vein wall, and increased blood coagulability (Figure 4-12).

The most common sites for thrombus formation are the deep veins of the legs (90%) and the pelvic veins. At some point the thrombus breaks loose and travels to and lodges in one of the pulmonary arteries.

A pulmonary embolism produces an area of the lung that is ventilated but underperfused. This results in an increase in physiologic dead space ventilation. Reflex bronchoconstriction occurs in the affected area and is thought to result from three factors. The release of histamine or serotonin from the clot contributes to bronchoconstriction, hypocarbia constricts bronchial smooth muscle, and the activation of thrombin from the clot constricts peripheral airways. The vagus nerve is stimulated, which slows the heart rate.

If the thrombus lodges in a large or medium-size artery, there may be insufficient collateral bronchial circulation. If this occurs, there may be significant tissue underperfusion, and pulmonary infarction.

Following are the most common predisposing factors[37, 99, 115]:

Venostasis
  Prolonged bed rest
  Obesity (20% increase above standard)
  Advanced age
  Burns
  Pregnancy and postpartum period
Venous injury
  Surgery, particularly on legs, pelvis, abdomen, and thorax
  Fractures or injury of pelvis or legs
Increased blood coagulability
  Malignancy
  Oral contraceptives high in estrogen (over 100 μg per pill)
  Polycythemia vera
Disease
  Lung disease, especially chronic
  Heart disease, especially congestive heart failure, myocardial infarction, atrial fibrillation, or rheumatic heart disease
  History of thromboembolism, thrombophlebitis, or vascular surgery
  Infection
  Diabetes mellitus

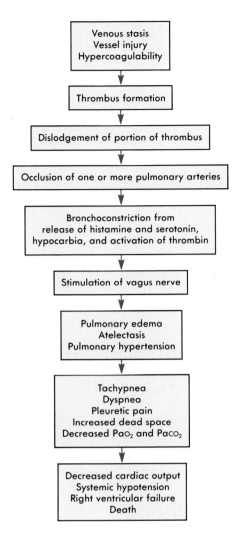

```
┌─────────────────────────┐
│    Venous stasis        │
│    Vessel injury        │
│   Hypercoagulability    │
└─────────────────────────┘
            ↓
┌─────────────────────────┐
│   Thrombus formation    │
└─────────────────────────┘
            ↓
┌─────────────────────────────────┐
│ Dislodgement of portion of thrombus │
└─────────────────────────────────┘
            ↓
┌─────────────────────────────────────┐
│ Occlusion of one or more pulmonary arteries │
└─────────────────────────────────────┘
            ↓
┌─────────────────────────────────────┐
│        Bronchoconstriction from      │
│  release of histamine and serotonin, │
│  hypocarbia, and activation of thrombin │
└─────────────────────────────────────┘
            ↓
┌─────────────────────────────┐
│  Stimulation of vagus nerve │
└─────────────────────────────┘
            ↓
┌─────────────────────────┐
│    Pulmonary edema      │
│     Atelectasis         │
│  Pulmonary hypertension │
└─────────────────────────┘
            ↓
┌─────────────────────────┐
│      Tachypnea          │
│       Dyspnea           │
│     Pleuretic pain      │
│  Increased dead space   │
│ Decreased PaO₂ and PacO₂ │
└─────────────────────────┘
            ↓
┌─────────────────────────┐
│ Decreased cardiac output│
│  Systemic hypotension   │
│ Right ventricular failure│
│        Death            │
└─────────────────────────┘
```

FIGURE 4-12
Pathogenesis of pulmonary embolism.

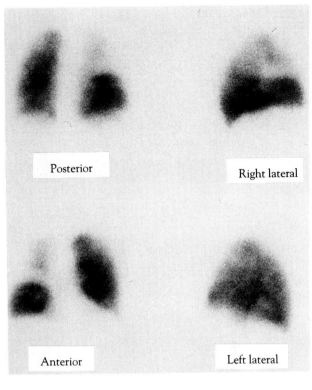

Posterior   Right lateral

Anterior   Left lateral

FIGURE 4-13
Lung scan showing pulmonary embolism. Note decreased perfusion of right upper lobe indicative of pulmonary embolism. (Courtesy R. Keith Wilson, M.D., Baylor College of Medicine, Houston, Tex; From Thompson).[99]

COMPLICATIONS

Cardiac dysrhythmias	Pulmonary hypertension
Cor pulmonale	Atelectasis
Hypotension	Chest congestion

DIAGNOSTIC STUDIES AND FINDINGS

Diagnostic Test	Findings
Chest x-ray	Unilateral diaphragm elevation, enlarged main pulmonary artery associated with decreased vascular markings on one side, unilateral pulmonary effusion, occasional wedge-shaped area of consolidation
Lung scans	Rapid, relatively safe and easy screening tests for establishing the diagnosis (Figure 4-13); if the patient has a chronic lung disease, asthma, or congestive heart failure, the lung scan is of little diagnostic value; two scans are commonly used sequentially: perfusion lung scan and ventilation lung scan; comparison of scans may be diagnostic of pulmonary embolism *Perfusion lung scan* This study involves the intravenous injection of serum albumin tagged with tracer amounts of a radioisotope; the radioactive particles pass through the right side of the heart and lodge in the pulmonary capillary bed; significant diagnostic findings reveal an area deficient in radioactivity, indicating a perfusion deficit

Diagnostic Test	Findings
	Ventilation lung scan
	The patient initially breathes a radioactive gas through a carefully sealed system for several minutes; during this time the lungs are scanned by a gamma camera
	Shows decreased ventilation in the area of the embolus
Pulmonary angiography	Although it is the most specific diagnostic procedure, pulmonary angiography also has the most risk; the two diagnostic criteria of this technique are intraarterial filling defects and complete obstruction of a pulmonary artery branch
ECG	The following classic signs help to differentiate pulmonary embolism from myocardial infarction: right axis deviation, incomplete or complete right bundle-branch block, tall peaked P waves, S wave in lead I, a Q wave in lead III, T wave insertion, ST segment depression, and T wave changes: peaked and inverted
Laboratory tests	
Serum assays	Serum assays (looking for the triad of elevated LDH and bilirubin with a normal SGOT and WBC [less than 15,000], and elevated fibrin split products [FSP])
ABGs	Pa_{O_2} <80 mm Hg in association with hyperventilation leads to Pa_{CO_2} >40 mm Hg; alveolar arterial oxygen tension gradient (PA-a) o_2 increased

MEDICAL MANAGEMENT

GENERAL MANAGEMENT

Oxygen therapy: Administer oxygen by mask or cannula to maintain blood gas levels.

Bed rest for first 2 or 3 days: Following that, mobilization should be gradually increased.

DRUG THERAPY

Anticoagulants: Main purpose of this therapy is supportive

Heparin: Halts clot propagation, enabling endogenous fibrinolytic mechanisms to remove the clot. Heparin may be administered by continuous intravenous infusion or by intermittent intravenous injections. **Initial bolus loading dose:** 500-1000 U subcutaneously q 8-12 h; **Continuous infusion:** 20 U/kg/h or 800-1500 U/h; **Intermittent bolus doses:** 70-100 U/kg q 4 h using a heparin lock. Clotting time is monitored by the partial thromboplastin time (PTT).

Warfarin (Coumadin): Should be started before the heparin is terminated. **Oral dose:** 5-10 mg daily. Warfarin may be used for 6 months up to life in some cases. Clotting time should be monitored by the prothrombin time (PT).

Fibrinolytic enzymes: Some authors believe fibrinolytic therapy to be superior to heparin therapy. The two drugs of choice are: Urokinase (Abbokinase, Breokinase): 4400 U/kg IV over 10 min, followed by 4400 U/kg/h for 12 h; thrombin time (TT) or PTT should be monitored after 2 h. Streptokinase (Kabikinase, Streptase): 2500 U IV over 20-30 min followed by 1000 U/h over 24-72 h; TT or PTT should be monitored after 2 h. The main side effects of these two drugs are bleeding and allergic reactions. Dextran: Dextran is a carbohydrate polymer available in two preparations, dextran 40 and dextran 70. Dextran has antithrombotic effects, which are attributed to a decrease in platelet aggregability, alterations in factor VIII activity, and interference with fibrin formation. Dextran 70 has been shown to be as effective as low-dose heparin. Major side effects of dextran are anaphylaxis, volume overload, renal failure, and excessive bleeding. Dextran is a suitable alternative to low-dose heparin when the latter is contraindicated.

SURGERY

Surgical therapy of pulmonary embolism infrequently indicated: When there are multiple emboli, umbrella filter (Mobin-Uddin umbrellas) may be surgically placed in inferior vena cava; other techniques are surgical removal of the embolus, which requires cardiopulmonary bypass, and interruption of blood flow through inferior vena cava via ligation.

1   ASSESS

ASSESSMENT	OBSERVATIONS
Respiratory	Respiratory distress: tachypnea, labored breathing, dyspnea, coughing, shallow breathing, restlessness, confusion, cyanosis, pleuritic pain Breath sounds: crackles or pleural friction rub
Cardiovascular	Positive Hamman's sign with calf tenderness Tachycardia Accentuated pulmonic component of second heart sound (S_2P) S_3 and S_4 gallop rhythms Murmurs Chest pain
Psychosocial	Apprehension, fear of suffocation

2   DIAGNOSE

NURSING DIAGNOSIS	SUBJECTIVE FINDINGS	OBJECTIVE FINDINGS
Impaired gas exchange related to ventilation/perfusion abnormalities	Complains of SOB; expresses need for supplemental oxygen	Crackles (rales), dyspnea, tachypnea, cyanosis $Pa_{O2} <80$ mm Hg $Pa_{CO2} <40$ mm Hg pH >7.45 Confusion, restlessness
Ineffective breathing pattern related to substernal pain	Complains of pain when breathing; complains of inability to breathe; expresses need for oxygen	Dyspnea, tachypnea, use of accessory muscles, cyanosis $Pa_{O2} <80$ mm Hg $Pa_{CO2} <40$ mm Hg pH >7.45 Shallow breathing, diminished chest wall movement
Potential for injury (bleeding) related to increased risk of bleeding from anticoagulant therapy	Reports increased bruising of skin	Anticoagulant therapy Altered clotting factors
Anxiety related to suffocation	Expresses apprehension; expresses fear of suffocation	Tachypnea, tachycardia, scared facial expression

3   PLAN

Patient goals

1. Patient's gas exchange will be improved.
2. Patient's breathing pattern will be effective without pain.
3. Patient will not exhibit signs of bleeding.
4. Patient's anxiety will be relieved.
5. Patient will demonstrate understanding of home care and follow-up instructions.

→ > >

4 IMPLEMENT

NURSING DIAGNOSIS	NURSING INTERVENTIONS	RATIONALE
Impaired gas exchange related to ventilation/perfusion abnormalities	Observe rate, depth of respirations, use of accessory muscles, dyspnea, diaphoresis, air hunger, tachycardia.	Determines adequacy of gas exchange and guides therapeutic interventions.
	Auscultate lungs for rhonchi, crackles, and wheezes.	Determines adequacy of gas exchange and detects atelectasis.
	Assess level of consciousness, listlessness, and irritability.	Decreased level of consciousness may indicate hypoxia.
	Observe skin color and capillary refill.	Determines circulatory adequacy.
	Monitor ABGs.	Determines acid-base balance and need for oxygen.
	Monitor CBC.	Detects amount of hemoglobin to carry oxygen and presence of infection.
	Monitor chest x-rays.	Shows extent of lung involvement.
	Observe sputum for color, amount, and character.	Indicates whether bleeding is occurring in lungs.
	Administer oxygen as ordered.	Improves gas exchange; decreases work of breathing.
	Maintain airway patency by assisting the patient to cough or by suctioning.	Facilitates gas flow to and from alveoli.
	Pace activities to patient's tolerance.	Decreases oxygen demand.
	Assist patient to turn and deep breathe.	Facilitates gas exchange.
Ineffective breathing pattern related to substernal pain	Inspect thorax for symmetry of respiratory movement.	Determines adequacy of breathing pattern.
	Measure tidal volume and vital capacity.	Indicates volume of air moving in and out of lungs.
	Assess for substernal pain.	Decreases inspiratory volume.
	Assess emotional response.	Hyperventilation from anxiety may alter breathing pattern.
	Elevate head of bed to semi-Fowler's position.	Optimizes diaphragmatic contraction.
	Encourage use of adaptive breathing techniques.	Decreases the work of breathing.
	Assist patient to use relaxation techniques.	Relieves anxiety and decreases work of breathing.

NURSING DIAGNOSIS	NURSING INTERVENTIONS	RATIONALE
Potential for injury (bleeding) related to increased risk of bleeding from anticoagulant therapy	Check PTT or PT and clotting functions or coagulation factors daily.	Indicates adequacy of anticoagulant therapy.
	Observe for bleeding in stools, urine, and sputum.	Indicates excessive anticoagulant therapy.
	Observe skin for bruising.	Indicates bleeding.
	Administer anticoagulants as ordered.	Prevents formation of additional thrombi.
	Do not administer aspirin-containing products.	Provides additional, unwanted anticoagulation.
	Maintain bed rest.	Protects patient from injury and decreases work of breathing.
	Elevate head of bed 45° to 60°.	Facilitates diaphragmatic contraction.
	Do not use knee gatch.	Applies pressure behind knee, which may promote venous stasis.
	Provide antiembolic stockings.	Promotes venous return.
	Administer stool softeners/laxatives as ordered.	Prevents straining to prevent rectal bleeding.
Anxiety related to fear of suffocation	Assess verbal and nonverbal signs of anxiety.	Determines type and extent of interventions required to reduce anxiety.
	Assist patient to identify coping skills used successfully in the past.	Facilitates problem solving.
	Encourage patient to ask questions and express feelings.	May relieve anxiety, helps patient put thoughts into perspective.
	Provide accurate information about pulmonary embolism.	Knowledge may decrease anxiety.
	Provide oxygen as ordered.	Decreases work of breathing.
Knowledge deficit	See Patient Teaching.	

5 EVALUATE

PATIENT OUTCOME	DATA INDICATING THAT OUTCOME IS REACHED
Gas exchange is improved.	ABGs are within normal limits (Pa_{O_2} = 80-100 mm Hg, Pa_{CO_2} = 35-45 mm Hg, pH = 7.35-7.45). Chest x-ray clear.
Breathing pattern is effective.	Vital capacity measurements including tidal volume and minute volumes are optimal for patient. Patient is breathing without difficulty or pain.
Injury did not occur.	No signs of bleeding noted.
Anxiety is relieved.	Patient able to breathe without difficulty or pain. Patient no longer apprehensive.
Knowledge deficit resolved.	Patient demonstrates knowledge of disease process and home care management.

PATIENT TEACHING

1. Teach the patient the importance of prescribed medications that are currently being used to treat the pulmonary embolism: name, dosage, purpose, time of administration, and side effects.
2. Teach preventive measures to all high-risk patients preoperatively and initiate interventions postoperatively that will help to prevent pulmonary embolism.
3. Teach strategies for persons at high risk to prevent venous pooling, which may lead to thrombophlebitis.
4. Changes in the health status of a patient recovering from pulmonary embolism must be reported immediately to the patient's health care provider. Changes include chest pain, shortness of breath, tachypnea, blood-tinged sputum, and blood in the stool or urine.

Pulmonary Edema

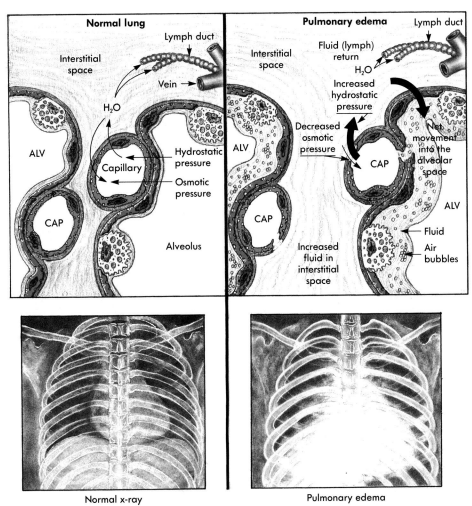

Normal lung

Pulmonary edema

Normal x-ray

Pulmonary edema

Pulmonary edema is the accumulation of serous fluid in the interstitium and alveoli of the lung.

Pulmonary edema may result from cardiogenic and noncardiogenic causes. Cardiogenic pulmonary edema usually accompanies underlying cardiac disease in which the failure of the left ventricle causes pooling of fluid to back up into the left atrium and into pulmonary veins and capillaries. The most common cause of pulmonary edema is increased capillary hydrostatic pressure from left ventricular failure. Noncardiogenic pulmonary edema results from damage to the capillaries' endothelium and blockage of lymphatic vessels. Damage to the endothelium increases capillary permeability, allowing fluid high in protein to escape into the interstitial spaces and alveoli. Blockage of lymphatic vessels interrupts the removal of excess fluid from the interstitial space, resulting in the accumulation of fluid in the interstitial spaces. Figure 4-14 shows the pathogenesis of pulmonary edema. Pulmonary edema is acute and extensive and may lead to death unless treated rapidly.

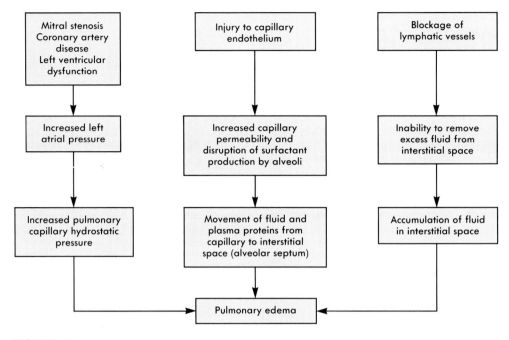

FIGURE 4-14
Causes of pulmonary edema.

PATHOPHYSIOLOGY

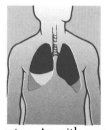 Hydrostatic and oncotic pressures are the major forces that affect movement of fluid across the capillary membranes. The normal hydrostatic pressure in the pulmonary capillaries is approximately 7 to 10 mm Hg.[8] The alveolar-capillary wall is permeable to fluid and small solutes. As with any capillary, the movement of fluid from the vascular space into the lung tissue is governed by Starling forces (Figure 4-15). The intravascular hydrostatic pressure is the major force that moves fluid out of the intravascular space into tissue. In other capillaries of the body, intravascular hydrostatic pressure is opposed to some degree by the tissue hydrostatic pressure. The lung tissue, however, exerts negligible opposing pressure. Thus the net pressure of force across the pulmonary vascular wall can be considered equal to the intravascular hydrostatic pressure. The plasma oncotic pressure caused primarily by serum proteins is the major force promoting retention of fluid in the intravascular space.[112] The plasma oncotic pressure is approximately 25 mm Hg. Therefore the alveoli tend to stay dry because the pressures oppose fluid movement into the interstitium and alveoli. A continuous filtration of small volumes of fluid cross the normal alveolar-capillary wall into the interstitial space of the alveolar wall and are removed through the lymph system.[112]

Hydrostatic pressure in the pulmonary capillaries must increase to about 25 to 30 mm Hg for pulmonary edema to occur when the capillary permeability is normal and the alveolar system is intact.

Pulmonary edema occurs in two stages: engorgement or interstitial edema followed by fluid movement or alveolar edema. In the first stage, interstitial edema causes engorgement of the perivascular and peribronchial spaces. Three adaptive mechanisms exist to prevent the second stage, alveolar edema. One adaptive mechanism is lymphatic drainage, which increases six to ten times normal to accommodate for a sustained increase in hydrostatic pressure. Second, the concentration of protein in the interstitial spaces falls because of an increase of water and solutes entering the interstitial space around the alveolar vessels.[8] This leads to an oncotic pressure difference between the plasma and the interstitial fluid, resulting in resorption of fluid into the circulation. The third adaptive mechanism is the capacity of the interstitial spaces in the lung, which contain up to 500 ml of edema fluid before edema symptoms become severe.

Once engorgement reaches its limits and the adaptive mechanisms are overwhelmed, alveolar edema occurs and fluid moves into the alveolar spaces. Blood plasma pours into the alveoli faster than coughing or the adaptive mechanisms can clear it.[77] The result of this process is acute pulmonary edema, which causes interference with the diffusion of oxygen, tissue hypoxia, and asphyxia. Without emergency treatment, respiratory failure occurs.

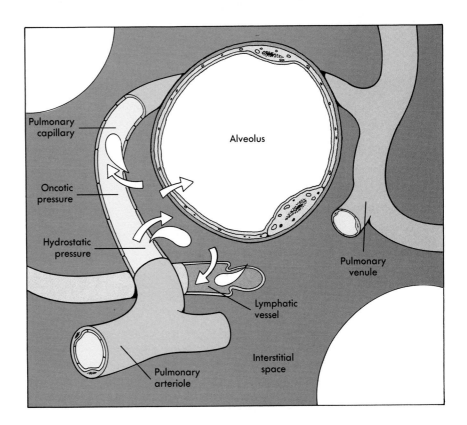

FIGURE 4-15
Starling forces governing movement of fluid out of and into the vascular spaces. The opposing pressures within the pulmonary capillary are the hydrostatic pressure and the oncotic pressure. The hydrostatic pressure is a pushing pressure generated by the pumping of the heart. The oncotic pressure is a pulling pressure and is generated by plasma proteins.

CAUSES OF PULMONARY EDEMA

Cause	Precipitating Event
Cardiogenic	
Increased capillary hydrostatic pressure	Myocardial infarction, mitral stenosis, fluid overload, pulmonary venocclusive disease
Noncardiogenic	
Increased capillary permeability	Inhaled or circulation toxins, irradiation, oxygen toxicity
Lymphatic insufficiency	Silicosis, lymphangitis, carcinoma
Decreased interstitial pressure	Rapid removal of pleural effusion or pneumothorax, hyperinflation
Decreased colloid osmotic pressure	Overtransfusion, hypoproteinemia
Unknown etiology	High altitude, heroin, neurogenic causes

Reprinted with permission from West JB: Pulmonary pathophysiology: the essentials, ed 2, Baltimore, 1982, Williams & Wilkins Co.

DIAGNOSTIC STUDIES AND FINDINGS

Diagnostic Test	Findings
Chest x-ray	Bilateral interstitial and alveolar infiltrates
	Prominent interlobular septa (Kerley-B lines) at the periphery of the lung bases
Laboratory tests	
ABGs	Pao_2 and $Paco_2$ variable; respiratory alkalosis or acidosis may occur
Cardiac monitoring	Tachycardia, dysrhythmias
Hemodynamic monitoring	PCWP increased 14 to 20 mm Hg in mild cases and 25 to 30 mm Hg in severe cases

MEDICAL MANAGEMENT

GENERAL MANAGEMENT

Rotation of tourniquets (infrequently used): Manually or by machine; pressure applied to three limbs at a time; cuff inflation slightly above patient's diastolic blood pressure; cuff inflated for 45 minutes followed by 15 minutes free of compression.

Oxygenation: High flow by Venturi mask at 50% concentration or intermittent positive-pressure breathing treatment; short-term intubation with mechanical ventilatory support if patient unable to maintain adequate arterial blood gas levels and adequate tidal volume.

DRUG THERAPY

D5W IV: With microdrip tubing running at keep-open rate for medication infusion.

Narcotic analgesics: Morphine sulfate, 10-15 mg IV, to reduce anxiety, slow respirations, and reduce venous return.

Diuretics: Furosemide (Lasix), loading dose at 40 mg IV over 1-2 min, increasing to 80 mg IV after 1 h; Ethacrynic acid (Edecrin), loading dose of 59 mg slow IV push (may be repeated once if needed); monitor serum potassium level.

Bronchodilators: Aminophylline, 250-500 mg (diluted in 50 mg IV solution) IV over 15-20 min; other drugs to treat underlying cause of pulmonary edema, e.g., cardiac drugs for cardiac-related problem.

1 ASSESS

ASSESSMENT	OBSERVATIONS
Respiratory	Nasal flaring; orthopnea; tachypnea; labored noisy breathing; diaphoresis; crackles; wheezes; noisy, wet breathing; cough productive of frothy, blood-tinged sputum; persistent cough; decreased vital capacity; decreased minute volume; increased intrapulmonary shunting; confusion, restlessness
Cardiovascular	Bounding pulse Decreased cardiac output; restlessness; lethargy; tachycardia; hypotension; weight gain PCWP increased: 14 to 20 mm Hg in mild cases, 25 to 30 mm Hg in severe cases
Psychosocial	Fear of suffocation; dying Anxiety

2 DIAGNOSE

NURSING DIAGNOSIS	SUBJECTIVE FINDINGS	OBJECTIVE FINDINGS
Fluid volume excess related to fluid accumulation in pulmonary vessels	Expresses inability to catch breath	Jugular venous distention Increased PAP Edema of extremities SOB Orthopnea Pulmonary congestion on chest x-ray Decreased urine output Restlessness, anxiety

NURSING DIAGNOSIS	SUBJECTIVE FINDINGS	OBJECTIVE FINDINGS
Impaired gas exchange related to alveolar-capillary membrane changes	Complains of SOB; expresses need for supplemental oxygen	Crackles (rales) Decreased breath sounds Dyspnea Tachypnea Pa_{O_2} <70 mm Hg Diffuse infiltrates on chest x-ray Confusion, somnolence Restlessness
Ineffective airway clearance related to tracheobronchial secretions	Complains of difficulty breathing	Rhonchi, crackles (rales), cyanosis, tachypnea, cough, dyspnea
Activity intolerance related to imbalance between oxygen supply and demand	Reports fatigue and SOB	SOB during activity; unable to perform ADL without fatigue and dyspnea
Anxiety related to dyspnea	Expresses worry about his condition and distress about the dyspnea	Appears scared, tense Dyspnea, tachypnea

3   PLAN

Patient goals

1. The patient's fluid volume will be within normal limits.
2. The patient's gas exchange will be improved.
3. The patient's airways will be patent.
4. The patient will be able to perform usual activities without fatigue or dyspnea.
5. The patient's anxiety will be relieved.
6. The patient will demonstrate understanding of home care and follow-up instructions.

4   IMPLEMENT

NURSING DIAGNOSIS	NURSING INTERVENTIONS	RATIONALE
Fluid volume excess related to fluid accumulation in pulmonary vessels	Weigh patient.	Detects fluid gain or loss.
	Measure intake and output.	Provides data on fluid balance.
	Monitor pulmonary artery pressures.	Provides data on fluid balance.
	Assess skin turgor.	Edema indicates fluid excess.
	Observe urine concentration.	Dilute urine may indicate excess fluids.
	Monitor hematocrit and hemoglobin.	Decreased values may indicate hemodilution.
	Assess neck veins.	Distention indicates fluid excess.

→ 〉 〉

NURSING DIAGNOSIS	NURSING INTERVENTIONS	RATIONALE
	Assess breath sounds.	Crackles may indicate pulmonary edema.
	Monitor serum electrolytes.	Detects electrolyte imbalances that may develop with fluid shifts.
	Administer diuretics as ordered.	Removes fluid via kidney tubules.
	Restrict fluid and sodium.	Prevents additional fluid excess.
	Administer cardiotonics, e.g., digoxin, as ordered.	Improves cardiac contractions for more efficient pumping.
	Assist patient to identify ways to prevent fluid excess.	May prevent recurrence and involves patient in care.
Impaired gas exchange related to alveolar-capillary membrane changes	Observe rate, depth of respirations, use of accessory muscles.	Determines adequacy of gas exchange and guides therapeutic interventions.
	Auscultate lungs for rhonchi, crackles, and wheezes.	Determines adequacy of gas exchange and detects atelectasis.
	Assist level of consciousness, listlessness, and irritability.	Decreased level of consciousness may indicate hypoxia.
	Observe skin color and capillary refill.	Determines circulatory adequacy.
	Monitor ABGs.	Determines acid-base balance and need for oxygen.
	Monitor CBC.	Detects amount of hemoglobin to carry oxygen and presence of infection.
	Monitor chest x-rays for Kerley-B lines.	Shows extent of fluid in lungs.
	Monitor side effects and blood levels of bronchodilators.	Guides medication use.
	Monitor changes in activity tolerance.	Activity may induce breathlessness.
	Administer oxygen as ordered.	Improves gas exchange; decreases work of breathing.
	Pace activities to patient's tolerance.	Decreases oxygen demand.
Ineffective airway clearance related to tracheobronchial secretions	Auscultate lungs for rhonchi, crackles, or wheezing.	Determines adequacy of gas exchange and extent of airway obstructed with secretions.
	Assess characteristics of secretions: quantity, color, consistency, odor.	Detects presence of fluid in lungs.
	Assess patient's hydration status: skin turgor, mucous membranes, tongue, intake and output over 24 hours, Hct.	Determines fluid balance.

NURSING DIAGNOSIS	NURSING INTERVENTIONS	RATIONALE
	Monitor theophylline levels if appropriate.	Determines blood level of theophylline (normally between 10-20 mEq/L).
	Assist patient with coughing as needed.	Removes secretions.
	Perform endotracheal or tracheostomy tube suctioning as needed.	Stimulates cough reflex and removes secretions.
	Position patient in proper body alignment for optimal breathing pattern (head of bed up 45°; if tolerated up to 90°).	Secretions move by gravity as position changes. Elevating head of bed moves abdominal content away from diaphragm to enhance diaphragmatic contraction.
	Administer expectorants/bronchodilators as ordered.	Facilitates mobilization of secretions.
	Assist patient with oral hygiene as needed.	Removes taste of secretions.
Activity intolerance related to imbalance between oxygen supply and demand	Observe response to activity.	Determines extent of tolerance.
	Identify factors contributing to intolerance, e.g., stress, side effects of drugs.	Guides selection of therapeutic interventions.
	Assess patient's sleep patterns.	May document a causative factor.
	Plan rest periods between activities.	Reduces fatigue by providing increased hours of sleep/rest.
	Encourage use of adaptive breathing techniques during activity.	Decreases work of breathing.
	Perform activities for patient until he/she is able to perform them.	Meets patient's need without causing fatigue.
	Provide progressive increase in activity as tolerated.	Slowly increase the number of and endurance of activities.
Anxiety related to dyspnea	Assess patient's level of anxiety (mild, moderate, severe, panic).	Determines type and extent of interventions required to reduce anxiety.
	Remain with the patient.	Reduces anxiety.
	Use short, simple sentences.	Facilitates patient's understanding.
	Encourage patient to ask questions and express feelings.	May relieve anxiety, helps patient put thoughts into perspective.
	Provide accurate information about pulmonary edema.	Knowledge can decrease anxiety.
	Provide comfort measures, e.g., back rub.	Facilitates relaxation; may decrease respiratory rate.

→ > >

NURSING DIAGNOSIS	NURSING INTERVENTIONS	RATIONALE
	Provide oxygen as ordered.	Decreased work of breathing.
	Administer morphine as ordered.	Reduces anxiety.
Knowledge deficit	See Patient Teaching.	

5 EVALUATE

PATIENT OUTCOME	DATA INDICATING THAT OUTCOME IS REACHED
Fluid volume is within normal limits.	Chest x-ray shows no evidence of fluid accumulation. PAP within normal limits. Breath sounds are clear. Weight has returned to value before pulmonary edema.
Gas exchange is within normal limits for patient.	Pa_{O_2} = 80-100 mm Hg Pa_{CO_2} = 35-45 mm Hg Arterial pH = 7.35-7.45 Breath sounds are clear.
Airways are patent.	Clear breath sounds. Breathing occurs without obstruction. Blood gas values are within normal limits.
Usual activities are performed without dyspnea or fatigue.	Patient demonstrates ability to perform usual daily activities without dyspnea or fatigue.
Anxiety has been resolved.	Patient reports lessened anxiety.
Knowledge deficit resolved.	Patient demonstrates knowledge of disease process and home care management.

PATIENT TEACHING

1. Teach the patient the importance of restricting salt intake and limiting fluid intake.
2. Teach the patient the importance of weighing self daily.
3. Provide the patient and family with information about pulmonary edema, assessment of the patient's capabilities and responses, and actions to take during an acute episode of dyspnea.
4. Teach the patient the importance of prescribed medications: name, dosage, purpose, time of administration, and side effects.
5. Provide the patient and family with information regarding care, cleaning, and maintenance of inhalation or oxygen equipment being used in the hospital or to be used at home, as well as the signs of oxygen toxicity.
6. Teach relaxation and stress reduction techniques.
7. Teach patient and family effective coughing techniques.

Pulmonary Hypertension

Pulmonary hypertension is defined as an elevation of mean pulmonary artery pressure above 15 mm Hg and systolic pulmonary artery pressure above 30 mm Hg under resting conditions.

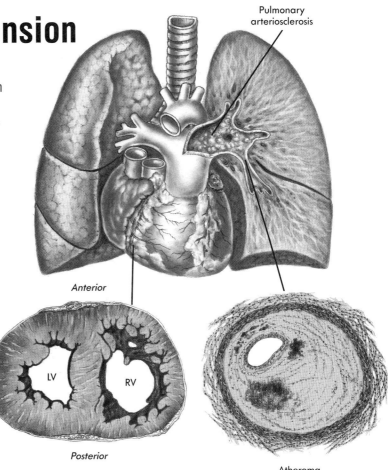

Anterior

LV   RV

Posterior

Right ventricular hypertrophy

Atheroma

Pulmonary hypertension can result from progressive disease of pulmonary vessels or lung parenchyma. The pulmonary circulation is unique in four respects: (1) it is a low-pressure, low-resistance system (resistance is 5 times less than the systemic circulation); (2) it is exposed to alveolar air; (3) it receives the entire cardiac output; and (4) it empties into the left atrium.[77]

Unexplained pulmonary hypertension (previously called primary pulmonary hypertension) is a disease of unknown origin that includes a variety of vascular lesions, rather than a specific disease. Familial cases have been reported, suggesting a genetic abnormality of pulmonary vasculature.[112] Secondary pulmonary hypertension has an identifiable etiology for the high pulmonary blood pressure.

The disease may occur at any age. In children it occurs equally between boys and girls whereas in adults it predominantly affects young women in their thirties. The ratio of adult females to males is 5:1. Many patients who are diagnosed with severe unexplained pulmonary hypertension die within 3 years after diagnosis.[112] Patients die from progressive right ventricular failure, pulmonary hemorrhage, and syncope.[77]

PATHOPHYSIOLOGY

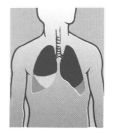

In primary hypertension, small pulmonary arteries become narrow or obliterated as a result of hypertrophy of smooth muscle in the vessels walls and formation of fibrous lesions around the vessels. The mechanisms that cause these changes are unknown. Vessel narrowing increases resistance and causes primary hypertension. Pressures in the left ventricle, which receives blood from the lungs, remains normal, but pressures generated in the lungs are transmitted to the right ventricle, which supplies blood to the pulmonary arteries. Eventually the right ventricle fails due to the force it must exert to pump blood into the narrowed pulmonary arteries.

Secondary pulmonary hypertension has four causes. Figure 4-16 shows the pathogenesis of pulmonary hy-

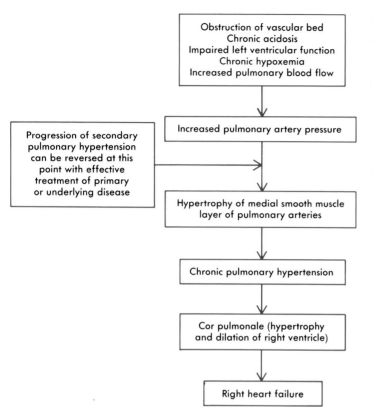

Obstruction of vascular bed
Chronic acidosis
Impaired left ventricular function
Chronic hypoxemia
Increased pulmonary blood flow

↓

Increased pulmonary artery pressure

Progression of secondary pulmonary hypertension can be reversed at this point with effective treatment of primary or underlying disease

↓

Hypertrophy of medial smooth muscle layer of pulmonary arteries

↓

Chronic pulmonary hypertension

↓

Cor pulmonale (hypertrophy and dilation of right ventricle)

↓

Right heart failure

FIGURE 4-16
Pathogenesis of pulmonary hypertension and cor pulmonale. (From McCance.)[73]

pertension. The first is elevated left ventricular filling pressures, such as occurs with coronary artery disease and mitral valve disease. When pressures on the left side of the heart are elevated, the pulmonary artery pressures rises proportionally to maintain normal blood flow. The second cause of secondary pulmonary hypertension is increased blood flow through the pulmonary circulation (left-to-right shunts), such as occurs with ventricle septal defect or patent ductus arteriosus. The third cause is obstruction of the pulmonary vascular bed by a pulmonary embolus, and the fourth cause is vasoconstriction of the vascular bed usually caused by hypoxemia, acidosis, or both.[73] In chronic lung disease, chemical mediators from products of the inflammatory process contribute to vasoconstriction in addition to the hypoxia. In the intimal lining of the pulmonary arteries and arterioles a concentric proliferation of cells develops, which eventually leads to fibrosis; the intima then assumes a concentric laminar appearance. In other forms of pulmonary hypertension the artery and/or arteriole are entirely obliterated. Medial lining of the pulmonary arteries hypertrophies in varying degrees of severity and is usually pronounced in infants and children. The vasoconstriction of the pulmonary vessels increases the force required by the right ventricle to pump blood through the lungs. Over time the right ventricle hypertrophies and further increases its systolic pressure.[61,112]

The system loses its ability to adapt to stress factors such as increased blood flow or hypoxia. Thus hypoxic vasoconstriction is both a cause and a result of pulmonary hypertension.[17]

In early stages the symptoms of right-sided heart failure from lung disease (cor pulmonale) occur only during increased stress on the heart. In later stages cor pulmonale is consistently present, as evidenced by jugular venous distention, hepatomegaly, and peripheral edema.[77,112]

COMPLICATIONS

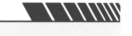

Cor pulmonale

DIAGNOSTIC STUDIES AND FINDINGS

Diagnostic Test	Findings
Chest x-ray	Shows normal lungs
	Enlargement of main pulmonary vessels; pulmonary branches may taper rapidly showing decreased vascularity in the peripheral third of the lung fields
ECG	Right axis deviation or evidence of right ventricular hypertrophy or RBBB
Cardiac catheterization	Elevated pulmonary artery systolic and diastolic pressures with normal PCWP
	Cardiac output frequently decreased
Laboratory tests	
ABGs	Pao_2 <80 mm Hg
	$Paco_2$ may be increased or decreased depending on the cause of the pulmonary hypertension

MEDICAL MANAGEMENT

Medical treatment for pulmonary hypertension is supportive and symptomatic since there is no cure. There is some hope for survival, however, with a lung transplant.

GENERAL MANAGEMENT

Pulmonary artery pressure measurement; cardiac monitoring; oxygenation—administer in concentrations ranging from 24% to 40% unless contraindicated by underlying disease; sodium-restricted diet; bed rest during acute episodes.

DRUG THERAPY

Vasodilators: Prostacyclin determines the reversibility of pulmonary hypertension. If found to be reversible, then treatment with calcium channel blockers or peripheral vasodilators.
Calcium channel blockers: Nifedipine (Procardia), initial 10 mg tid PO; usual effective dose range 10 to 20 mg tid PO. Verapamil hydrochloride (Calan, Isoptin), initial dose 5 to 10 mg given IV bolus over 2 minute period. Repeat dose if necessary 30 minutes after first dose.
Peripheral vasodilator: Hydralazine (Apresoline), 10-50 mg PO qid; Sodium nitroprusside (Nipride), (0.5-10 mg/kg/min IV).

SURGERY

Bilateral or unilateral lung transplant or heart and lung transplants have been performed when heart failure is advanced in unexplained pulmonary hypertension.

1 ASSESS

ASSESSMENT	OBSERVATIONS
Respiratory	Dyspnea on exertion and at rest Crackles, decreased breath sounds at periphery Cyanosis Tachypnea
Cardiovascular	Dizziness, syncope, some patients have precordial chest pain Pulmonic valve (S_2) closure may be accentuated Murmurs of tricuspid insufficiency, pulmonic insufficiency, or pulmonic outflow obstruction may be audible Peripheral edema Distended jugular veins
Psychosocial	Apprehension, fear

2 DIAGNOSE

NURSING DIAGNOSIS	SUBJECTIVE FINDINGS	OBJECTIVE FINDINGS
Impaired gas exchange related to alveolar-capillary membrane changes	Complains of SOB	Hypoxia Pa_{O_2} <60 mm Hg Dyspnea, cyanosis, tachypnea, irritability, restlessness

→ > >

NURSING DIAGNOSIS	SUBJECTIVE FINDINGS	OBJECTIVE FINDINGS
Activity intolerance related to dyspnea	Reports decrease in activity Reports dyspnea during activity	Decreased activity, DOE
Anxiety related to change in health status	Expresses fears	Tachypnea, tachycardia
Hopelessness related to poor prognosis of disease	Reports feeling depressed about lack of treatment options	Sad appearance, withdrawn

3 PLAN

Patient goals

1. Patient's gas exchange will be improved.
2. Patient will be able to perform usual activities without fatigue or dyspnea.
3. Patient's anxiety will be relieved.
4. Patient's hopelessness will be lessened.
5. Patient or significant other will demonstrate understanding of home care and follow-up instructions.

4 IMPLEMENT

NURSING DIAGNOSIS	NURSING INTERVENTIONS	RATIONALE
Impaired gas exchange related to alveolar-capillary membrane changes	Observe rate, depth of respirations, use of accessory muscles, dyspnea, diaphoresis, air hunger, tachycardia.	Determines adequacy of gas exchange.
	Auscultate lungs for rhonchi, crackles, and wheezes.	Determines adequacy of gas exchange and detects atelectasis.
	Assess level of consciousness, listlessness, and irritability.	Decreased level of consciousness may indicate hypoxia.
	Observe skin color and capillary refill.	Determines circulatory adequacy.
	Monitor ABGs.	Determines acid-base balance and need for oxygen.
	Monitor CBC.	Detects amount of hemoglobin to carry oxygen and presence of infection.
	Monitor chest x-rays.	Shows extent of pulmonary vessel involvement.
	Monitor changes in activity tolerance.	Activity may induce breathlessness.
	Administer oxygen as ordered.	Improves gas exchange; decreases work of breathing.
	Maintain airway patency by assisting the patient to cough or by suctioning.	Facilitates gas flow to and from alveoli.

NURSING DIAGNOSIS	NURSING INTERVENTIONS	RATIONALE
	Administer vasodilators as ordered.	Reduces vascular resistance to lower PAP.
	Pace activities to patient's tolerance.	Decreases oxygen demand.
Activity intolerance related to dyspnea	Observe response to activity.	Determines extent of tolerance.
	Assess patient's sleep patterns.	Lack of sleep may be contributing to activity intolerance.
	Plan rest periods between activities.	Reduces fatigue by increasing the number of hours of rest/sleep.
	Encourage use of adaptive breathing techniques during activity.	Decreases work of breathing.
	Perform activities for patient until he/she is able to perform them.	Meets patient's need without causing fatigue.
	Provide oxygen as needed.	Decreases work of breathing during activity.
	Keep frequently used objects within reach.	Provides convenient use for patient; decreases oxygen demand.
	Problem solve with patient to determine methods of conserving energy while performing tasks, e.g., sit on stool while shaving; dry skin after bath by wrapping in terry cloth robe instead of drying skin with a towel.	Identifies ways to conserve energy, thereby using less oxygen and producing less carbon dioxide.
Anxiety related to change in health status	Assess patient's level of anxiety (mild, moderate, severe, panic).	Determines type and extent of interventions required to reduce anxiety.
	Assist patient to identify coping skills used successfully in the past.	Facilitates problem-solving.
	Encourage patient to ask questions and express feelings.	May relieve anxiety, helps patient put thoughts into perspective.
	Provide accurate information about pulmonary hypertension.	Knowledge can decrease anxiety.
	Provide comfort measures, e.g., back rub.	Facilitates relaxation; may decrease respiratory rate.
	Provide oxygen as ordered.	Decreases work of breathing.
	Remain with patient during anxiety attack.	Provides support.
	Limit visitors as necessary.	Visitors may contribute to anxiety.

→ > >

NURSING DIAGNOSIS	NURSING INTERVENTIONS	RATIONALE
Hopelessness related to poor prognosis of disease	Interview patient to determine patient's perceptions.	Need to validate diagnosis.
	Observe for apathy, despondency, indecision, loss of interest, loss of pleasure, negativism, sadness.	Indicates feelings of hopelessness.
	Encourage patient to verbalize frustrations, fears, anger, and/or depression.	Help patient examine own feelings.
	Assist patient to identify strengths.	Focusing on positive qualities may restore sense of hope.
	Encourage patient not to make unreasonable demands on self.	Decreases frustration.
	Discuss options for increasing support network.	Decreases isolation and loneliness.
	Assist patient to identify precipitating events that increase hopelessness feelings.	Helps patient deal with feelings of hopelessness.
	Assist patient to identify alternatives for dealing with precipitating events.	Promotes independence; may prevent precipitating event from causing hopelessness in future.
	Explore consequences for identified alternatives and solutions.	Assists in resolving future crises.
Knowledge deficit	See Patient Teaching.	

5 EVALUATE

PATIENT OUTCOME	DATA INDICATING THAT OUTCOME IS REACHED
Gas exchange is improved.	ABGs are within normal limits (Pa_{O2} = 80-100 mm Hg, Pa_{CO2} = 35-45 mm Hg, pH = 7.35-7.45). Patient is breathing without difficulty.
Able to perform activities without fatigue.	Completes ADL without dyspnea.
Anxiety is relieved.	Patient reports lessened anxiety with reduced SOB.
Hopelessness is lessened.	Patient reports feeling more hopeful.
Knowledge deficit is resolved.	Demonstrates knowledge of pulmonary hypertension and home care management.

PATIENT TEACHING ▪▪▪▪▪▪▪▪▪▪▪▪▪▪▪▪▪▪▪▪▪▪▪▪▪▪▪▪▪▪▪▪

1. Teach the patient adaptive breathing techniques.
2. Teach the patient the importance of prescribed medications such as vasodilators—name, dosage, purpose, time of administration, and side effects.
3. Inform the patient that a change in health status must be reported to the patient's health care provid-

ers. Indicators of change may include change in sputum characteristics or color, decreased activity tolerance, increased cough or chest fullness, noisy wet breathing, or leg or ankle edema.
4. Teach the patient adaptive exercises and relaxation and stress reduction techniques.

Cor Pulmonale

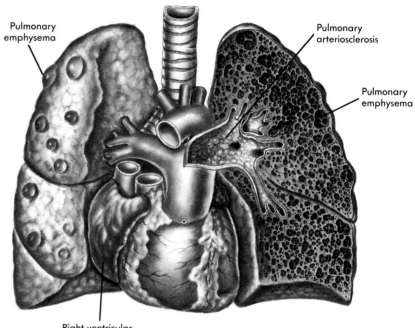

Pulmonary emphysema

Pulmonary arteriosclerosis

Pulmonary emphysema

Right ventricular hypertrophy

Cor pulmonale is a condition of hypertrophy and dilation of the right ventricle of the heart resulting from a disease process that affects the function or structure of the lung or its vasculature. This may occur with or without heart failure.

Cor pulmonale occurs as a secondary process following a primary pulmonary disease. The four most common types of disorders leading to cor pulmonale are obstructive lung diseases, vascular diseases, restrictive lung diseases, and chest wall disorders.

Obstructive lung diseases
  Chronic bronchitis
  Emphysema
  Asthma
  Cystic fibrosis
  Bronchiectasis

Vascular diseases
  Thromboembolism
  Primary pulmonary hypertension
Restrictive lung diseases
  Atelectasis
  Pneumonia
  Interstitial fibrosis
  Sarcoidosis
Chest wall disorders
  Kyphoscoliosis

COPD accounts for about 75% of cases of cor pulmonale in the United States.[99]

PATHOPHYSIOLOGY

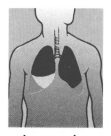

The pulmonary circulation is normally a low-pressure, low-resistance system that may increase output, without increasing pulmonary pressure, to increase cardiac output. As pulmonary vascular resistance of the small arterioles and arteries increases in some types of disease, pulmonary hypertension results (Figure 4-17).

Both anatomic and functional alterations in the pulmonary blood vessels increase the pressure required to pump blood through the lungs, which can result in cor pulmonale. Anatomic changes reduce the size of the pulmonary vascular bed, which in turn requires increased pressure for the circulation of blood. Functional alterations in the lungs are associated with both hypoxia and hypercapnia. Chronic hypoxia leads to vasoconstriction, while hypercapnia creates respiratory acidosis, causing pulmonary arteriolar vasoconstriction. The pulmonary vascular resistance caused by either anatomic or functional alterations leads to pulmonary hypertension. The right ventricle must exert more pressure to circulate blood through the pulmonary arteries. This additional work load of the right ventricle eventually leads to right ventricular hypertrophy and cor pulmonale with or without right-sided congestive heart failure.[81]

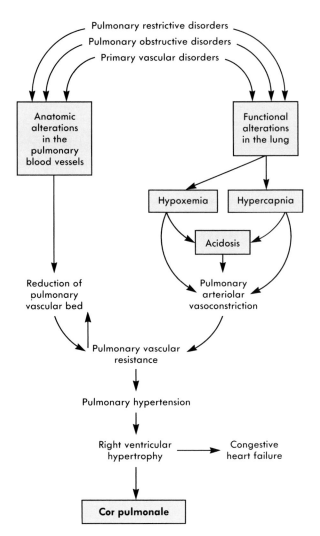

FIGURE 4-17
Etiology and pathogenesis of cor pulmonale. (From Price.)[81]

COMPLICATIONS

Pulmonary edema
Pulmonary infarction

DIAGNOSTIC STUDIES AND FINDINGS

Diagnostic Test	Findings
Chest x-ray	Right ventricular hypertrophy
Echocardiogram	Right ventricular enlargement
ECG	Arrhythmias resulting from hypoxia; RBBB; right axis deviation; right ventricular hypertrophy
Laboratory tests	
ABGs	Decreased Pao_2 in range of 40 to 60 mm Hg; $Paco_2$ in range of 45 to 70 mm Hg
CBC	Elevated hemoglobin level and hematocrit value and polycythemia resulting from chronic hypoxia

MEDICAL MANAGEMENT

The underlying pulmonary and cardiac diseases must be treated first.

GENERAL MANAGEMENT

Oxygenation: Administered in concentrations ranging from 24% to 40% unless contraindicated by underlying pulmonary disease; 85% to 95% arterial oxygen saturation or arterial oxygen tension greater than 55 mm Hg.[47]

Sodium-restricted diet

DRUG THERAPY

Diuretics: Initial diuresis can lower pulmonary artery pressure by decreasing total blood volume; careful monitoring of serum electrolytes needed when administering diuretics; Furosemide (Lasix), 20-80 mg/d to maximum of 600 mg/d.

Bronchodilators: Concomitant administration of theophylline and terbutaline recommended to improve airway obstruction and reduce afterload on right and left sides of heart, thereby improving cardiac output.[47] Theophylline (Theo-Dur, Theolair, Elixophyllin, others), 16 mg/kg divided into 3 or 4 doses; Terbutaline (Brethine, Bricanyl), 2.5-5 mg PO tid.

Anti-infective agents: Antibiotics administered after Gram stain analysis of sputum specimens.

1 ASSESS

ASSESSMENT	OBSERVATIONS
Respiratory	Evidence of other chronic lung diseases; dyspnea; cough; cyanosis; wheezing; crackles
Cardiovascular	Pitting edema, weight gain, distended neck veins; loud pulmonic secondary sound on cardiac auscultation; gallop rhythm and occasional murmur resulting from functional insufficiency of tricuspid and pulmonic valves PAP: systolic pressure above 30 mm Hg; diastolic pressure above 15 mm Hg
Gastrointestinal	Anorexia, nausea, hepatomegaly, ascites
Psychosocial	Apprehension, fear

2 DIAGNOSE

NURSING DIAGNOSIS	SUBJECTIVE FINDINGS	OBJECTIVE FINDINGS
Impaired gas exchange related to alveolar-capillary membrane changes	Complains of SOB	Crackles (rales), wheezing, decreased breath sounds, dyspnea, tachypnea, Pao_2 <60 mm Hg Cough Restlessness

NURSING DIAGNOSIS	SUBJECTIVE FINDINGS	OBJECTIVE FINDINGS
Fluid volume excess related to fluid accumulation in pulmonary vessels	Reports inability to catch breath	Weight gain, distended neck veins, pitting edema in extremities, shortness of breath, orthopnea, pulmonary congestion on chest x-ray, decreased to absent breath sounds, restlessness, anxiety Elevated PAP Systolic pressure >30 mm Hg Diastolic pressure >15 mm Hg
Activity intolerance related to fatigue and dyspnea	Reports decrease in activity and decrease in energy	Decreased activity, DOE
Anxiety related to difficulty in breathing	Reports SOB Expresses apprehension, fear	SOB, restlessness

3 PLAN

Patient goals

1. Patient's gas exchange will be improved.
2. Patient's fluid volume will be within normal limits.
3. Patient will be able to perform usual activities without fatigue or dyspnea.
4. Patient's anxiety will be relieved.
5. Patient will demonstrate understanding of home care and follow-up instructions.

4 IMPLEMENT

NURSING DIAGNOSIS	NURSING INTERVENTIONS	RATIONALE
Impaired gas exchange related to alveolar capillary membrane changes	Observe rate, depth of respirations, use of accessory muscles, dyspnea, diaphoresis, air hunger, tachycardia.	Determines adequacy of gas exchange and guides therapeutic interventions.
	Auscultate lungs for crackles and wheezes.	Determines adequacy of gas exchange.
	Assess level of consciousness, listlessness, and irritability.	Decreased level of consciousness may indicate hypoxia.
	Observe skin color and capillary refill.	Determines circulatory adequacy.
	Monitor ABGs.	Determines acid-base balance and need for oxygen.
	Monitor CBC.	Detects amount of hemoglobin to carry oxygen and presence of infection.
	Administer oxygen as ordered.	Improves gas exchange; decreases work of breathing.

NURSING DIAGNOSIS	NURSING INTERVENTIONS	RATIONALE
	Maintain airway patency by assisting the patient to cough or by suctioning.	Facilitates gas flow to and from alveoli.
	Assist patient to Fowler's position.	Optimizes diaphragmatic contraction.
	Administer bronchodilators as ordered.	Facilitates gas flow to and from alveoli.
Fluid volume excess related to fluid accumulation in pulmonary vessels	Weigh patient.	Detects fluid gain or loss.
	Measure intake and output.	Provides data on fluid balance.
	Assess skin turgor.	Edema indicates fluid excess.
	Measure PAP.	Indicates increase or decrease in pulmonary edema.
	Assess neck veins.	Distention indicates fluid excess.
	Administer diuretics as ordered.	Removes fluid via kidney tubules.
	Restrict fluid and sodium.	Prevents additional fluid excess.
	Assist patient to identify ways to prevent fluid excess.	May prevent recurrence and involves patient in care.
Activity intolerance related to fatigue and dyspnea	Observe response to activity.	Determines extent of tolerance.
	Identify factors contributing to intolerance, e.g., stress, side effects of drugs.	Guides selection of therapeutic interventions.
	Plan rest periods between activities.	Reduces fatigue.
	Encourage use of adaptive breathing techniques during activity.	Decreases work of breathing.
	Provide oxygen as needed.	Decreases work of breathing during activity.
	Perform activities for patient until he/she is able to perform them.	Meets patient's need without causing fatigue.
	Provide progressive increase in activity as tolerated.	Slowly increase the number of and endurance of activities.
	Keep frequently used objects within reach.	Provides convenient use for patient; decreases oxygen demand.
Anxiety related to difficulty in breathing	Assess patient's level of anxiety (mild, moderate, severe, panic).	Determines type and extent of interventions required to reduce anxiety.
	Assist patient to identify coping skills used successfully in the past.	Facilitates problem solving.

NURSING DIAGNOSIS	NURSING INTERVENTIONS	RATIONALE
	Encourage patient to ask questions and express feelings.	May relieve anxiety, helps patient put thoughts into perspective.
	Provide accurate information about cor pulmonale and procedures.	Knowledge can decrease anxiety.
	Provide oxygen as ordered.	Decreases work of breathing.
	Remain with patient; use calm, reassuring voice.	Provides support.
Knowledge deficit	See Patient Teaching.	

5 EVALUATE

PATIENT OUTCOME	DATA INDICATING THAT OUTCOME IS REACHED
Airway is patent.	Airways are clear and breathing occurs without secretions. Clear breath sounds. Arterial blood gas values are normal for patient's condition. Chest x-ray is clear. Cough has subsided.
Fluid volume is within normal limits.	PAP within normal limits. Breath sounds clear. No evidence of distended neck veins or pitting edema. Weight has returned to value before cor pulmonale.
Performs usual activities without fatigue or dyspnea.	Patient performs self-care activities.
Anxiety is resolved.	Patient able to breathe without difficulty; appears calm.
Knowledge deficit resolved.	Patient demonstrates knowledge of disease process and home care management.

PATIENT TEACHING

The primary education is directed toward the patient's disease state; refer to patient education for specific primary disease.

1. Teach the patient the importance of restricting salt intake and limiting fluid intake.
2. Teach the patient to weigh self daily.
3. Provide the patient and family with information regarding chronic lung diseases, assessment of the patient's capabilities and responses, and actions to take during an acute episode.
4. Teach the patient the importance of avoiding environmental pollutants and not smoking.
5. Teach the patient the importance of prescribed medications: name, dosage, purpose, time of administration, and side effects.
6. Provide the patient and family with information regarding the care, cleaning, and maintenance of inhalation or oxygen equipment being used in the hospital or to be used at home, as well as the signs of oxygen toxicity.

Lung Cancer

Lung cancer is an uncontrolled growth of anaplastic cells in the lung.

The incidence of lung cancer for white men rose from 82.7 per 1000 in 1982 to 84.2 in 1984. The incidence rate for white women and black men and women rose also. The American Cancer Society estimated 1550 new cases of lung cancer in 1989.[1]

Tobacco smoke, particularly from cigarettes, is the major factor responsible in the rise in incidence of lung cancer. Cigarette smokers have at least a 10 times greater risk of developing lung cancer than do nonsmokers.[77] The use of filtered cigarettes reduces the risk of lung cancer. Following cessation of cigarette smoking, after 10 years the ex-smoker's risk of developing lung cancer returns to that of the nonsmoker.[109] Asbestos exposure is a potent risk factor for bronchogenic carcinoma. Asbestos exposure and cigarette smoke act synergistically; an asbestos worker who smokes has a 50- to 100-fold increased chance of developing lung cancer. Also, exposure to radon daughters, which emit radioactive gas, may act synergistically with cigarette smoke, resulting in a risk 50 to 100 times greater than that of the normal population. Exposure to radon occurs near uranium mining operations in the western United States and also when homes are built on or near hard rock formations.[109]

PATHOPHYSIOLOGY

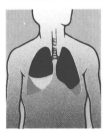

Cancer develops when the genes responsible for sequential cell division, called proto-oncogenes, change to a type of cell called oncogenes. This change causes cancer cells to divide indiscriminately without regard to the needs of the body. Also the cells produced are undifferentiated so that they do not function normally.

There are three types of pulmonary neoplastic disease: benign tumors, primary malignant tumors (lung cancer), and metastatic malignant tumors. Of the four types of cancer—carcinoma, sarcoma, lymphoma, leukemia—it is the carcinoma arising from epithelial cells that affects the lungs.

The cell origin of the various types of bronchogenic carcinoma remains a controversial issue. One currently popular theory is that the four major cell types (adeno-

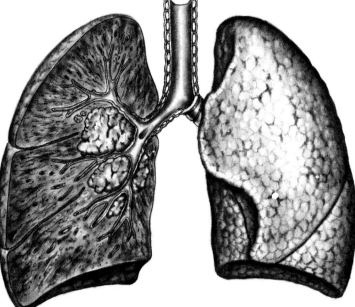

carcinoma, squamous, large cell, and small cell) originate from a common stem cell (Figure 4-18 and Table 4-6). Adenocarcinoma appears to be increasing in frequency and is probably the most common, accounting for approximately 40% of cases.[77] Adenocarcinoma arises in peripheral lung tissue or in areas scarred from pulmonary infarction, infection, or idiopathic fibrosis. This form of lung cancer metastasizes to the pleura easily.[98] Squamous cell carcinoma accounts for about 30% of all lung cancer. It arises in the ciliated epithelium of central airways. These tumor cells usually cause metaplastic or dysplastic changes in adjacent bronchial mucosa. Squamous cell carcinomas produce local signs and symptoms of airway occlusion with lung collapse distal to the occlusion. This tumor spreads first to intrathoracic sites and tends to cavitate more than other types of lung cancer.[98]

COMPLICATIONS

Atelectasis
Pneumonia
Lung abscess
Metastasis to brain, bones, contralateral lung, liver, adrenal gland, and lymph nodes

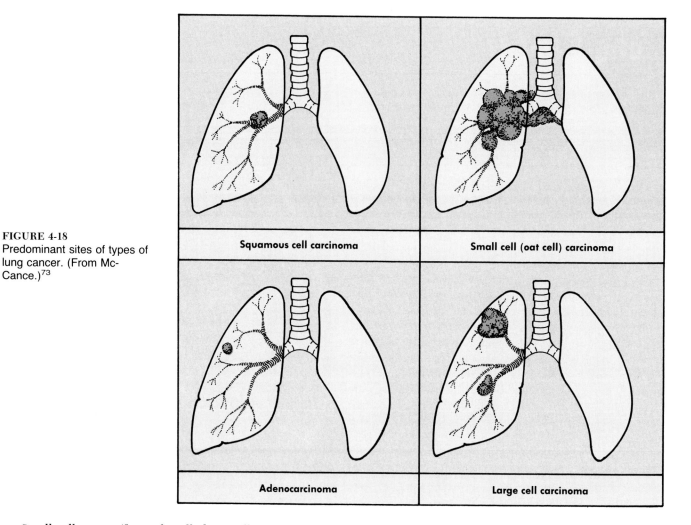

FIGURE 4-18
Predominant sites of types of lung cancer. (From Mc-Cance.)[73]

Small cell cancer (formerly called oat cell carcinoma) accounts for approximately 20% of lung cancers. This tumor type arises from Kulchitsky cells of the airways or from neuroendocrine cells elsewhere in the body. The usual cancer staging does not apply to this cancer because it spreads to regional nodes, other intrathoracic structures, and distant sites before it is diagnosed. The classification for this carcinoma is either limited stage or extensive stage disease. In limited stage disease, the carcinoma spreads to structures in the ipsilateral hemithorax, mediastinum, and ipsilateral supraclavicular nodes. About one third of small cell carcinomas fall into this category. The remaining two thirds are extensive-stage carcinomas in which the cancer has spread to distant sites. Few patients in this category live more than 5 years after diagnosis despite chemotherapy and radiation therapy.

Less common primary malignant tumors of the lung include large cell carcinoma and bronchioloalveolar cell carcinoma (a subset of adenocarcinoma), which account for 5% to 8% of lung cancers. Rare cell types include giant cell carcinoma, clear cell carcinoma, and pulmo-nary blastoma, which account for less than 2% of lung cancers. Bronchial adenomas and carcinoid tumors are classified as benign lung tumors, although they have a rare but significant tendency to metastasize.[77]

All types of lung cancer have lymphatic metastasis early in the course of the disease, beginning in the bronchial and mediastinal nodes and extending upward to the supraclavicular nodes and downward to nodes below the diaphragm and to the liver and adrenal gland.

The prognosis for persons with lung cancer is correlated with tumor cell type. Those with well-differentiated squamous cell cancer have the best chance of survival; those with undifferentiated small cell cancer have the poorest. Peripheral tumors are more curable than central lesions. The presence of lymph node metastases and distant metastases reduces the chance of cure. The stage of disease, patient's performance status, and immunologic state of the patient are important prognostic signs. Patients with gross supraclavicular adenopathy, a malignant pleural effusion, massive local extension, or distant metastases usually survive less than 1 year.

TNM CLASSIFICATION OF LUNG CANCER

Tumor definitions

TX Tumor proved by cytology but not visualized by radiograph or bronchoscopically.

TO No evidence of tumor.

TIS Carcinoma in situ.

TI Tumor 3 cm or less in greatest dimension, surrounded by lung or visceral pleura, without invasion proximal to lobar bronchus.

T2 Tumor greater than 3 cm in diameter, or invading viseral pleura, or with atelectasis or obstructive pneumonitis extending to the hilum. Proximal extent of tumor at least 2 cm from carina.

T3 Tumor with direct extension into chest wall, diaphragm, mediastinal pleura, or pericardium without involvement of mediastinal viscera. Tumor within 2 cm of carina but not involving carina.

T4 Tumor invading mediastinal viscera or carina, or with malignant pleural effusion.

Nodal involvement

NO No nodal metastasis.

N1 Metastasis to peribronchial or ipsilateral mediastinal or subcarinal lymph nodes.

N2 Metastasis to ipsilateral mediastinal or subcarinal lymph nodes.

N3 Metastasis to contralateral mediastinal or hilar nodes or any scalene or supraclavicular node.

Metastases

MO No known metastasis.

MI Distant metastasis present.

From Miller Y and Johnston M: Lung cancer. In Mitchell RS, Petty TL, and Schwarz MI, editors: Synopsis of clinical pulmonary disease, ed 4, St Louis, 1989, The CV Mosby Co., pp. 330-331.

STAGE GROUPING OF TNM SUBSETS

Occult carcinoma	TX	NO	MO
Stage O	TIS	NO	MO
Stage 1	T1	NO	MO
	T2	NO	MO
Stage II	T1	N1	MO
	T2	N1	MO
Stage IIIa	T3	NO	MO
	T3	N1	MO
	T1-3	N2	MO
Stage IIIb	Any T	N3	MO
	T4	Any N	MO
Stage IV	Any T	Any N	M1

From Miller Y and Johnston M: Lung cancer. In Mitchell RS, Petty TL, and Schwarz MI, editors: Synopsis of clinical pulmonary disease, ed 4, St Louis, 1989, The CV Mosby Co., pp. 330-331.

PROGNOSIS BY STAGE

Clinical Stages*	5-Year Survival (%)
I	45-50
II	25-30
IIIa	15-20
IIIb	5
IV	2

These survival figures are for tumors that are clinically staged rather than surgically staged. Because clinical staging typically underestimates the extent of disease, survival for surgically staged disease is better.

From Miller Y and Johnston M: Lung cancer. In Mitchell, RS, Petty TL, and Schwarz MI, editors: Synopsis of clinical pulmonary disease, ed 4, St. Louis, 1989, The CV Mosby Co., pp 330-331.

Table 4-6

CHARACTERISTICS OF LUNG CANCER

Tumor type	Growth rate	Metastasis	Means of diagnosis	Clinical manifestations and treatment
Squamous cell carcinoma	Slow	Late; mostly to hilar lymph nodes	Biopsy, sputum analysis, bronchoscopy, electron microscopy, immunohistochemistry	Cough, sputum production, airway obstruction; treated surgically
Small cell (oat cell) carcinoma	Very rapid	Very early; to mediastinum or distally in lung	Radiography, sputum analysis, bronchoscopy, electron microscopy, immunohistochemistry, and clinical manifestations (cough, chest pain, dyspnea hemoptysis, localized wheezing)	Airway obstruction caused by pneumonitis, signs and symptoms of excessive hormone secretion; treated by chemotherapy and ionizing radiation to thorax and central nervous system
Adenocarcinoma	Moderate	Early	Radiography, fiberoptic bronchoscopy, electron microscopy	Pleural effusion; treated surgically
Large cell carcinoma	Rapid	Early and widespread	Sputum analysis, bronchoscopy, electron microscopy (by exclusion of other cell types)	Chest wall pain, pleural effusion, cough, sputum production, hemoptysis, airway obstruction caused by pneumonia (if airways involved); treated surgically

DIAGNOSTIC STUDIES AND FINDINGS

Diagnostic Test	Findings
Chest x-ray (lateral and posteroanterior views), chest tomography, and **computed tomographic scanning**	A common radiographic finding is the solitary pulmonary nodule, by definition less than 3 cm in diameter and completely surrounded by lung tissue; larger lesions are termed masses; the importance of the solitary nodule is that it represents the most curable group of lung tumors, with a 5-year survival rate of 70%-90% if metastasis is absent; squamous cell carcinomas may cavitate in the lung; alveolar infiltrates may represent bronchioloalveolar carcinoma, and interstitial markings with Kerley-B lines can be caused by lymphatic spread of a tumor, either primary (in the lung) or metastatic; dense, central, concentric, or "popcorn" calcification seen on plain x-ray or conventional tomography is a reliable sign that a nodule is benign
Radioisotope scanning	
Lung	Reveals size, shape, and position of lesion
Brain and bone	Evidence of metastases
Laboratory tests	
Sputum collection for cytology, bronchoscopy with biopsy, brushings, or washings, and percutaneous biopsy under fluoroscopy	Cells gathered for histologic examination show evidence of malignancy
Scalene node biopsy	Evidence of spread to scalene nodes
Mediastinoscopy	Evidence of spread to ipsilateral and contralateral mediastinal lymph nodes

MEDICAL MANAGEMENT

After deciding that a patient is physiologically a candidate for resection, the physician determines the extent of disease by staging. The box on p. 161 presents the new TNM (T, tumor; N, nodal involvement; M, metastasis) staging system.

GENERAL MANAGEMENT

Radiation therapy: Sole modality for patient who has clinically resectable lesion but is medically nonoperable and for patient with locally advanced, nonresectable tumor without demonstrable distant metastases but with symptoms such as cough, wheezing, obstructive infection, hemoptysis, pain, dysphagia, or superior vena cava syndrome; may be used preoperatively or postoperatively.[1]

SURGERY

Lobectomy

Pneumonectomy: For centrally located lesions.

Segmental and wedge resection: Based on patient tolerance and absence of spread.

DRUG THERAPY

For small cell lung cancer

Antineoplastic agents:
Cyclophosphamide (Cytoxan), 40-50 mg/kg IV in individually determined doses over several days and then adjusted to lower maintenance dosage; PO 1-5 mg/kg/d; Methotrexate (Mexate), 2.5-5 mg/kg/d PO or parenterally; Doxorubicin (Adriamycin), 60-75 mg/m^2 at intervals of 21 days or 30 mg/m^2/day for 3 days repeated every 4 wk; Vincristine sulfate (Oncovin; VCR), 2 mg/m^2 for children, 1.4 mg/m^2 for adults; Carmustine (BCNU), 200 mg/m^2 IV q 6 wk; Procarbazine (Mastulane), 2-4 mg/kg/d po initially and then 4-6 mg/kg/day until maximum response occurs; maintain at 1-2 mg/kg/day; Hexamethylmelamine (HXM), in combination therapy; dose individually determined. These agents only slightly useful in non-small cell cancer; partial regression with cisplatin-based regimens.

1 ASSESS

ASSESSMENT	OBSERVATIONS
Respiratory	Chronic cough, nonproductive or productive; wheezing; chest tightness; hemoptysis; dyspnea; hoarseness, chest pain, clubbed fingers, orthopnea, tachypnea
Nutritional	Fatigue, weight loss, anorexia
Psychosocial	Fear, apprehension
Vital signs	Elevated temperature, tachypnea

2 DIAGNOSE

NURSING DIAGNOSIS	SUBJECTIVE FINDINGS	OBJECTIVE FINDINGS
Ineffective airway clearance related to bronchial obstruction secondary to tumor invasion	Complains of difficulty breathing	Wheezing, tachypnea, productive or nonproductive cough, fever, dyspnea, labored or irregular breathing
Altered nutrition: less than body requirements related to fatigue and dyspnea	Reports decreased appetite and fatigue	Decrease in food and fluid intake Dyspnea
Activity intolerance related to generalized weakness	Complains of fatigue, SOB	SOB during activity Decreased activity level
Dysfunctional grieving related to loss associated with cancer, its treatment, or threat of loss of life	Expresses hopelessness, expresses guilt about smoking	Decreased verbalization, appears sad and withdrawn, crying

3 PLAN

Patient goals

1. Patient's airways will be patent.
2. Patient's nutritional status will be improved.
3. Patient will be able to perform usual activities without fatigue or dyspnea.
4. Patient will demonstrate progress in the grieving process.
5. Patient will demonstrate an understanding of follow-up care.

4 IMPLEMENT

NURSING DIAGNOSIS	NURSING INTERVENTIONS	RATIONALE
Ineffective airway clearance related to bronchial obstruction secondary to tumor invasion	Auscultate lungs for rhonchi, crackles, or wheezing.	Determines adequacy of gas exchange and extent of airway obstructed with secretions.
	Assess symmetry of chest expansion, depth, and rate of inspiration and use of accessory muscles.	Indicates ease of gas exchange.
	Assess characteristics of secretions: quantity, color, consistency, odor. Note hemoptysis.	Detects presence of infection or bleeding. Infection is indicated by increased, thick and/or yellow secretions that may have a foul odor.
	Assess patient's hydration status: skin turgor, mucous membranes, tongue, intake and output over 24 hours, Hct.	Determines needs for fluids. Fluids are needed if skin turgor is poor, mucous membranes and tongue are dry, intake >output and/or hematocrit is elevated.
	Monitor ABGs.	Determines acid-base balance and need for oxygen.
	Monitor chest x-rays.	Shows extent and location of lung involvement.
	Monitor results of sputum cytology.	Determines presence of cancer cells.
	Assist patient with coughing as needed.	Coughing removes secretions.
	Position patient in proper body alignment for optimal breathing pattern (head of bed up 45°; if tolerated up to 90°).	Secretions move by gravity as position changes. Elevating head of bed moves abdominal content away from diaphragm to enhance diaphragmatic contraction.
	Administer humidified oxygen as ordered.	Supplies supplemental oxygen and reduces the work of breathing.
	Assist patient with ambulation/position changes (turning side to side).	Secretions move by gravity as position changes.
	Increase room humidification.	Humidifies secretions to facilitate their elimination.
	Assist patient is using blow bottles, incentive spirometry.	Requires deep breathing to prevent atelectasis by filling alveoli with air.
	Encourage increased fluid intake to 1½ to 2L/day unless contraindicated.	Liquifies and thins secretions so they can be expectorated easier.
	Assist patient with oral hygiene as needed.	Removes taste of secretions.

→ > >

NURSING DIAGNOSIS	NURSING INTERVENTIONS	RATIONALE
Altered nutrition: less than body requirements related to fatigue and dyspnea	Assess dietary habits and needs.	Helps to individualize the diet.
	Weigh patient weekly.	As nutrition improves, the patient's weight will increase.
	Auscultate bowel sounds.	Documents gastrointestinal peristalsis.
	Assess psychologic factors, e.g., depression, anger.	Identifies effect of psychologic factors that may decrease food and fluid intake.
	Monitor albumin and lymphocytes.	Indicates adequate visceral protein needed for the immune system
	Measure mid-arm circumference and triceps skinfold.	Indicates protein and fat stores, which indicate presence of malnutrition.
	Provide oxygen while eating as ordered.	Reduces dyspnea by reducing the work of breathing.
	Encourage oral care before meals.	Removes taste of sputum that may reduce appetite.
	Provide frequent small feedings.	Lessens fatigue.
	Administer antiemetics before meals.	Reduces nausea that may be interfering with eating.
	Provide foods in appropriate consistency for eating.	Requires less energy to eat soft foods and liquids, thereby reducing oxygen requirement.
	Provide high-protein diet.	Supports immune system.
	Administer vitamins as ordered.	Supplements diet.
Activity intolerance related to generalized weakness	Observe response to activity.	Determines extent of tolerance.
	Identify factors contributing to intolerance, e.g., stress, side effects of drugs.	When causative factors for weakness can be identified, then interventions can be planned to counteract their effect.
	Assess patient's sleep patterns.	May document a causative factor of weakness.
	Plan rest periods between activities.	Reduces fatigue by providing additional rest.
	Perform activities for patient until he/she is able to perform them.	Meets patient's need without causing fatigue.
	Provide progressive increase in activity as tolerated.	Slowly increases the number of and endurance of activities as tolerance allows to promote as much independence as possible.

NURSING DIAGNOSIS	NURSING INTERVENTIONS	RATIONALE
	Provide oxygen as needed.	Decreased work of breathing during activity.
	Instruct patient/family member in use of equipment.	Ensures proper use and decreases frustration of users.
	Keep frequently used objects within reach.	Provides convenient use for patient; decreases oxygen demand.
	Problem solve with patient to determine methods of conserving energy while performing tasks, e.g., sit on stool while shaving; dry skin after bath by wrapping in terry cloth robe instead of drying skin with a towel.	Identifies ways to conserve energy, thereby using less oxygen and producing less carbon dioxide.
Dysfunctional grieving related to loss associated with cancer, its treatment, or threat of loss of life	Assess appetite, weight loss, sleep patterns, mobility, and constipation.	Depression may be indicated by decreased appetite, weight loss, inability to sleep or sleeping more than usual, decreased activity, and/or constipation.
	Assess presence and quality of support system.	Determines if persons are available to patient and if they are supportive, ambivalent, or disruptive.
	Monitor changes in communication patterns with others.	Changes to withdrawal or silence may indicate depression.
	Monitor expressions such as worthlessness, anxiety, powerlessness, abandonment, or exhaustion.	Indicates patient's state of mind and guides the nurse's communication with patient.
	Monitor ongoing coping such as withdrawal, denial, rationalization, compliance, dependency.	Provides data on patient's current coping strategies.
	Encourage eating a balanced diet, regular sleeping habits, active or passive exercise, and comfort measures.	Ensures that physiologic needs are met while patient is unable to do so independently.
	Accept patient's behavior at current level.	Develops trust as the basis for all other interventions.
	Listen and accept verbalized anger without personalizing reaction.	Fosters constructive expression of anger and negative feelings.
	Assist patient to use physical expression geared to his physical capabilities, e.g., walking, punching a pillow.	Physical activity can be used as a means to express anger.
	Encourage patient to keep a "gripe list"; discuss list with patient if patient agrees.	Allows patient to write and verbalize anger.

→ > >

NURSING DIAGNOSIS	NURSING INTERVENTIONS	RATIONALE
	Encourage patient to identify, redefine situation, obtain needed information, generate alternatives, and focus on solutions.	Supports coping, problem solving, and decision making.
	Respect patient's need for privacy.	Allows patient and others to grieve together.
	Use humor with patient as appropriate.	Can improve mood and self view.
	Administer antidepressants as ordered.	Improves depressive mood.
Knowledge deficit	See Patient Teaching.	

5 EVALUATE

PATIENT OUTCOME	DATA INDICATING THAT OUTCOME IS REACHED
Airway is patent.	Airways are clear and breathing occurs without secretions. Clear breath sounds. Chest x-ray is clear. Cough has subsided.
Nutritional status has improved.	Weight gain. Patient is eating a balanced diet. Albumin = 3.2-4.5 g/dl Lymphocytes = 2100 or 35-40% per ml^3 blood Triceps skinfold = 12.0 mm (men), 23.0 mm (women) Midarm circumference = 32.7 cm (men), 29.2 cm (women)
Patient performed usual activities without fatigue or dyspnea	Patient performs self-care activities.
Progress is demonstrated in moving through grief process.	Patient talks about diagnosis and treatment options.
Learning is demonstrated.	Patient demonstrates an understanding of follow-up care.

PATIENT TEACHING

1. Encourage patient to stop smoking and encourage family members to stop also.
2. Teach importance of exercising to tolerance each day.
3. Teach name, action, dosage, frequency of administration, and side effects of medications.
4. Encourage eating a diet high in protein and calories.
5. Identify resources in the community, such as the American Cancer Society and the American Lung Association, that can assist the patient and family with information, support groups, and equipment needs.
6. Instruct the patient and family to notify the physician if the patient experiences any side effects from medications or signs of recurrence such as shoulder or arm pain, difficulty in memory, fatigue, weight loss, increased coughing or hemoptysis.

Pneumoconioses (Occupational lung disease)

Industrial and work-related lung diseases are caused by inhaling inorganic dusts or gaseous or particulate matters in the air. They are referred to as **pneumoconioses** (*pneuma* lung; *konia* dust; *osis,* condition). The three major pneumoconioses are silicosis, asbestosis, and coal workers' pneumoconiosis.

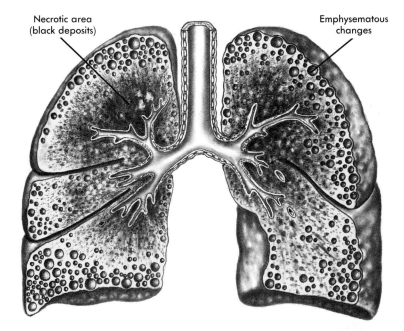

Necrotic area (black deposits)

Emphysematous changes

PATHOPHYSIOLOGY

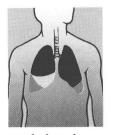

Fine particles and gaseous agents entering the lung encounter little, if any resistance. Once inhaled, particulate matters are deposited on various areas of the respiratory tract. Particles deposited on the mucous surfaces of the nose and upper airways are readily moved toward the pharynx, from which they are swallowed or coughed out.

The ciliated pseudostratified epithelium is covered by a mucus blanket. The rhythmic beating of the epithelium moves inhaled particles along. The speed of the mucus movement has been estimated to be between 10 and 20 mm/minute. Thus 90% of the deposited material is physically cleared in less than 1 hour.[42,77,99]

The irritating effects of certain particles and gases increase mucus production. With repeated exposures the mucous glands hypertrophy and secrete more mucus in response to a variety of inhaled irritants. This may result in a type of chronic bronchitis.

Bronchioles and alveoli have no epithelium, mucous glands, or goblet cells; therefore particles deposited in their lumen are not as easily removed. Alveolar clearance involves more complex pathways of cellular and fluid transport. Phagocytic cells in the alveoli play the major role in disposing of the particles reaching this part of the respiratory tract. In addition, alveolar sur-

factant and fluid produced from capillary transudation help in moving the particles to the lymph channels. Disposal of particles from the alveoli is a very slow process, and the respiratory membrane remains exposed to their harmful effects until they are removed. Coating of the particles by surfactant and certain chemical reactions, as well as some enzymatic actions, reduce their harmful effects.

Once phagocytized, the particles are processed by the metabolic and enzymatic apparatus of the alveolar macrophages. The phagocytic effectiveness of these cells is influenced by many exogenous and endogenous factors. Sometimes the offending agents impair the function of these cells.

When the primary defense mechanisms fail to control the agents' harmful effects, the secondary cellular and humoral defense mechanisms are brought into action. These mechanisms result in inflammation, which consists of dilation and increased permeability of capillaries, exudation of fluid, and infiltration of white blood cells.[42,77,99]

SILICOSIS

Silicosis is a progressive pulmonary disease marked by nodular lesions, which often progress to fibrosis. This disease often shows no symptoms. It is caused by the inhalation and pulmonary deposition of crystalline silicon dioxide dust, mostly from quartz.

Industrial sources of silica in its pure form include the manufacture of ceramics (flint) and building materials (sandstone). It occurs in mixed form in the production of construction materials such as cement. Silica is found in powder form in paints, porcelain, scouring soaps, and wood fillers. It may also be found in the mining of gold, coal, lead, zinc, and iron. Sources of free silica dust include industries such as mining, quarrying, tunneling, stone cutting, and abrasive industry as well as pottery and tile manufacturing. The development of silicosis depends on the size of the silica particle, its concentration in the air, length of exposure, and susceptibility of the individual. Very heavy exposure, as sometimes occurs in sandblasters, may result in a more acute form of silicosis after brief exposure.[42,77,99]

PATHOPHYSIOLOGY

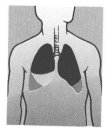

The silica particles deposited in the alveoli are 1 to 3 μm in diameter. These are phagocytized by the macrophages. In the process, part of these macrophages containing the particles is damaged. Cellular enzymes dispersing in cytoplasm cause death of the macrophages and release of their contents, including the silica particles. When the cell dies, the enzymes as well as other bioactive substances within the cell are released into the lung parenchyma. These substances stimulate inflammatory and fibrogenic response in the lung. More macrophages are attracted to the area and are also killed. The pathologic process continues even after the environmental exposure has ceased.

The characteristic pathologic changes are the silicotic nodules, which are fibrotic lesions. In simple silicosis the nodules may measure 2 to 3 mm in diameter and are unevenly scattered throughout the lungs. They are surrounded by distorted lung tissue, which may show emphysematous changes. As the disease state progresses, these changes are characteristic of progressive massive fibrosis (PMF) and indicate complicated silicosis. With progressive massive fibrosis, the upper lobes may show evidence of emphysema, sometimes with large bullous changes.

ASBESTOSIS

Asbestos, the name given to a number of fibrous silicates, is mined principally in Canada, South Africa, and Russia. Raw asbestos is first processed to release asbestos fibers from the parent rock and then transported for use in a variety of industries. In the United States most asbestos is used for fireproofing purposes. Workers in these industries may be exposed to asbestos dust. Symptoms of asbestosis are delayed from 20 to 40 years after exposure.

PATHOPHYSIOLOGY

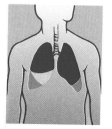

Asbestosis is caused by deposition of small asbestos particles on bronchioles or alveolar walls where they are ingested by macrophages. This swells the alveolar wall by a process that is not fully understood.

Fibrosis in asbestosis, unlike silicosis, is nonnodular, involves mostly the lower lungs, and often has pleural thickening, plaque formation, and pleural calcification. Pleural effusion, sometimes bloody, is a fairly common form of pleural reaction.

Bronchogenic carcinoma often occurs with asbestosis, primarily because of the combined effect of asbestos and cigarette smoking. Heavy smokers who are also exposed to asbestos have 80 to 90 times the risk of nonsmokers for having bronchogenic carcinoma.[42,77,99]

COAL WORKERS' PNEUMOCONIOSIS (BLACK LUNG)

Coal workers' pneumoconiosis (CWP) is a chronic pathologic condition resulting from prolonged exposure to coal dust.

Although carbon is not a fibrogenic agent, with massive and prolonged exposure the clearance mechanisms of the lung are overwhelmed, and coal dust accumulates in terminal air spaces, resulting in pulmonary problems.

The incidence of pneumoconiosis in anthracite mining is much higher than in soft (bituminous) coal mining. An estimated 10 to 12 years of mining work is needed for the development of this disease.[42,77,99]

PATHOPHYSIOLOGY

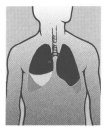

After the deposition of coal dust in the respiratory bronchioles and alveoli, the first reaction is phagocytosis of the particles by increasing numbers of macrophages, which move to the terminal bronchioles. An excessive dust load overwhelms the pulmonary clearing mechanism. Fibroblasts appear in this area, laying a thin network of reticulin fibers without significant collagen formation. The aggregations of macrophages and dust particles enmeshed in reticulin fibers are called coal macules because they appear as black dots on the lung sections. These spots are often linked with dilation of respiratory bronchioles, called focal centrilobular emphysema. These changes are often seen in simple CWP. The complicated form of the disease is marked by massive fibrosis, involving mostly the upper lobes.

COMPLICATIONS

Pulmonary hypertension
Cor pulmonale
Secondary infection such as tuberculosis

NURSING CARE

Nursing diagnoses for patients with pneumoconiosis include Ineffective Breathing Pattern related to pulmonary fibrosis; Ineffective Airway Clearance related to increased bronchial secretions; Impaired Gas Exchange related to alveolar-capillary membrane changes secondary to dust inhalation; and Potential for Infection related to bronchial obstruction and mucopurulent sputum.

DIAGNOSTIC STUDIES AND FINDINGS[42,77,99]

Diagnostic Test	Findings
Chest x-ray	*Silicosis* The initial manifestation of silicosis is the development of small nodules on the chest x-ray; at this point in the disease the patient is usually asymptomatic; exposure to silica may have been going on for 10 to 20 years With the development of massive fibrosis, the upper lobes show evidence of volume loss; the lower lobes show emphysematous changes In complicated silicosis, massive densities may be seen in the fields; progressive changes from simple nodular form to massive fibrosis may take place within 5 years *Asbestosis* Asbestosis is manifest as interstitial markings with reticular density, predominantly involving the lower lung fields; sometimes a marked honeycomb pattern is present; the lung volume is often diminished; common pleural changes include thickening, plaques, calcification, and effusion *Coal workers' pneumoconiosis* CWP usually does not appear until the worker has been exposed to coal dust for approximately 10 years; the x-ray shows the presence of small opacities or nodular densities through the lung fields; these lesions are usually confined to the upper lung fields; the nodular densities are often smaller and less defined than those of silicosis
Pulmonary function tests	These may be normal in early disease; as the diseases progress, abnormalities may be seen; these changes may indicate both obstructive and restrictive lung damage; test findings may include decreases in FVC, FEV_1, reduced diffusing capacity of CO (DL_{CO}), reduced total lung capacity (TLC), and static lung compliance
Laboratory tests ABGs	These are normal early in the diseases; as the diseases progress, decreased Po_2 and increased Pco_2 may occur; Hypoxemia may become severe
WBC	Leukocytosis

EXAMPLES OF CURRENTLY ACCEPTABLE THRESHOLD LIMITS OF DUST

Substance	Amount of respirable particles per cubic foot of air or per cc
Crystalline silica	0.1 mg/cc
Amorphous silica	0.1 mg/cc
Silica gel	5.0
Diatomaceous earth	10.0
Asbestos	
Amosite	0.5 fibers/cc
Chrysotile	0.5
Crocidolite	0.2
Other	2.0
Talc	2.0
Portland cement	10.0
Coal dust	2.0

From Mitchell R: Pneumoconiosis. In Mitchell RS, Petty TL, and Swhwarz MI, editors: Synopsis of clinical pulmonary disease, ed 4, St. Louis, 1989, The CV Mosby Company, p 335.

MEDICAL MANAGEMENT

GENERAL MANAGEMENT

Prevention of secondary infections; chest physical therapy; steam inhalation; oxygen by cannula, 1 to 2 L/min; increased fluids.

DRUG THERAPY

None specific; treat complications of disease such as infection, pulmonary hypertension, and cor pulmonale.

SURGERY

Biopsy: May be necessary for diagnostic evaluation.

PATIENT TEACHING

1. Teach patient how to perform pursed-lip breathing and abdominal breathing exercises to reduce the work of breathing.
2. Teach name, action, purpose, frequency of administration, and side effect of medications.
3. Encourage patient to get influenza vaccine.
4. Teach patient and family the importance of avoiding environmental pollutants and not smoking.
5. Teach patient and family the signs of complications of pneumoconioses such as dyspnea, cough, worsening expectoration, and hemoptysis.
6. Teach patient that protective hoods should be used at work when dust production is heavy. Exposure to crystalline silica, asbestos, or coal dust may occur during mining or quarrying for the material. In addition individuals who work in foundries; who are involved in abrasive blasting, stone cutting, or other masonry work; or who work in areas where glass, pottery, or porcelain is manufactured may be at risk for silicosis.

CHAPTER 5

Infectious Respiratory Diseases

The respiratory system has several defense mechanisms against infection. The first line of defense is in the large airways, which are lined with ciliated columnar cells; each cell contains as many as 300 cilia. Interspersed among these cells are mucus-secreting cells. The sticky mucous membranes trap pathogens, which are propelled toward the trachea by cilia that beat about 1000 times a minute. Coughing and sneezing expel the antigens from the body.

As a second line of defense, the lungs contain alveolar macrophages, phagocytic cells that recognize and destroy foreign material. The alveolar macrophages also remove old cells and participate in immune system response.

> The respiratory tract is the most common site of infections and respiratory infections are the most common category of disease.

Despite these protective mechanisms, the respiratory tract is the most common site of infections, and respiratory tract infections are the most common category of disease. In fact, over one half of all visits to primary care physicians are related to respiratory infections. The Centers for Disease Control estimates that pneumonia and lower respiratory infections affect 29.321 million persons annually and account for 52,000 deaths. At least 160 million upper respiratory infections are diagnosed yearly, 3,300 of which result in death.

One of the primary ingredients for pathogenic growth is host susceptibility. Persons with chronic lung diseases and immune deficiency disorders are particularly susceptible to respiratory infections. Also more susceptible are individuals who are poorly nourished, the elderly, and the very young. However, other factors that contribute to host susceptibility account for the high rate of respiratory infections among healthy populations. These factors include duration of exposure and pathogenic virulence. Infection can occur with prolonged close contact, even with an organism that is not highly contagious. In contrast, a single contact with an extremely virulent pathogen can also cause illness.

The transmission rate of respiratory infections varies considerably. With pathogens that are highly contagious, precautions are required to prevent spread of the disease. To limit disease transmission, some respiratory infections, such as tuberculosis, are reportable to public health authorities.

Pneumonia and Pneumonitis

Lobar pneumonia
(right upper lobe)

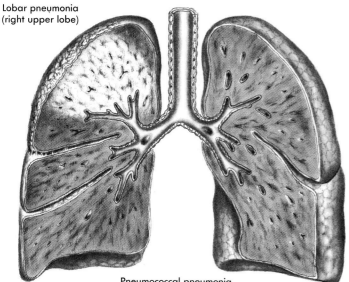

Pneumococcal pneumonia

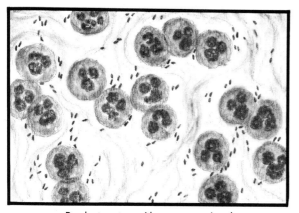

Purulent sputum with pneumococci and
polymorphonuclear leukocytes

Pneumonia is an inflammatory process of the respiratory bronchioles and the alveolar spaces that is caused by infection. **Pneumonitis** is non-infectious bronchial and alveolar inflammation. Together, these terms are used to refer to inflammatory processes of the parenchyma of the lung.

Pneumonia is the most common cause of death from infectious disease in North America. It is also considered to be the major source of disease and death in critically ill patients.[67,99] Despite the use of antibiotics, pneumonia still accounts for 27.7 of every 100,000 deaths.[77,99]

Pneumonia may be caused by bacteria, viruses, *Mycoplasma*, fungi, and parasites. Currently about half of pneumonia cases are caused by bacteria and half by virus. Up to 96% of bacterial pneumonia cases are caused by the organisms described below. Because most of the organisms require specific therapy, it is important to identify the agent causing the disease.

Pneumonia occurs most often during the winter and early spring and in persons 60 years or older. The disease usually resolves within 2 to 3 weeks.[99]

BACTERIAL PNEUMONIA

Streptococcus pneumoniae **(pneumococcal) pneumonia.** S. *pneumoniae* (hemolytic streptococcus type A), a gram-positive diplococcus, is by far the most common and important cause of bacterial pneumonia, accounting for 90% of cases. The infection usually involves extensive consolidation of part or all of the parenchyma of the lobe. S. *pneumoniae* pneumonia is often seen in infants and the elderly and in patients with sickle cell disease, congestive heart failure, alcoholism, or diabetes mellitus. A vaccine is now available and is 80% to 90% effective against this type of pneumonia in adults.[42,77,96,112]

Staphylococcus aureus **pneumonia.** S. *aureus*, a

gram-positive coccus, causes a necrotizing infection. It may cause pneumonia in infants and the elderly and commonly causes pneumonia as a complication of influenza or in hospitalized patients as a secondary infection after surgery, tracheostomy, coma, or immunosuppressive therapy. It accounts for 3% to 5% of bacterial pneumonia.[77,96,112]

Haemophilus influenzae (type B) pneumonia. *H. influenzae,* a gram-negative bacillus, causes lobar-type pneumonia, bronchopneumonia, or bronchiolitis in adults. It accounts for 1% of bacterial pneumonia.[42,77,112]

VIRAL PNEUMONIA

Influenza A is the most common type of viral pneumonia. It is transmitted by respiratory droplet, causing an interstitial infection that adversely affects many respiratory defense mechanisms and predisposes the person to secondary bacterial pneumonia.

MYCOPLASMA PNEUMONIA

Infection with *M. pneumoniae,* which is most common in school-age children and young adults, spreads among family members. Transmission is believed to be by infected respiratory secretions. *M. pneumoniae* causes an interstitial infection.

ASPIRATION PNEUMONIA SYNDROME

Aspiration pneumonia syndrome occurs most commonly as a result of aspiration when the patient is in an altered state of consciousness owing to a seizure, use of drugs or alcohol, anesthesia, acute infection, or shock. It may also occur when the anatomy is altered by esophageal stricture, tracheal fistula, a nasogastric tube, or a tracheotomy. Aspiration pneumonia may be acquired through foreign body aspiration. Nonbacterial aspiration pneumonia may follow aspiration of toxic materials such as toxic fluids and inert substances; bacterial aspiration pneumonia may occur as a secondary problem.

The causative agents of bacterial pneumonia include the gram-positive coccus *Staphylococcus aureus,* the gram-negative coccus *Escherichia coli,* and the gram-negative bacilli *Klebsiella pneumoniae, Pseudomonas aeruginosa, Proteus,* and *Enterobacter.*

All of these bacterial aspiration pneumonias have a poor prognosis even with antibiotic therapy. They may cause extensive lung damage resulting in lung abscess or empyema. Mortality is 70% with *P. aeruginosa,* 45% with *E. coli,* 25% to 50% with *K. pneumoniae,* and 15% to 50% with *S. aureus.*[77,80,96,112]

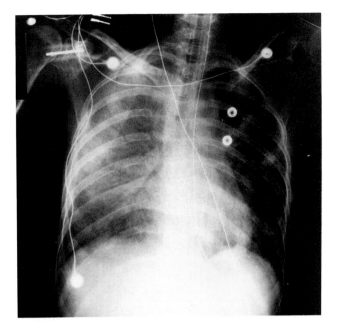

FIGURE 5-1
Chest x-ray of patient with pneumonia. Note infiltrate of right middle and lower zones with air bronchogram seen; right heart border not obliterated. Also note monitor electrodes, gown snaps, endotracheal tube, and ventilator tubing. (Courtesy R. Keith Wilson, M.D., Baylor College of Medicine, Houston, Tex; From Thompson.)[99]

PATHOPHYSIOLOGY

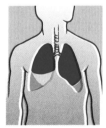

The pathophysiology depends on the etiologic agent. Most bacterial pneumonia is marked by an intraalveolar suppurative exudate with consolidation. Lobar pneumonia causes consolidation of the entire lobe (Figure 5-1). Bronchopneumonia causes a patchy distribution of infectious areas around and involving the bronchi. A chest roentgenogram of bronchopneumonia shows patchy segmental or subsegmental infiltration in one or more dependent lobes.[99]

Mycoplasmal and viral pneumonias produce interstitial inflammation with accumulation of an infiltrate in the alveolar walls. There is no consolidation or exudate.

Fungal, mycobacterial, and staphylococcal pneumonias are marked by patchy distribution of granulomas that may undergo necrosis with the development of cavities.

The most extensively studied type of pneumonia is pneumococcal or streptococcal pneumonia. The bacteria are thought to reach the alveoli in mucus or saliva. In the alveoli they undergo four predictable phases[51]:

Engorgement (first 4 to 12 hours). Serous exudate pours into alveoli from the dilated, leaking blood vessels.

Red hepatization (next 48 hours). The lung assumes a red granular appearance as red blood cells, fibrin, and polymorphonuclear leukocytes fill the alveoli.

Gray hepatization (3 to 8 days). The lung assumes a grayish appearance as the leukocytes and fibrin consolidate in the involved alveoli.

Resolution (7 to 11 days). Exudate is lysed and reabsorbed by macrophages, restoring the tissue to its original structure.

These stages represent the course of untreated pneumococcal pneumonia; with the use of antibiotics the course should run 3 to 5 days.

Viral pneumonia affects the tissues differently. The inflammatory response in the bronchi damages the ciliated epithelium. The lungs are congested and in some cases hemorrhagic. The inflammatory response is composed of mononuclear cells, lymphocytes, and plasma cells in proportions that vary with the type of virus causing the disease. In severe types of viral pneumonia the alveoli contain hyaline membranes. Characteristic intracellular viral inclusions may be seen in adenovirus, cytomegalovirus, respiratory syncytial virus, or varicella virus infections.

Aspiration pneumonia presents a still different physiologic response, which is based on the pH of the aspirated substance. If the pH is 2.5 or above, little necrosis results. However, if the pH is below 2.5, atelectasis occurs, followed by pulmonary edema, hemorrhage, and type II cell necrosis. The alveolar-capillary "membrane" may be damaged, leading to exudation and in severe cases ARDS.[75]

COMPLICATIONS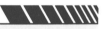

Pleurisy	Pulmonary edema
Atelectasis	Superinfection pericarditis
Empyema	Meningitis
Lung abscess	Arthritis

DIAGNOSTIC STUDIES AND FINDINGS

Diagnostic Test	Findings
Laboratory tests	
Sputum examination	Sputum from lower respiratory tract needed for assessment; if necessary, may be obtained by needle aspiration, transtracheal aspiration, fiberoptic bronchoscopy, or open lung biopsy; sputum *must* be examined before initiation of antibiotic therapy
	Macroexamination for odor, consistency, amount, color
	Microexamination, including Gram stain, for etiologic agent, neutrophilia, increased epithelial cells, presence of other organisms
	Sputum culture for organism identification; although routinely performed, culture thought to be only 50% sensitive for pneumococcal disease and only 35%-50% sensitive for pneumonia caused by *Haemophilus influenzae*[75]
Blood cultures	May be transient bacteremia in pneumococcal pneumonia
Acid-fast stains and cultures	To rule out tuberculosis
Serum specimen for cold agglutinins	Test requires 10 ml of clotted blood; used for differential diagnosis of viral or mycoplasmal infections; cold agglutinins present in about 50% of diseases caused by these two agents
White blood cell count	Leukocytosis (15,000-25,000/mm^3); neutrophilia (normal or low WBC count in mycoplasmal or viral infection)
ABGs	Pao$_2$ <80 mm Hg
Chest x-ray	Presence of density changes involving primarily lower lobes (see Figure 5-1)
Lung function studies	Volumes: congestion and collapse of alveoli; decreased lung volumes
	Pressures: in increased airway resistance and decreased compliance
	Gas exchange: shunting as a result of hypoxemia

Table 5-1 ⎯⎯⎯〜〜〜⎯

ANTIBIOTIC THERAPY FOR PNEUMONIA

Organism	Agent of First Choice	Adult Daily Dose	Duration (Days)	Alternate Agents
Streptococcus pneumoniae				
Mild	Penicillin	Penicillin V, 500 mg PO q 6 h	7-10	Erythromycin 500 mg q 6 h
Fulminant	Penicillin	Penicillin G, 2×10^6 U q 6 h	7	Cefazolin 1 g q 8 h Vancomycin 1 g q 12 h
Streptococcus pyogenes (group A)	Penicillin G	2×10^6 U q 4 h	14-21	Cefazolin*
Staphylococcus aureus				
Nonbacteremic	Nafcillin	1.5-2 g q 4-6 h	21	Cefazolin*
Bacteremic	Nafcillin	1.5-2 g q 4-6 h	28	Vancomycin†
Anaerobic mouth flora (Peptostreptococci, *Bacteroides melaninogenicus*)	Penicillin	2×10^6 U q 4 h followed by penicillin V 0.5-1 g q 6 h	10-14 14-30	Clindamycin 600 mg q 8 h followed by 300 mg q 6 h
Mycoplasma penumoniae	Erythromycin	250 mg q 6 h	21	Tetracycline 250 mg q 6 h
Legionella spp.	Erythromycin	1 g q 6 h IV followed by 250 mg q 6 h PO	7-14 14-21	Rifampin 300 mg q 8 h PO
Escherichia coli	Third-generation cephalosporin‡	1-2 g q 8 h	14	Imipenem 500 mg q 6 h Aztreonam 1 g q 8 h
Providencia spp. or *Morganella*	Third-generation cephalosporin‡	2 g q 8 h	14	TMP/SMX ‖
Chlamydia psittaci	Tetracycline	500 mg q 6 h	14	
Francisella tularensis	Streptomycin *plus* tetracycline	1 g q 12 h IM 500 mg q 6 h	14	TMP/SMX ‖
Yersinia pestis	Streptomycin *plus* tetracycline	1 g q 12 h	21	
Haemophilus influenzae	Cefuroxime	0.75 g q 8 h	14	Third-generation cephalosporin‡ aztreonam TMP/SMX ‖
Klebsiella pneumoniae	Third-generation cephalospirin‡	2 g q 8 h	21	TMP/SMX ‖ aztreonam or aminoglycoside¶
Pseudomonas aeruginosa	Antipseudomonas penicillin§ or aztreonam *plus* aminoglycoside**	18g IV 2 g q 8 h	21	Imipenem 500 mg q 6 h *plus* aminoglycoside
Acinetobacter calcoaceticus	Ticarcillin *plus* tobramycin**	3 g q 4 h 2 mg/kg q 8 h **	14-21	Imipenem 500 mg q 6 h
Serratia marcescens	TMP/SMX	15 mg/75 mg/kg/day in 3 doses	14-21	Third-generation cephalosporin‡ *plus* aminoglycoside *or* imipenem††
Enterobacter spp.	TMP/SMX	15 mg/75 mg/kg/day in 3 doses	14-21	Imipenem 500 mg q 6 h *plus* aminoglycoside

From Rakel[82]
*Cefazolin - 1 g q 8 h.
†Vancomycin - 500 mg q 6 h or 1 g q 12 h.
‡Cefotaxime - 2 g q 2 h , ceftriaxone 2 g q 8 h , ceftriaxone 2 g q 12 h , ceftazidime 1-2 g q 8 h .
‖ TMP/SMX - 15 mg/kg of trimethoprim, 75 mg/kg sulfamethoxazole per day given as three divided doses.
¶ Gentamicin - 2 mg/kg q 8 h , tobramycin 2 mg/kg q 8 h , amikacin 5 mg/kg q 8 h .
§Anti-*Pseudomonas* penicillin - azlocillin, piperacillin, ticarcillin 3 g q 4 h; adjust dose of ticarcillin if creatinine clearance less than 30 ml/min. Aztreconam 2 g q 8 h .
**Adjust dose depending on renal function status.
††Imipenem 0.25 to 1 g q 6 h; adjust dose in presence of renal failure.

MEDICAL MANAGEMENT

GENERAL MANAGEMENT

Humidification: Humidifier or nebulizer if secretions are thick and copious.

Oxygenation: If patient has Pa_{O_2} <60 mm Hg, Venturi mask or nasal prongs commonly used.

Physiotherapy: Role in hastening resolution of pneumonia uncertain; patient should be encouraged at least to cough and deep breathe to maximize ventilatory capabilities.[75]

Hydration: Monitoring of intake and output; supplemental fluids to maintain hydration and liquefy secretions.

SURGERY

Thoracentesis with chest tube insertion: May be necessary if secondary problem such as empyema occurs.

DRUG THERAPY

Antiinfective agents: See Table 5-1 for complete list of antiinfective agents.

Assessment observations vary, depending on the type of pneumonia. A general assessment is given below, followed by specific variations.

1 ASSESS

ASSESSMENT	OBSERVATIONS
Respiratory	Tachypnea; retractions; labored breathing; dyspnea; nasal flaring; crackles; pleural friction rub; diminished breath sounds over area of consolidation; hypoventilation; labored or irregular breathing; breathing tiring for patient; percussion tone dull over area of consolidation
Vital signs	Fever, tachypnea, tachycardia
Streptococcal, pneumococcal	Sudden onset; chest pain; chills; fever; headache; cough; rust-colored sputum; crackles and possibly friction rub; hypoxemia as blood is shunted away from area of consolidation; cyanosis
Staphylococcal	Many of same signs as streptococcal; sputum copious and salmon colored
Haemophilus	Commonly follows upper respiratory infection; low-grade fever; croupy cough; malaise; arthralgias; yellow or green sputum
Viral	Symptoms generally mild; cold symptoms; headache; anorexia; fever; myalgia; irritating cough that produces mucopurulent or bloody sputum
Mycoplasmal	Gradual onset; headache; fever; malaise; chills, cough severe and nonproductive; decreased breath sounds and crackles

2 DIAGNOSE

NURSING DIAGNOSIS	SUBJECTIVE FINDINGS	OBJECTIVE FINDINGS
Ineffective airway clearance related to mucopurulent sputum	Reports difficulty breathing	Cough (may be productive or non-productive), crackles and rhonchi, fever, dyspnea, tachypnea
Ineffective breathing pattern related to inflammatory process and pleuritic pain	Reports SOB, painful respirations	Dyspnea, shallow respirations, cough, tachypnea, asymmetric chest movements
Impaired gas exchange related to alveolar-capillary membrane changes secondary to inflammation	Complains of SOB	Hypoxia (Pa_{O2} <80 mm Hg), cyanosis, irritability, restlessness, diminished to absent breath sounds
Hyperthermia related to inflammatory process	Reports feeling hot, thirsty	Fever; warm, dry skin
Altered nutrition: less than body requirements related to anorexia and dyspnea	Reports inadequate intake, reports feeling too tired to eat, SOB	Weight loss, inadequate food and fluid intake, fatigue, dyspnea
Activity intolerance related to generalized weakness	Complains of fatigue, SOB	SOB during activity, decreased activity level
Anxiety related to dyspnea	Expresses worry about his condition, expresses distress about dyspnea	Appears scared, tense

3 PLAN

Patient goals

1. The patient's airways will be patent.
2. The patient's breathing pattern will be effective and without pain.
3. The patient's gas exchange will be improved.
4. The patient's temperature will be within normal limits.
5. The patient's nutritional status will be improved.
6. The patient will be able to perform usual activities without fatigue or dyspnea.
7. The patient's anxiety will be relieved.
8. The patient will demonstrate understanding of home care and follow-up instructions.

4   IMPLEMENT

NURSING DIAGNOSIS	NURSING INTERVENTIONS	RATIONALE
Ineffective airway clearance related to mucopurulent sputum	Auscultate lungs for crackles, consolidation, and pleural friction rub.	Determines adequacy of gas exchange and extent of airways obstructed with secretions.
	Assess characteristics of secretions: quantity, color, consistency, odor.	Presence of infection is suspected when secretions are thick, yellow or rust colored, and/or foul smelling.
	Assess patient's hydration status: skin turgor, mucous membranes, tongue, intake and output over 24 h, Hct.	Determines need for fluids. Fluids needed if skin turgor poor, tongue and mucous membranes are dry, intake <output, and/or hematocrit is elevated.
	Monitor chest x-rays.	Shows extent and location of lung involvement.
	Monitor sputum Gram stain, and culture and sensitivity reports.	Identifies microorganisms present so that appropriate antiinfective agents can be prescribed.
	Assist patient with coughing as needed.	Coughing removes secretions, prevents atelectasis.
	Administer antiinfective agents as ordered.	Interrupts growth of microorganisms.
	Position patient in proper body alignment for optimal breathing pattern (head of bed up 45°, if tolerated up to 90°).	Secretions move by gravity as position changes. Elevating head of bed moves abdominal contents away from diaphragm to enhance diaphragmatic contraction.
	Keep environment allergen free (e.g., dust, feathers, smoke) according to individual needs.	Prevents allergic reactions that may cause bronchial irritation.
	Assist patient with ambulation/position changes (turning side to side).	Secretions move by gravity as position changes.
	Increase room humidification.	Humidifies and loosens secretions to facilitate their expectoration.
	Perform chest physiotherapy (e.g., percussion, vibration) and postural drainage.	Applying percussion and vibration to chest loosens secretions so they can be expectorated.
	Assist patient in using blow bottles, incentive spirometry.	Requires deep breathing to expand alveoli.
	Avoid suppressing cough reflex unless cough is frequent and nonproductive.	Cough reflex needed to mobilize secretions, but excessive nonproductive coughing leads to fatigue.

NURSING DIAGNOSIS	NURSING INTERVENTIONS	RATIONALE
	Encourage increased fluid intake to 1 ½ to 2 L/day unless contraindicated.	Liquefies secretions so that they are easier to expectorate.
	Assist patient with oral hygiene as needed.	Removes taste of secretions.
Ineffective breathing pattern related to inflammatory process and pleuritic pain	Observe changes in respiratory rate and depth.	Determines adequacy of breathing pattern.
	Inspect thorax for symmetry of respiratory movement.	Determines adequacy of breathing pattern.
	Observe breathing pattern for SOB, labored breathing, use of accessory muscles and intercostal retractions.	Identifies increased work of breathing.
	Measure V_T and VC.	Indicates volume of air moving in and out of lungs.
	Assess emotional response.	Detects use of hyperventilation as a cause of altered breathing pattern.
	Assess for pain.	Often is a cause of altered breathing pattern and pleuritic pain.
	Position patient in optimal body alignment in semi-Fowler's position for breathing.	Elevating head of the bed moves abdominal contents away from the diaphragm to enhance diaphragmatic contraction.
	Assist patient to use relaxation techniques.	Relieves anxiety and reduces muscle tension.
	Medicate with analgesic without depressing respirations.	Analgesics reduce pain that may be interfering with breathing pattern.
Impaired gas exchange related to alveolar-capillary membrane changes secondary to inflammation	Auscultate lungs for crackles, consolidation, and pleural friction rub.	Determines adequacy of gas exchange and detects areas of consolidation and pleural friction rub.
	Assess LOC, listlessness, and irritability.	These signs may indicate hypoxia.
	Observe skin color and capillary refill.	Determines circulatory adequacy, which is necessary for gas exchange to tissues.
	Monitor ABGs.	Determines need for oxygen.
	Monitor CBC.	Detects amount of hemoglobin present to carry oxygen and presence of infection.
	Administer antiinfective agents as ordered.	Interrupts growth of microorganisms.

NURSING DIAGNOSIS	NURSING INTERVENTIONS	RATIONALE
	Administer oxygen as ordered.	Improves gas exchange; decreases work of breathing.
	Pace activities to patient's tolerance.	Decreases oxygen demand.
Hyperthermia related to inflammatory process	Measure temperature.	Indicates if a fever exists and its extent.
	Assess skin temperature and color.	Warm, dry, flushed skin may indicate a fever.
	Monitor WBC count.	Leukocytosis indicates an inflammatory and/or infectious process are present.
	Measure intake and output.	Determines fluid balance and need to increase intake.
	Encourage fluid intake orally or intravenously as ordered.	Replaces fluids lost by insensible loss and perspiration.
	Administer antipyretics as ordered.	Reduces fever through action on the hypothalamus.
	Provide/encourage frequent oral hygiene.	Maintains moist mucous membranes.
	Increase air circulation in the room with a fan.	Facilitates heat loss by convection.
	Give a tepid sponge bath.	Facilitates heat loss by evaporation.
	Apply an ice bag covered with a towel to the axilla and/or groin.	Facilitates heat loss by conduction.
	Cover the patient with a sheet only.	Prevents chilling; shivering will further increase the metabolic rate.
	Place patient on a hypothermia blanket as ordered.	Facilitates heat loss by conduction.
	Administer antiinfective agents as ordered.	Interrupts growth of microorganisms.
Altered nutrition: less than body requirement related to anorexia and dyspnea	Assess dietary habits and needs.	Helps to individualize the diet.
	Weigh patient weekly.	Improved nutrition will result in weight gain.
	Auscultate bowel sounds.	Documents GI peristalsis needed for digestion.
	Assess psychologic factors, e.g., depression, that might decrease food and fluid intake.	Identifies effect of psychologic factors on food intake.

NURSING DIAGNOSIS	NURSING INTERVENTIONS	RATIONALE
	Monitor albumin and lymphocytes.	These lab values indicate adequate visceral protein, which is low when nutrition is inadequate.
	Measure mid-arm circumference.	This measurement indicates protein stores.
	Measure triceps skinfold.	This measurement indicates fat stores.
	Provide oxygen while eating as ordered.	Oxygen reduces dyspnea during meals so that more food may be eaten.
	Encourage oral care before meals.	Removes taste of sputum that may reduce appetite.
	Provide foods in appropriate consistency for eating. Soft or liquid foods may be preferred.	Requires less energy to eat soft foods and liquids, thereby reducing oxygen requirement.
	Provide high-protein diet.	Supports immune system to fight infection.
	Administer vitamins as ordered.	Supplements diet and promotes healing.
Activity intolerance related to generalized weakness	Observe response to activity.	Determines extent of tolerance.
	Identify factors contributing to intolerance, e.g., stress, side effects of drugs.	Eliminating contributing factors may resolve activity intolerance.
	Assess patient's sleep patterns.	Lack of sleep may lead to fatigue.
	Plan rest periods between activities.	Reduces fatigue and facilitates ventilation.
	Perform activities for patient until patient is able to perform them.	Meets patient's need without causing fatigue.
	Provide oxygen as needed.	Decreases work of breathing during activity.
	Keep frequently used objects within reach.	Provides convenient use for patient; decreases oxygen demand.
Anxiety related to dyspnea	Assess patient's level of anxiety (mild, moderate, severe, panic).	Determines the kinds of interventions needed to reduce anxiety.
	Assist patient to identify events that precipitated anxiety in the past and how patient dealt with them.	Facilitates problem solving; reviews coping skills used in the past.
	Encourage patient to acknowledge and express feelings.	May relieve anxiety; helps patient put thoughts into perspective.

NURSING DIAGNOSIS	NURSING INTERVENTIONS	RATIONALE
	Provide accurate information about pneumonia.	Knowledge can decrease anxiety.
	Provide comfort measures, e.g., back rub.	Facilitates relaxation; may decrease respiratory rate.
	Provide oxygen as ordered.	Decreases work of breathing.
Knowledge deficit	See Patient Teaching.	

5 EVALUATE

PATIENT OUTCOME	DATA INDICATING THAT OUTCOME IS REACHED
Airway is patent.	Airways are clear and breathing occurs without obstruction. Breath sounds are clear. Chest x-ray is clear. Cough has subsided. Temperature is normal for patient.
Breathing pattern is effective without pain.	ABGs are within normal limits (Pa_{O_2} = 80-100 mm Hg). Vital capacity measurements are optimal for patient. Cough has subsided. Breathing pattern is effective without pain.
Gas exchange is within normal limits for patient.	Pa_{O_2} = 80-100 mm Hg Arterial pH = 7.35-7.45 Breath sounds are clear.
Temperature is within normal limits.	Temperature = 38° C (98.6° F) Skin is warm and moist.
Nutritional status is within normal limits.	Weight gain. Food and fluid intake have improved.
Patient performs usual activities without fatigue or dyspnea.	Patient performs self-care activities.
Anxiety is reduced.	Patient reports anxiety is reduced to a manageable level. Patient appears relaxed.
Learning is demonstrated.	Patient demonstrates knowledge of self-care management, disease process, compliance with treatment regimen, and how to prevent recurrence.

PATIENT TEACHING

1. Teach the patient deep breathing and coughing techniques.
2. Teach the patient and family facts about prescribed medication, including the action, dosage, frequency of administration, and side effects.
3. Provide the patient and family with information regarding the specific type of pneumonia the patient has, treatment, anticipated response, possible complications, and probable disease duration.
4. Inform the patient and family that a change in health status must be reported to health care providers. Indicators of change may include a change in sputum characteristics or color, decreased activity tolerance, fever despite the antibiotic intake, increasing chest pain, or a feeling that things are not getting better.
5. Teach the patient the importance of drinking large quantities of fluids.
6. Teach the patient adaptive breathing exercises.
7. Instruct the patient in relaxation techniques.
8. Teach the patient the importance of rest during the day in addition to a full night's sleep.
9. Inform the patient that eating a balanced diet each day is important in maintaining the immune system.
10. Teach the patient the importance of avoiding smoke and fumes that irritate the bronchi.
11. Advise patient to obtain influenza and pneumococcal vaccines at the prescribed times to increase immunity.

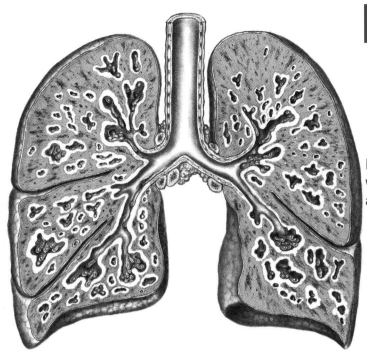

Bronchiectasis

Bronchiectasis is the chronic dilation of bronchi with eventual destruction of the bronchial elastic and muscular elements.

PATHOPHYSIOLOGY

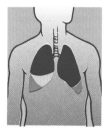

Bronchiectasis is a chronic disease of the bronchi and bronchioles characterized by irreversible dilation associated with chronic infection and inflammation of the bronchial tree. It usually is preceded by respiratory infection that causes the bronchial mucosa to be replaced by fibrotic scar tissue. It is not known whether bronchiectasis begins as an infection or if it results from abnormal structure of the bronchial walls.[42]

There are three types of bronchiectasis: saccular, cylindrical, and varicose. Figure 5-2 shows the three forms of bronchiectasis. Saccular bronchiectasis occurs in large bronchi that become large and balloon-like. Cylindrical bronchiectasis involves medium-sized bronchi, which usually are symmetrically dilated. This type of bronchiectasis may occur as a complication of pneumonitis, but disappears after a few months.[77] In varicose bronchiectasis, constrictions and dilations deform the bronchi.[73]

Most cases of bronchiectasis are acquired as a result of repeated or prolonged episodes of pneumonitis, especially those complicating pertussis or influenza during childhood; gastrointestinal reflux; and recurrent sinusitis.[77] Bronchiectasis also occurs later in life in asso-

ciation with a variety of infections such as tuberculosis and bacterial pneumonia and congenital disorders such as cystic fibrosis. Figure 5-3 outlines the pathogenesis of bronchiectasis.

The incidence of this acquired disorder has decreased greatly since the development of antibiotics and aggressive management of pulmonary infections. Before the use of antibiotics, pulmonary infections sometimes lingered, and a second pulmonary obstruction occurred distal to the buildup of sputum and bronchial secretions. The chronic obstruction and tissue stretching eventually progress to the destruction of bronchial elasticity and actual malfunctioning of bronchial muscle tone.

Children are at high risk for the development of bronchiectasis. This is because their bronchi are small and soft and easily damaged by prolonged overinflation caused by infection or bronchial foreign body obstruction. The prevalence of childhood bronchiectasis is decreasing because of the use of antibiotics, but it is still seen in children with cystic fibrosis and immune deficiency diseases.[25,77]

Although disease onset, especially in children, may follow a single episode of pulmonary disease, most adults have a history of numerous pulmonary infections such as pneumonia and a chronic bronchitis type of cough. Delayed resolution of any type of pulmonary disease should raise suspicion of bronchiectasis.

COMPLICATIONS

Chronic bronchitis
Pneumonia with or without
 atelectasis
Cor pulmonale
Metastatic brain abscess

Empyema
Amyloidosis
Respiratory failure

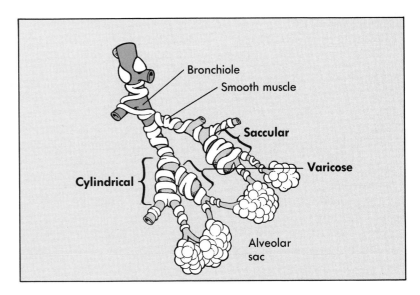

FIGURE 5-2
Types of bronchiectasis. (From McCance).[73]

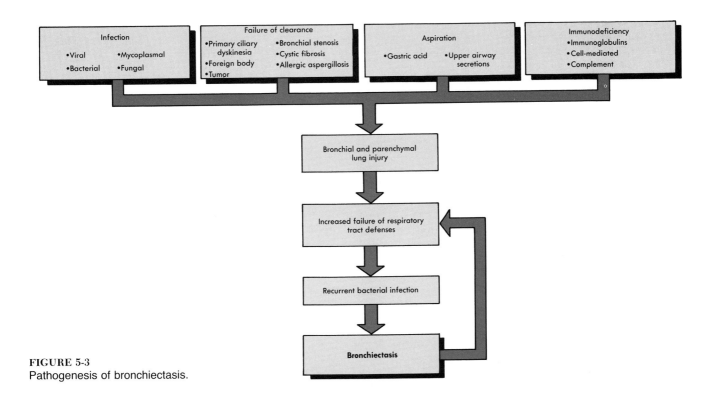

FIGURE 5-3
Pathogenesis of bronchiectasis.

DIAGNOSTIC STUDIES AND FINDINGS

Diagnostic Test	Findings
Pulmonary function studies	Spirometry may reveal a decreased FEV_1 and a decreased FVC; many patients with mild to moderate bronchiectasis will have no abnormality detectable by routine spirometry and ABG analysis
Chest x-ray	Clear but may show patches of inflammation with increased pulmonary markings at the lung bases
Bronchography	Definitive diagnostic procedure of bronchiectasis; bronchography outlines walls of bronchi and clearly shows bronchiectatic areas
Laboratory studies	
Complete blood count (CBC)	With severe hypoxia, may show polycythemia secondary to pulmonary insufficiency
Sputum examination	Gross examination shows that the sputum has three layers (sediment, fluid, and foam); a sputum smear is done to rule out tuberculosis and identify secondary bacterial infections such as those caused by pneumococci, *Pseudomonas*, and *Enterobacter*; large numbers of white blood cells and bacteria that mostly include pharyngeal flora, including anaerobic organisms, are usually seen; the decision on choice of antibiotics in the treatment of the intercurrent infection depends on the result of culture and sensitivity studies of sputum

MEDICAL MANAGEMENT

The goal of medical management is to maintain maximum ventilation by controlling infections and removing secretions.

DRUG THERAPY

Mucolytic agents: Acetylcysteine (Mucomyst), nebulization q 2-6 h with 20% solution (1-10 ml) or 10% solution (2-20 ml).

Antiinfective agents: Antibiotic therapy should be specific to the organism identified in the sputum evaluation.

Bronchodilators: Ipratropium bromide (Atrovent), 40-80 μg q 6 h; Theophylline used in rare cases, long acting, 200 mg q 12 h increased in a few days to 300 mg q 12 h.

SURGERY

Bronchial resection: May rarely be performed on patients with isolated areas of bronchiectasis that do not respond to conservative treatment; this disease must be localized enough to permit complete resection without inadvertently compromising pulmonary function.

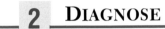 ASSESS

ASSESSMENT	OBSERVATIONS
Respiratory	Breath sounds: crackles and rhonchi over lower lobes Breathing patterns: may be labored with prolonged expiration; increased dyspnea Cough: chronic with production of large quantities of purulent sputum (coughing and sputum production may become worse with changes in posture and activity) Hemoptysis in 50% of cases Chest wall may have retractions during breathing and decreased expiratory excursion
Cardiovascular	In advanced cases, cyanosis and clubbing of fingers
Generalized response	Weight loss, night sweats, fever, gradual emaciation may be indications of disease progression with possible secondary infections

2 DIAGNOSE

NURSING DIAGNOSIS	SUBJECTIVE FINDINGS	OBJECTIVE FINDINGS
Ineffective airway clearance related to mucopurulent sputum	Reports difficulty breathing	Productive cough (often foul smelling), crackles and rhonchi, labored breathing with prolonged expiration, fever, dyspnea, hemoptysis
Ineffective breathing pattern related to bronchial obstruction and inflammatory process	Reports difficulty breathing	Dyspnea, productive cough, chest wall retractions
Altered nutrition: less than body requirements related to anorexia and dyspnea	Reports inadequate intake and anorexia	Weight loss, inadequate food and fluid intake
Activity intolerance related to generalized weakness and dyspnea	Complains of fatigue and SOB	SOB during activity, decreased activity level
Fear related to hemoptysis and possibility of chronic disease	Expresses fear when hemoptysis occurs, expresses fear of developing chronic respiratory disease	Appears scared, tense, worried

→ > >

3 PLAN

Patient goals

1. Patient's airways will be patent.
2. Patient's breathing pattern will be effective without fatigue or dyspnea.
3. Patient's nutritional status will be improved.
4. Patient will be able to perform usual activities without fatigue or dyspnea.
5. Patient's fears will be relieved.
6. Patient will demonstrate understanding of home care and follow-up instructions.

4 IMPLEMENT

NURSING DIAGNOSIS	NURSING INTERVENTIONS	RATIONALE
Ineffective airway clearance related to mucopurulent sputum	Auscultate lungs for rhonchi and crackles.	Determines adequacy of gas exchange and extent of airways obstructed with secretions.
	Assess characteristics of secretions: quantity, color, consistency, odor.	Detects presence of infection if sputum becomes thicker and changes from white to yellow.
	Assess patient's hydration status: skin turgor, mucous membranes, tongue, intake and output over 24 h, Hct.	Fluid needed if skin turgor is poor, tongue and mucous membranes are dry, intake < output, and/or Hct is elevated.
	Evaluate results of pulmonary functions tests.	Indicates extent of decline in pulmonary function due to airway obstruction.
	Monitor chest x-rays.	Shows extent and location of lung involvement.
	Monitor sputum smear and culture and sensitivity reports.	Identifies microorganisms present and which antibiotics are effective; rules out tuberculosis.
	Assist patient with coughing as needed.	Coughing removes secretions.
	Avoid vigorous coughing.	Vigorous coughing may spread infection.
	Perform endotracheal or tracheostomy tube suctioning as needed.	Stimulates cough reflex and removes secretions.
	Assist patient with ambulation/position changes (turning side to side).	Secretions move by gravity as position changes.
	Position patient in proper body alignment for optimal breathing pattern (head of bed up 45°, if tolerated up to 90°).	Secretions move by gravity as position changes. Elevating head of bed moves abdominal contents away from diaphragm to enhance diaphragmatic contraction.

NURSING DIAGNOSIS	NURSING INTERVENTIONS	RATIONALE
	Increase room humidification.	Humidifies secretions to facilitate their expectoration.
	Administer mucolytic agents as ordered (e.g., Mucomyst).	Facilitates liquefying of secretions so they can be expectorated.
	Administer antiinfective agents as ordered.	Interrupts growth of microorganisms.
	Administer bronchodilators as ordered.	Dilates bronchi to facilitate airway clearance.
	Perform chest physiotherapy (e.g., percussion, vibration) and postural drainage.	Applying percussion and vibration loosens secretions so they can be expectorated.
	Assist patient in using blow bottles, incentive spirometry.	Requires deep breathing to clear airways.
	Keep environment allergen free (e.g., dust, feathers, smoke) according to individual needs.	Prevents allergic reactions to bronchial irritation.
	Avoid suppressing cough reflex unless cough is frequent and nonproductive.	Cough reflex needed to mobilize secretions.
	Encourage increased fluid intake to 1 1/2 to 2 L/day unless contraindicated.	Liquefies secretions so that they can be expectorated.
	Assist patient with oral hygiene as needed.	Removes taste of secretions.
Ineffective breathing pattern related to bronchial obstruction and inflammatory process	Observe changes in respiratory rate and depth.	Determines adequacy of breathing pattern.
	Inspect thorax for symmetry of respiratory movement.	Determines adequacy of breathing pattern.
	Measure tidal volume and vital capacity.	Indicates volume of air moving in and out of lungs. The volume is decreased by obstructed airways.
	Administer mucolytic agents as ordered, e.g., acetylcysteine (Mucomyst).	Liquefies secretions to relieve bronchial obstruction.
	Administer antiinfectives as ordered.	Interrupts growth of microorganisms to reduce infections and inflammatory process.
	Encourage use of blow bottles or incentive spirometry.	Facilitates deep breathing to open airways.

NURSING DIAGNOSIS	NURSING INTERVENTIONS	RATIONALE
Altered nutrition: less than body requirements related to anorexia and dyspnea	Assess dietary habits and needs.	Helps to individualize the diet.
	Weigh patient weekly.	Improved nutrition will result in weight gain.
	Auscultate bowel sounds.	Documents presence of gastrointestinal peristalsis needed for digestion.
	Assess psychologic factors, e.g., depression, that might decrease food and fluid intake.	Identifies effect of psychologic factors on food intake.
	Monitor albumin and lymphocytes.	Indicates visceral protein, which is low when nutrition is inadequate.
	Encourage oral care before meals.	Removes taste of sputum that may reduce appetite.
	Provide frequent small feedings.	Lessens fatigue to eat small meals.
	Provide foods in appropriate consistency for eating. Soft or liquid foods may be preferred.	Requires less energy to eat soft foods and liquids thereby reducing oxygen requirement.
	Provide high-protein diet.	Supports immune system to fight infection.
	Avoid very hot and very cold foods.	May induce cough spasms.
	Administer vitamins as ordered.	Supplements diet, promotes healing.
	Avoid gas-forming foods and carbonated drinks.	These foods limit movement of diaphragm and hamper abdominal breathing.
Activity intolerance related to generalized weakness and dyspnea	Observe response to activity.	Determines extent of tolerance.
	Identify factors contributing to activity intolerance, e.g., stress, side effects of drugs.	Eliminating contributing factors may resolve activity intolerance.
	Assess patient's sleep patterns.	Lack of sleep may be causative factor.
	Plan rest periods between activities.	Reduces fatigue.
	Encourage use of adaptive breathing techniques during activity.	Decreases work of breathing.
	Perform activities for patient until patient is able to perform them.	Meets patient's need without causing fatigue and dyspnea.
	Provide progressive increase in activity as tolerated.	Gradually increasing activities fosters maximum independence without causing weakness and dyspnea.

NURSING DIAGNOSIS	NURSING INTERVENTIONS	RATIONALE
	Keep frequently used items within reach.	Provides convenient use of items for patient; decreases oxygen demand.
	Problem solve with patient to determine methods of conserving energy while performing tasks, e.g., sit on stool while shaving; dry skin after bath by wrapping in terry cloth robe instead of drying skin with a towel.	Identifies ways to conserve energy, thereby using less oxygen and producing less carbon dioxide.
Fear related to hemoptysis and possibility of chronic disease	Validate source(s) of fear with patient.	Ensures congruence between nurse and patient in trying to resolve fear.
	Assess vital signs.	Determines effect of fear on heart and respiratory rates.
	Encourage patient to discuss contributing factors to fear and actions to allay fear.	Facilitates problem solving; reviews coping skills used in the past.
	Explain the disease process involved with bronchiectasis and encourage patient to ask questions.	Knowledge can decrease fear.
	Provide oxygen as ordered.	Decreases work of breathing.
	Accept patient's fears.	Facilitates problem solving, supports therapeutic relationship.
Knowledge deficit	See Patient Teaching.	

5 EVALUATE

PATIENT OUTCOME	DATA INDICATING THAT OUTCOME IS REACHED
Airway is patent.	Airways are clear and breathing occurs without obstruction. Breath sounds are clear.
Breathing pattern is effective without anorexia or dyspnea.	Vital capacity (VC) and forced expiratory volume (FEV_1) are optimal for patient. Breathing occurs without difficulty; no chest wall retractions or dyspnea noted.
Nutritional status is improved.	Weight gain. Patient eating balanced diet without dyspnea. Serum albumin and leukocytes are within normal limits.
Fear is decreased.	Patient expresses fears. Patient discusses plans to maintain health.
Learning is demonstrated.	Patient demonstrates knowledge of home care, disease process, and compliance with treatment regimen.

PATIENT TEACHING

1. Teach adaptive breathing techniques such as pursed-lip and abdominal breathing.
2. Teach effective coughing techniques and importance of coughing and deep breathing.
3. Encourage use of postural drainage at home as long as needed.
4. Teach importance of not smoking and avoiding fumes and smoke during active disease state.
5. Instruct about the medications prescribed, including the name, action, dosage, frequency, and side effects.
6. Encourage eating a high-protein, high-caloric diet to help immune system fight infection.
7. Instruct about importance of drinking 2000-3000 ml (2-3 quarts) of fluids daily.
8. Discuss symptoms to report to physician: chest pain, difficulty breathing, hemoptysis, fever, and cold or flu.
9. Explain need to avoid persons with respiratory infections, avoid crowds, avoid chilling, and stay warm.
10. Teach importance of getting immunizations to prevent illness, e.g., influenza.

Pleurisy (Pleuritis)

Pleurisy is an inflammation of the visceral and parietal pleura. It is also referred to as dry pleurisy or fibrinous pleurisy.

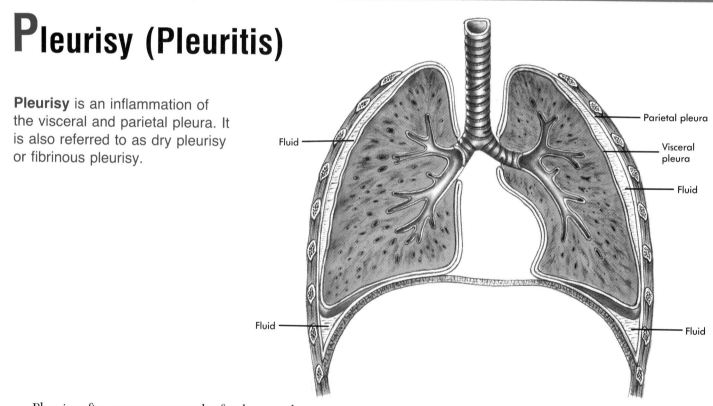

Pleurisy often occurs as a result of pulmonary bacterial infections such as pneumonia or pulmonary infarction, viral infections of the intercostal muscles, transport of an infectious agent or neoplastic cells directly to the pleura by the bloodstream or lymphatics, pleural trauma, asbestos-related pleural diseases, or early stages of tuberculosis or lung tumor. The size of the affected area varies greatly. The disease onset is usually sudden, and the diagnosis is easily made based on the characteristic pleuritic pain and pleural friction rub.[25,42,112]

PATHOPHYSIOLOGY

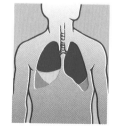

The visceral pleura attaches to the lung's surface, whereas the parietal pleura lines the costal, diaphragmatic, mediastinal, and cervical regions of the thoracic cavity. Under normal circumstances these membranes slide easily over each other to reduce friction during breathing.

During the development of pleurisy the pleura becomes edematous and congested, an exudate collects on the pleural surface, and cell infiltration occurs. The exudate develops from plasma proteins leaking from damaged vessels. It may be reabsorbed into the fibrous tissue, causing pleural adhesions. The buildup of the fibrinous exudate causes the pleural surfaces to rub roughly together. This causes the audible pleural friction rub.

The pain felt in pleurisy is caused by stretching of the inflamed pleura. The pain is usually felt in the chest wall and occasionally the abdominal wall. If the pleuritic area is along the diaphragm border, pain is referred to the shoulder.[25,42,112]

DIAGNOSTIC STUDIES AND FINDINGS

Diagnostic Test	Findings
Chest x-ray	Limited value in diagnosing pleurisy; diagnostic if fluid accumulates as in pleural effusion
Laboratory tests	
WBC	Increased leukocytes with bronchopulmonary infection
ABGs	Pao_2 <70 mm Hg pH <7.35

COMPLICATIONS

Atelectasis
Empyema

MEDICAL MANAGEMENT

GENERAL MANAGEMENT

Treatment of underlying disease or problem

DRUG THERAPY

Local anesthetics: Paravertebral infiltration of anesthetic to block intercostal nerves.

Narcotic analgesics: Analgesics to relieve discomfort; narcotics such as meperidine (Demerol), 50-75 mg q 4-6 h IM or IV, or morphine, 15 mg q 4-6 h IM, to decrease pain while patient takes deep breaths and coughs.

Analgesic-antipyretics: Acetaminophen (Tylenol), 600 mg q 4-6 h.

1   ASSESS

ASSESSMENT	OBSERVATIONS
Respiratory	Auscultation during late inspiration and early expiration reveals dry rubbing sound (may not occur until 24-36 h after onset of pain); history of pain with deep breath or coughing; with diaphragmatic pleurisy, pain referred to shoulder; respirations rapid and shallow; breath sounds diminished; if pleural effusion develops, pain subsides and fever and dry cough occur
Vital signs	Fever, tachypnea

→ > >

2 DIAGNOSE

NURSING DIAGNOSIS	SUBJECTIVE FINDINGS	OBJECTIVE FINDINGS
Ineffective breathing pattern related to pain on inspiration and expiration	Reports pain on inspiration and on coughing	Dyspnea, tachypnea, shallow respirations, pleural friction rub
Impaired gas exchange related to alveolar-capillary membrane changes secondary to inflammation of the pleura	Complains of SOB	Hypoxia (Pa_{O_2} <70 mm Hg), pleural friction rub, irritability, restlessness
Fear related to development of a secondary pulmonary disease	Expresses fear of never getting well, expresses fear of developing chronic respiratory disease	Scared facial expression

3 PLAN

Patient goals

1. Patient's breathing pattern will be effective without pain.
2. Patient's gas exchange will be improved.
3. Patient's fear will be relieved.
4. Patient will demonstrate understanding of home care and follow-up instructions.

4 IMPLEMENT

NURSING DIAGNOSIS	NURSING INTERVENTIONS	RATIONALE
Ineffective breathing pattern related to pain on inspiration and expiration	Auscultate lungs for rhonchi or crackles and pleural friction rub.	Determines adequacy of breathing pattern.
	Observe changes in respiratory rate/depth.	Determines adequacy of breathing pattern.
	Inspect thorax for symmetry of respiratory movement.	Determines adequacy of breathing pattern.
	Observe breathing pattern for SOB.	Identifies increased work of breathing.
	Review chest x-rays.	Indicates presence of pleural effusion.
	Assess for pain.	Pleural friction rub may cause pain, which would limit inspiration.
	Turn patient at least q 2 h.	Drains secretions by gravity.
	Position patient on affected side.	Optimizes breathing pattern and splints chest.

NURSING DIAGNOSIS	NURSING INTERVENTIONS	RATIONALE
	Encourage patient to cough; assist patient by splinting affected side when coughing.	Facilitates deep breathing and mobilization of secretions to prevent atelectasis and pneumonia.
	Medicate with analgesic without depressing respirations.	Reduces pain that may be interfering with breathing pattern.
	Apply heat to affected area of chest.	Relieves pain by relaxing muscles and increasing circulation; probably stimulates release of endorphins.
Impaired gas exchange related to alveolar-capillary membrane changes secondary to inflammation of the pleura	Auscultate lungs for rhonchi, crackles, and pleural friction rub.	Determines adequacy of gas exchange and detects atelectasis and pleurisy.
	Assess level of consciousness, listlessness, and irritability.	These signs may indicate hypoxia.
	Observe skin color and capillary refill.	Determines circulatory adequacy, which is necessary for gas exchange to tissues.
	Monitor ABGs.	Determines need for oxygen.
	Monitor CBC.	Detects amount of hemoglobin present to carry oxygen and presence of infection.
	Administer oxygen as ordered.	Improves gas exchange; decreases work of breathing.
	Maintain airway patency by splinting chest when helping patient cough or by suction.	Removes secretions that can obstruct gas flow to and from alveoli.
	Pace activities to patient's tolerance.	Decreases oxygen demand.
	Assist patient to Fowler's position.	Optimizes diaphragmatic contraction.
	Assist patient to turn from affected side to back q 2 h.	Facilitates gas exchange, since perfusion of blood is greater on the dependent side.
Fear related to development of a secondary pulmonary disease	Validate source of fear with patient.	Ensures congruence between nurse and patient in trying to resolve fears.
	Assess vital signs.	Determines effect of fear on heart and respiratory rate.
	Encourage patient to discuss contributing factors to fear and actions to allay fear.	Facilitates problem solving; reviews coping skills used in the past.
	Explain pleurisy. Encourage patient to ask questions.	Knowledge can decrease fear.

→ ❯ ❯

NURSING DIAGNOSIS	NURSING INTERVENTIONS	RATIONALE
	Assist patient to use relaxation techniques.	Relieves muscle tension.
	Promote patient's control of situation when possible.	Provides some power and control.
	Accept patient's fears.	Facilitates problem solving, supports therapeutic relationship.
Knowledge deficit	See Patient Teaching.	

5 EVALUATE

PATIENT OUTCOME	DATA INDICATING THAT OUTCOME IS REACHED
Breathing pattern is effective without pain.	Breath sounds are clear with no evidence of pleural friction rub during inspiration or expiration. No pain on inspiration.
Gas exchange is within normal limits for patient.	Pa_{O2} = 80-100 mm Hg Arterial pH = 7.35-7.45 Breath sounds are clear.
Fear is resolved.	Patient discusses fears. Patient is able to describe causative factors for pleurisy.
Learning is demonstrated.	Demonstrates knowledge of home care disease process and compliance with treatment regimen.

PATIENT TEACHING

1. Teach importance of coughing and deep breathing to prevent respiratory infections.

2. Instruct patient on splinting the chest during the cough to decrease the pain.

Empyema

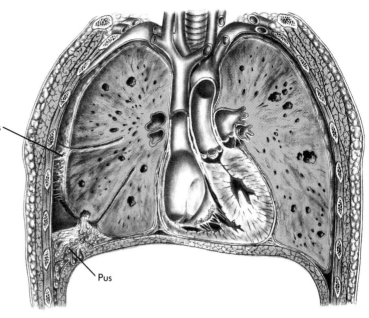

Empyema is the accumulation of infected purulent fluid in the pleural space.

The accumulation of purulent exudate in the pleural cavity may occur in several ways. The most common cause is direct extension from adjacent structures such as occurs in pneumonia, tuberculosis, pulmonary abscess, bronchiectasis, or esophageal rupture. Exudate accumulation may also occur from direct contamination such as that caused by penetrating chest wounds or chest surgery. Empyema is an uncommon but serious disorder that occurs most often in debilitated patients. If identified early and treated promptly with antibiotics, it can usually be controlled.[25,42]

PATHOPHYSIOLOGY

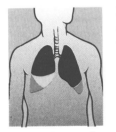

Both kinds of empyema, acute and chronic, may affect a small area of pleura or may involve the entire pleural cavity. In the acute stage the affected area appears inflamed and has a thin layer of exudate with a low leukocyte count. If untreated, the exudate thickens and pus may accumulate. The pleura may thicken, and adhesions may occur. Chronic empyema develops when there are recurrent infections or when treatment of a previous infection was incomplete. Treatment of chronic empyema is difficult because the pleura often becomes thickened and fibrous, and the lung may stick to the chest wall, decreasing ventilation. Pleural fibrosis with secondary limited ventilatory capacity may result. The multiloculated cavities within the pleural space fill with pus and are difficult to drain.[25,42]

COMPLICATIONS

Bronchopleural fistula	Pneumonia
Pneumothorax	

DIAGNOSTIC STUDIES AND FINDINGS

Diagnostic Test	Findings
Chest x-ray	Pleural fluid, usually unilateral, with associated lung lesion
Thoracentesis	Evidence of pus in pleural exudate (because pus is difficult to aspirate, 18-gauge or larger needle must be used)
Laboratory tests	
Laboratory examination of pleural exudate	Odor and general appearance; specific gravity; cell count; Gram stains; aerobic and anaerobic cultures (NOTE: When materials are sent for culture, all air must be expressed from syringe and sample must be quickly transported to laboratory for anaerobic evaluation)
pH of pleural fluid	Of special diagnostic value; fluid collected and analyzed in same manner as for ABGs (using capped, 5 to 10 ml heparinized syringe); pH less than 7.21 suggestive of empyema that necessitates chest tube drainage
ABGs	Pao_2 <70 mm Hg $Paco_2$ and pH would be within normal limits

MEDICAL MANAGEMENT

GENERAL MANAGEMENT

Oxygen support: May be necessary if signs of hypoxia are present.

Irrigation of pleural cavity with sterile solution: Periodically for patient with thoracotomy tube in place to flush out purulent and necrotic materials.

Bed rest: While patient is febrile and has drainage mechanism in process.

DRUG THERAPY

Antiinfective agents: Antibiotic therapy based initially on results of Gram stain; alterations made if necessary when culture results are available.

Fibrinolytic agents: Controversial; recommended by several researchers as method to decrease viscosity of pus and dissolve fibrin clots.

Trypsin (Granulex) as aerosol, 0.1 mg/0.82 ml with balsam of Peru and castor oil; spray bid to debride necrotic areas.

Streptokinase (Kabikinase, Steptase), 100,000 U/h IV over 24-72 h for adults; converts plasminogen to proteolytic enzyme fibrinolysin, which breaks down fibrin clots.

SURGERY

Thoracentesis: May be performed to drain purulent drainage if area is small and localized.

Thoracic drainage: Closed or open drainage system for large areas or quantities of collected pus; if intrapleural fluid and pus are thin and localized, large-diameter thoracotomy tube may be inserted and connected to closed system under water-seal drainage; open drainage possible only if there is no danger of lung collapse when atmospheric pressure enters pleural space; for open drainage, thoracotomy tube exits to room air and is covered with large, absorbent, sterile dressing. See pp. 264-268 for discussion of thoracic drainage systems.

Intrapleural aspiration and instillation of medications: Chest tube may be used to aspirate pleural drainage and as vehicle for instillation of antibiotics and fibrinolytic enzymes.

Thoracotomy: May be necessary for patients not effectively treated by tube drainage system; area with empyema is resected and thickened membrane is stripped by decortication to permit reexpansion of lung.

1 ASSESS

ASSESSMENT	OBSERVATIONS
History	Recent thoracic or abdominal surgery; blunt or penetrating chest trauma; esophageal fistula; lung infections; aspiration; recent thoracentesis; persistent fever despite administration of antibiotics
Physical assessment	
Respiratory	Nasal flaring; tachypnea; decreased chest wall movement; dyspnea; restlessness; decreased breath sounds; paradoxic breathing; dull percussion tone; decreased vital capacity and minute volume; ABGs must be assessed if signs of hypoxia are present
Vital signs	Fever, tachypnea, tachycardia

2 DIAGNOSE

NURSING DIAGNOSIS	SUBJECTIVE FINDINGS	OBJECTIVE FINDINGS
Ineffective breathing pattern related to pain on inspiration and expiration	Complains of SOB	SOB, DOE, tachypnea, labored or irregular breathing, nasal flaring, respiratory depth changes (shallow respirations), paradoxic breathing
Impaired gas exchange related to alveolar-capillary membrane changes secondary to inflammation of the pleura	Complains of SOB	Hypoxia (Pa_{O_2} <70 mm Hg), irritability, restlessness, absent or decreased breath sounds over affected area
Self-care deficit related to chest tube placement and fatigue	Expresses inability to independently perform self-care activities due to chest tubes and drainage container	Requires assistance with bathing, toileting, dressing, and grooming activities

3 PLAN

Patient goals

1. Patient's breathing pattern will be effective without pain.
2. Patient's gas exchange will be improved.
3. Patient will be able to perform self-care activities.
4. Patient will demonstrate understanding of home care and follow-up instructions.

4 IMPLEMENT

NURSING DIAGNOSIS	NURSING INTERVENTIONS	RATIONALE
Ineffective breathing pattern related to pain on inspiration and expiration	Observe changes in respiratory rate and depth.	Determines adequacy of breathing pattern.
	Inspect thorax for symmetry of respiratory movement.	Area affected by empyema does not rise symmetrically on inspiration.
	Observe breathing pattern for SOB, paradoxic breathing, or nasal flaring.	These altered breathing patterns indicate increased work of breathing.
	Review chest x-ray.	Indicates area of lung affected by empyema.
	Maintain chest tube drainage system (refer to care plan for patient with chest tube, p. 266-268).	Removes purulent exudate from the pleural space so that lung can reexpand.
	Position patient in optimal body alignment in semi-Fowler's position for breathing.	Elevating the head of bed moves abdominal contents away from diaphragm to enhance diaphragmatic contraction.

➜ ❯ ❯

NURSING DIAGNOSIS	NURSING INTERVENTIONS	RATIONALE
	Assist patient to use relaxation techniques.	Relieves anxiety, relaxes muscles to reduce tension.
	Encourage use of blow bottles or incentive spirometry.	Requires the patient to deep breathe, which helps to reexpand alveoli and prevents collapse of others.
Impaired gas exchange related to alveolar-capillary membrane changes secondary to inflammation of the pleura	Auscultate lungs for decreased breath sounds.	Determines adequacy of gas exchange and determines area affected by empyema.
	Assess level of consciousness, listlessness, and irritability.	These signs may indicate hypoxia.
	Observe skin color and capillary refill.	Determines circulatory adequacy, which is necessary for gas exchange to cells.
	Monitor ABGs.	Determines need for oxygen.
	Monitor CBC.	Detects amount of hemoglobin present to carry oxygen and presence of infection.
	Monitor changes in activity tolerance.	Activity may induce breathlessness, indicating inadequate oxygen.
	Administer antiinfective agents as ordered.	Interrupts growth of microorganisms.
	Administer oxygen as ordered.	Improves gas exchange; decreases work of breathing.
	Maintain airway patency by assisting the patient to cough or by suctioning.	Removes secretions that can obstruct gas flow to and from alveoli.
	Administer fibrinolytics as ordered.	Decreases viscosity of pus and dissolves fibrin clots of empyema.
	Pace activities to patient's tolerance.	Decreases oxygen demand.
Self-care deficit related to chest tube placement and fatigue	Assess patient's ability to perform self-care activities.	Determines which activities patient can do independently and which require assistance.
	Determine strengths and skills of patient.	Determines how willing and able patient is to perform self-care activities.
	Allow sufficient time for patient to accomplish tasks to fullest ability.	Allows patient to set own pace congruent with limitations.
	Perform self-care activities for patient as needed.	Completes self-care activities that patient cannot perform independently.

NURSING DIAGNOSIS	NURSING INTERVENTIONS	RATIONALE
	Develop an adequate high-protein, high-carbohydrate diet with sufficient fluid intake.	Reduces fatigue, provides energy for activities, promotes healing and provides fluids to liquefy secretions.
Knowledge deficit	See Patient Teaching.	

5 EVALUATE

PATIENT OUTCOME	DATA INDICATING THAT OUTCOME IS REACHED
Breathing pattern is effective without pain.	Breath sounds are clear bilaterally with no evidence of pain during inspiration or expiration.
Gas exchange is within normal limits for patient.	Pa_{O_2} = 80-100 mm Hg Breath sounds are clear.
Patient is able to perform self-care activities.	Performs bathing, dressing, toileting, and grooming activities without assistance.
Learning is demonstrated.	Demonstrates knowledge of home care, disease process, and compliance with treatment regimen.

PATIENT TEACHING

1. Teach the importance of positioning to facilitate ventilatory support, a 60-90 degree angle often is most comfortable.
2. Teach importance of deep breathing and coughing to keep lungs aerated and prevent complications.
3. Instruct patient to report the following symptoms to the physician: difficulty breathing, coughing up foul-smelling sputum, and pain on breathing.
4. If patient goes home with chest tube, teach patient and family to care for chest tube and drainage bottle.
5. Inform patient and family about empyema, that the healing process is slow and that repeated treatments, drainage, irrigation, and chest x-rays may be necessary.

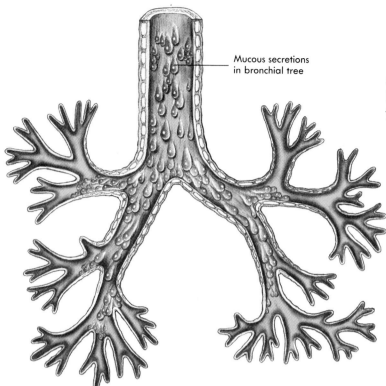

Mucous secretions
in bronchial tree

Acute Bronchitis

Acute bronchitis is an inflammation of the bronchi or trachea or both that results from irritation or infection.

PATHOPHYSIOLOGY

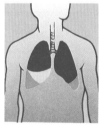

Congestion of the bronchial mucous membranes is the earliest physiologic change. This is followed by desquamation, or shedding, of the submucosa. The congestion and shedding process causes submucosal edema with leukocyte infiltration. This process in turn interferes with the normal function of the ciliated bronchial epithelium and the phagocytes. The result is a sticky or mucopurulent exudate that stays in the bronchi until coughed out.

Because the normally sterile bronchial system is contaminated, bacteria may move in to cause secondary bacterial infection. At the beginning of the disease process the sputum of a patient with acute bronchitis is normally mucoid. If the sputum becomes mucopurulent or purulent, a superimposed bacterial infection can be suspected (Table 5-2).[25,42]

COMPLICATIONS

Pneumonia
Respiratory failure

Acute bronchitis usually heals itself. It is most common in winter. Acute bronchitis may occur alone and also occurs with many chronic diseases such as bronchiectasis, emphysema, or tuberculosis. It may also be linked to systemic illnesses such as chickenpox, measles, and influenza. Once the disease is in process, exposure to air pollutants or physical disabilities such as malnutrition or fatigue may make it worse. If the patient already has a chronic disease such as pulmonary or cardiovascular disease, acute bronchitis may become serious.

In most cases infective acute bronchitis is viral, but bacterial causes (e.g., *Streptococcus pneumoniae*, *Haemophilus influenzae*) are also common. Irritative bronchitis may be caused by dust or fumes, such as from strong acids, ammonia, chlorine, bromide, or smoke.[25,42,75]

DIAGNOSTIC STUDIES AND FINDINGS

DIAGNOSTIC TEST	FINDINGS
Chest x-ray	Clear; no evidence of lung consolidation
Laboratory tests	
ABGs	Pao_2 <70 mm Hg
	$Paco_2$ >45 mm Hg
	pH <7.35
WBC count	Leukocytosis

Table 5-2

AGENTS COMMONLY CAUSING ACUTE BRONCHITIS AND PNEUMONITIS

Product	Industry	Injury
Aldehydes (acrylaldehyde, formaldehyde, and acetaldehydes)	Plastic, rubber, textiles, resins, disinfectants	Bronchitis, asthma
Ammonia	Fertilizer, explosives, refrigeration	Tracheobronchitis, pulmonary edema
Chlorine and hydrochloric acid	Bleaches, disinfectants, plastics, refining, dye making, organic chemical synthesis	Tracheobronchitis, pulmonary edema
Nitrogen dioxide	Fertilizer, dyes, explosives, farming, rockets, arc welding	Tracheobronchitis, pulmonary edema, bronchiolitis obliterans
Ozone	Arc welding, sewage and water treatment	Tracheobronchitis
Phosgene	Chemical industry, dyes, insecticides	Tracheobronchitis, pulmonary edema
Sulfur dioxide	Bleaching, smelting, paper manufacture, refrigeration	Tracheobronchitis, pulmonary edema (rare)

From Cherniack.[25]

MEDICAL MANAGEMENT

The goals of the treatment plan are to provide supportive therapy during the course of the self-limited disease and to prevent secondary infections.

GENERAL MANAGEMENT

Increase in fluid intake—up to 4000 ml/day to liquefy secretions and maintain hydration. Steam or cool mist vaporizer to humidify air surrounding patient.

DRUG THERAPY

Antitussive agents: Cough suppressants (use with extreme caution in patients with chronic lung disease): Hydrocodone bitartrate (Codone, Dicodid, Hycodan), 5-10 mg tid or qid; Codeine phosphate (tablets and in mixture form in numerous syrups), 10-20 mg q 4-6 h.

Nonnarcotic analgesic agents: Many agents available; following is incomplete list: dextromethorphan (Romilar, Benylin CM, Pertussin, Congespirin), 10-20 mg q 4 h or 30 mg q 6-8 h; noscapine (Tusscapine, Narcotine), 15-30 mg tid or qid; levopropoxyphene napsylate (Novrad), 50-100 mg q 4-6 h.

Bronchodilators: Terbutaline (Brethine, Bricanyl), 2.5-5 mg tid; theophylline (Aerolate, Theolair, Slo-Phyllin, Theo-Dur, Bronkodyl, Elixophyllin, others); dosage highly individualized based on serum theophylline levels; therapeutic level 10-20 μg/ml; 200-250 mg q 6 h or 1-2 timed-release preparations q 8-12 h (3.5-5 mg/kg).

Antiinfective agents: Antibiotics given when superimposed respiratory infection is suspected on basis of clinical evidence such as purulent sputum, high fever, and ill-appearing patient; antibiotics also indicated for patients with chronic obstructive lung disease. Doxycycline (Vibramycin), oxytetracycline (Terramycin), others, 250-500 mg PO qid; Ampicillin (Amcill, Omnipen, others), 250-500 mg PO qid.

Antipyretic-analgesics: To reduce fever and relieve malaise.

1 ASSESS

ASSESSMENT	OBSERVATIONS
Respiratory	Cough initially dry and nonproductive but may produce mucoid sputum within a few days; if cause is bacterial, midsternal chest pain, malaise, sore throat, diffuse crackles and rhonchi throughout chest; if patient already has chronic lung disease, sputum may change from clear to thin to thick to tenacious or purulent
Vital signs	Low-grade fever (38.3° to 38.9° [101° to 102° F]) Tachypnea Normal pulse and blood pressure

2 DIAGNOSE

NURSING DIAGNOSIS	SUBJECTIVE FINDINGS	OBJECTIVE FINDINGS
Ineffective airway clearance related to mucopurulent sputum	Complains of difficulty breathing	Cough (may be productive or nonproductive), crackles and rhonchi, labored breathing, fever, dyspnea
Ineffective breathing pattern related to inflammatory process and pain	Complains of SOB	Dyspnea, tachypnea, shallow respirations, cough, midsternal chest pain
Activity intolerance related to generalized weakness	Complains of fatigue and SOB	SOB during activity, decreased activity level

3 PLAN

Patient goals

1. Patient's airways will be patent.
2. Patient's breathing pattern will be effective without pain.
3. Patient will be able to perform usual activities without fatigue or dyspnea.
4. Patient will demonstrate understanding of home care and follow-up instructions.

4 IMPLEMENT

NURSING DIAGNOSIS	NURSING INTERVENTIONS	RATIONALE
Ineffective airway clearance related to mucopurulent sputum	Auscultate lungs for rhonchi and crackles.	Determines adequacy of gas exchange and extent of airway obstructed with secretions.
	Assess characteristics of secretions: quantity, color, consistency, odor.	Presence of infection is suspected when sputum is thick, yellow or green, and foul-smelling.

NURSING DIAGNOSIS	NURSING INTERVENTIONS	RATIONALE
	Assess patient's hydration status: skin turgor, mucous membranes, tongue, intake and output over 24 h, Hct	Determines need for fluids. Fluids needed if skin turgor is poor, tongue and mucous membranes are dry, intake < output, and/ or Hct is elevated.
	Assist patient with ambulation/position changes (turning side to side).	Secretions move by gravity as position changes.
	Increase room humidification.	Humidifies and thins secretions to facilitate their expectoration.
	Administer expectorants/bronchodilators as ordered.	Dilates bronchi to reduce work of breathing and facilitates mobilization of secretions.
	Administer antitussives.	Suppresses coughing; used when cough is nonproductive, is interfering with sleep, and is fatiguing for patient.
	Administer antiinfective agents.	Interrupts growth of microorganisms.
	Assist patient in using blow bottles, incentive spirometry.	Requires deep breathing to expand alveoli.
	Encourage increased fluid intake to 2 1/2 to 4 L/day unless contraindicated.	Liquefies secretions so that they are easier to expectorate.
	Assist patient with oral hygiene as needed.	Removes taste of secretions.
Ineffective breathing pattern related to inflammatory process and pain	Observe changes in respiratory rate and depth.	Determines adequacy of breathing pattern.
	Inspect thorax for symmetry of respiratory movement.	Determines adequacy of breathing pattern.
	Monitor ABGs.	Determines need for oxygen.
	Assess for pain.	Pain often is a causative factor that limits inhalation.
	Administer antiinfective agents.	Interrupts growth of microorganisms.
	Administer oxygen as ordered.	Improves gas exchange and decreases work of breathing.
	Medicate with analgesic without depressing respirations.	Reduces pain that may be interfering with breathing.
	Assist patient to use relaxation techniques.	Relieves anxiety and muscle tensions.

→ > >

NURSING DIAGNOSIS	NURSING INTERVENTIONS	RATIONALE
Activity intolerance related to generalized weakness	Observe response to activity.	Determines extent of tolerance.
	Assess patient's sleep patterns.	Lack of sleep may contribute to fatigue.
	Plan rest periods between activities.	Reduces fatigue.
	Perform activities for patient until patient is able to perform them.	Meets patient's need without causing fatigue.
	Provide progressive increase in activity as tolerated.	Gradually increasing activity fosters maximum independence without causing weakness.
	Keep frequently used objects within reach.	Provides convenient use for patient; decreases oxygen demand.
Knowledge deficit	See Patient Teaching.	

5 EVALUATE

PATIENT OUTCOME	DATA INDICATING THAT OUTCOME IS REACHED
Airway is patent.	Airways are clear and breathing occurs without obstruction. Breath sounds are clear.
Breathing pattern is effective without pain.	Arterial blood gases are within normal limits. Pa_{O2} = 80-100 mm Hg Pa_{CO2} = 35-45 mm Hg pH = 7.35-7.45
Patient performs usual activities without fatigue or dyspnea.	Patient performs self-care activities.
Learning is demonstrated.	Patient demonstrates knowledge of home care, disease process, and compliance with treatment regimen.

PATIENT TEACHING

1. Teach importance of drinking at least 2 quarts of fluids each day to help liquefy secretions.
2. Teach the importance of not smoking and of avoiding fumes or smoke when the disease is active.
3. Teach the importance of rest during the day in addition to a full night's sleep.
4. Instruct about the prescribed medications, including the name, dosage, action, frequency of administration, and side effects.
5. Inform the patient to avoid people with respiratory infections.
6. Teach the signs of secondary infection to report to the physician, such as a change in sputum characteristics or prolonged fever.

Lung Abscess

A lung abscess is a circum-scribed, suppurative inflammation followed by central necrosis.

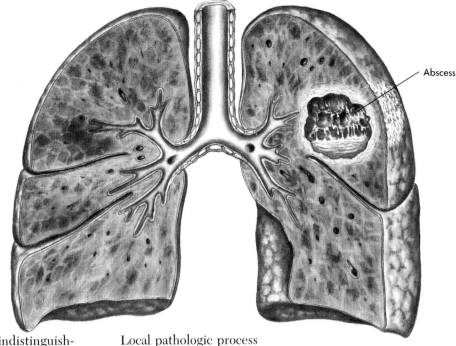

Abscess

In the early stages a lung abscess is indistinguishable from any localized pneumonitis. Only after a lung abscess has communicated with a bronchus and started to drain can the characteristic air-fluid level be seen on chest x-ray with the area of inflammation.[24]

The incidence of lung abscess has dropped significantly because of the availability of effective antibiotics and the increased willingness of people to seek medical care. Lung abscesses are generally caused by aspiration of infected material, which may occur during unconsciousness, general anesthesia, drunkenness, near-drowning, diabetic coma, or drug sedation. It can also occur as a result of poor oral hygiene, gum disease, infected tonsils, or aspiration of food. Bronchial carcinoma (squamous cell type) is also considered to be a common cause of lung abscess for male smokers over 55 years of age. Other less common causes of lung abscess include septic pulmonary emboli and abscess transfers from the liver. The following are predisposing factors.[25,77]

Massive inoculum
  Aspiration*
    Stupor, coma, seizure, intoxication
    Anesthesia
    Laryngeal dysfunction
  Dental and gingival infection*
  Hematogenous dissemination
    Intravenous drug abuse
    Right-sided endocarditis
    Septic phlebitis
    Osteomyelitis or other specific focus

Local pathologic process
  Obstructing neoplasm
  Foreign body
  Distortion by fibrosis
  Bronchostenosis
  Cysts, bullae
  Sequestration
  Contusion or trauma
  Gastric acid
Necrotizing vascular disorders
  Embolic infarction
  Vasculitis (Wegener's, rheumatoid arthritis, poly-arteritis)
  Necrosis within neoplasm
  Necrotizing conglomerate pneumoconiosis
  Chronic eosinophilic pneumonia
Impaired host resistance
  Alcoholism*
  Diabetes
  Chronic debilitating disease
  Malnutrition*
  Impaired humoral resistance
    Leukopenia
    Hypoglobulinemia
  Impaired tissue-mediated immunity
    Acquired immunodeficiency syndrome
    Radiation exposure
    Chemotherapy
    Steroid therapy
    Neoplasia; Hodgkin's disease, lymphomas

*Circumstances commonly associated with primary lung abscess.

PATHOPHYSIOLOGY

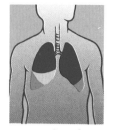

The site of the abscess is determined by the body's position at the time of the inhalation. The aspirated material moves to the most dependent position in the lung. Once it has settled, a fibrous granulation tissue forms around it and embeds itself in the parenchyma.

As the abscess develops, it fills with pus. Pressure develops, and the infected tissue ruptures into the bronchus. Drainage of foul-smelling, pus-filled, or bloody sputum results. The expectoration of purulent sputum may lead to partial healing and cavity formation. However, if the cavity does not drain adequately, small abscesses may form within the lung. The following is a partial list of etiologic organisms.[25]

Pyogenic aerobic bacteria
  Staphylococcus aureus
  Gram-negative bacilli (*Klebsiella*, *Proteus*, and others)
  Streptococcus pneumoniae
  Group A streptococci
  Legionella
Pyogenic anaerobes*
  Fusobacterium nucleatum and other species
  Bacteroides melaninogenicus, *B. fragilis*, and other species
  Peptostreptococci
  Treponema macrodentium
  Nocardia

Mycobacteria—*M. tuberculosis, M. kansasii, M. intracellulare,* and other species
Fungi
  Histoplasma
  Coccidioides
  Blastomyces
  Actinomyces
  Sporothrix
  Aspergillus
  Cryptococcus
  Phycomycetes
Parasites
  Entamoeba histolytica
  Paragonimus
  Echinococcus

COMPLICATIONS

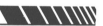

Pleural effusion
Empyema
Bloodstream dissemination, e.g., to the brain
Fatal pulmonary hemorrhage

*Primary lung abscess is caused by combinations of these anaerobes with *S. viridans*, *Neisseria* species, and other normal oral flora.

DIAGNOSTIC STUDIES AND FINDINGS

Diagnostic Test	Findings
Chest x-ray	Initially, lobar consolidation, which becomes globular as disease progresses; rupture of consolidation causes fluid level, which indicates communication with bronchus; when fluid level is apparent, diagnosis can be narrowed to either empyema with a bronchopleural fistula or a lung abscess
Laboratory tests	
WBC count	Leukocytosis common
Laboratory examination of pleural exudate	Odor and general appearance; specific gravity; cell count; Gram stains; aerobic and anaerobic cultures to determine infective organisms; therapeutic intervention based on agent identification (NOTE: When material is sent for culture, all air must be expressed from syringe and sample must be quickly transported to laboratory for an aerobic evaluation)
Bronchoscopy	Unnecessary if x-ray shows rapid resolution of abscess but may be needed to verify presence of abscess or determine its severity if patient's condition does not improve

MEDICAL MANAGEMENT

The ability of the lung abscess to heal depends primarily on its ability to drain adequately through the bronchus. With free drainage, resolution occurs. Without free drainage, and without prompt antibiotic therapy, the abscess may become chronic.

GENERAL MANAGEMENT

Postural drainage: Extremely important to drain abscess (see pp. 235-239 for techniques).

Percussion: To loosen secretions and enhance their removal.

DRUG THERAPY

Antiinfective agents

Antibiotic therapy directed at causative agent; should be monitored and perhaps changed, depending on patient's clinical response; should begin as soon as initial sputum specimens have been collected; drug of choice while awaiting test results is penicillin G, 1.2 million U PO qid, or 300,000-600,000 U IM q 6-8 h; if after 4-7 days patient is not improved and specific organisms are still not identified, medication may be changed to tetracycline (Achromycin, others), 500 mg PO qid; antibiotic therapy continued until all signs of abscess are resolved on serial chest roentgenograms.

SURGERY

Bronchoscopy: Occasionally necessary to remove thick, tenacious sputum.

Pulmonary resection: Necessary in rare cases if lung abscess does not respond to antibiotic therapy; single lesions removed by lobectomy and multiple lesions removed by pneumonectomy.

1   ASSESS

ASSESSMENT	OBSERVATIONS
Respiratory	Initial signs resembling pneumonia; cough producing bloody, purulent, foul-smelling sputum; general malaise; sporadic fever; pleuritic pain; dyspnea if abscess is large; dull percussion tone; decreased or absent breath sounds over abscess area; pleural friction rub; if abscess left untreated and becomes chronic, auscultation may detect only fine crackles or rhonchi; hypertrophic pulmonary osteoarthropathy (clubbing)
Nutritional	May be weight loss and anemia; anorexia
Vital signs	Fever, tachycardia
Psychosocial	Concern that there is infection that must be treated for extended period

→ > >

2 DIAGNOSE

NURSING DIAGNOSIS	SUBJECTIVE FINDINGS	OBJECTIVE FINDINGS
Ineffective airway clearance related to mucopurulent sputum	Reports difficulty breathing	Cough (may be productive or non-productive), crackles and rhonchi, fever, dyspnea
Ineffective breathing pattern related to inflammatory process and pleuritic pain	Reports SOB; pain when breathing	Dyspnea, shallow respirations, cough, pleural friction rub
Altered nutrition: less than body requirements related to anorexia and dyspnea	Reports inadequate intake and anorexia, complains of SOB	Weight loss, inadequate food and fluid intake
Activity intolerance related to generalized weakness	Complains of fatigue and SOB	SOB during activity, decreased activity level
Ineffective individual coping related to long-term therapy required	Expresses concern about infection requiring extended treatment and how home and work responsibilities will be managed	

3 PLAN

Patient goals

1. Patient's airways will be patent.
2. Patient's breathing pattern will be effective without pain.
3. Patient's nutritional status will be improved.
4. Patient will be able to perform usual activities without fatigue or dyspnea.
5. Patient will devise ways of coping with this illness.
6. Patient will demonstrate understanding of home care and follow-up instructions.

4 IMPLEMENT

NURSING DIAGNOSIS	NURSING INTERVENTIONS	RATIONALE
Ineffective airway clearance related to mucopurulent sputum	Auscultate lungs for rhonchi and crackles.	Determines adequacy of gas exchange and extent of airway obstructed with secretions.
	Assess characteristics of secretions: quantity, color, consistency, odor.	Presence of infection is suspected when secretions are thick, yellow, and/or foul-smelling.
	Assess patient's hydration status: skin turgor, mucous membranes, tongue, intake and output over 24 h, Hct.	Determines need for fluids. Fluids needed if skin turgor is poor, tongue and mucous membranes are dry, intake < output, and/or hematocrit is elevated.

NURSING DIAGNOSIS	NURSING INTERVENTIONS	RATIONALE
	Monitor chest x-rays.	Shows extent and location of lung involvement.
	Assist patient with coughing as needed.	Coughing removes secretions.
	Assist patient with ambulation/position changes (turning side to side).	Secretions move by gravity as position changes.
	Increase room humidification.	Humidifies and thins secretions to facilitate their expectoration.
	Perform chest physiotherapy (e.g., percussion, vibration) and postural drainage.	Applying percussion and vibration to the chest loosens secretions so they can be expectorated.
	Assist patient in using blow bottles, incentive spirometry.	Requires deep breathing to expand alveoli.
	Administer antiinfective agents as ordered.	Interrupts growth of microorganisms.
	Avoid suppressing cough reflex unless cough is frequent and nonproductive.	Cough reflex needed to mobilize secretions but excessive nonproductive coughing leads to fatigue.
	Encourage increased fluid intake to 1 1/2 to 2 L/day unless contraindicated.	Liquefies secretions so that they are easier to expectorate.
	Assist patient with oral hygiene as needed.	Removes taste of secretions.
Ineffective breathing pattern related to inflammatory process and pleuritic pain	Auscultate lungs for pleural friction rub.	Pleural friction rub produces pain during respiration.
	Observe changes in respiratory rate and depth.	Determines adequacy of breathing pattern.
	Inspect thorax for symmetry of respiratory movement.	Determines adequacy of breathing pattern.
	Review chest x-rays.	Indicates severity of lung involvement and location of consolidation.
	Assess for pleuritic pain.	Pleuritic pain during respiration prevents the patient from breathing deeply.
	Position patient in optimal body alignment in semi-Fowler's position for breathing.	Elevating head of bed moves abdominal contents away from the diaphragm to enhance diaphragmatic contraction.
	Assist patient to splint chest when coughing.	Facilitates deep breathing and mobilization of secretions.
	Medicate with analgesic without depressing respirations.	Analgesics reduce pain that may be interfering with breathing pattern.

NURSING DIAGNOSIS	NURSING INTERVENTIONS	RATIONALE
Altered nutrition: less than body requirements related to anorexia and dyspnea	Assess dietary habits and needs.	Helps to individualize the diet.
	Weigh patient weekly.	Improved nutrition will result in weight gain.
	Auscultate bowel sounds.	Documents presence of gastrointestinal peristalsis needed for digestion.
	Assess psychologic factors, e.g., depression, that might decrease food and fluid intake.	Identifies effect of psychologic factors on food intake.
	Monitor albumin and lymphocytes.	These lab values indicate adequate visceral protein, which is low when nutrition is inadequate.
	Measure midarm circumference.	This measurement indicates protein stores needed for tissue healing and to support immune system.
	Measure triceps skin fold.	This measurement indicates fat stores.
	Provide oxygen while eating as ordered.	Oxygen reduces dyspnea during meals so that more food may be eaten.
	Encourage oral care before meals.	Removes taste of sputum that may reduce appetite.
	Provide foods in appropriate consistency for eating. Soft or liquid foods may be preferred.	Requires less energy to eat soft foods and liquids, thereby reducing oxygen requirement.
	Provide high-protein diet.	Supports immune system to fight infection.
	Administer vitamins as ordered.	Supplements diet and promotes healing.
Activity intolerance related to generalized weakness	Observe response to activity.	Determines extent of tolerance.
	Identify factors contributing to intolerance, e.g., stress, side effects of drugs.	Eliminating contributing factors may resolve activity intolerance.
	Assess patient's sleep patterns.	Lack of sleep may contribute to weakness.
	Plan rest periods between activities.	Reduces fatigue.
	Encourage use of adaptive breathing techniques during activity.	Decreases work of breathing.
	Perform activities for patient until patient is able to perform them.	Meets patient's need without causing fatigue.

NURSING DIAGNOSIS	NURSING INTERVENTIONS	RATIONALE
	Provide progressive increase in activity as tolerated.	Gradually increases independence without causing weakness.
	Keep frequently used items within reach.	Provides convenient use of items for patient; decreases oxygen demand.
Ineffective individual coping related to long-term therapy required	Assess patient's psychologic status, e.g., fearful, anxious, angry, depressed.	Determines the patient's present feelings.
	Identify significant other from whom patient derives support.	Gives information about which persons are available to assist the patient with coping.
	Assess ability to understand events, provide realistic appraisal of situation.	Patient's perception about lung abscess will affect coping.
	Encourage patient to verbalize fears, anxieties, depression, and anger.	Talking about feelings is the first step in coping with disease state; begins problem-solving process.
	Assist patient to use problem-solving method to select methods of coping.	Guides patient through a process that can assist coping.
	Validate information by reflecting back what was heard.	Identifies inaccuracies, provides feedback for the patient.
Knowledge deficit	See Patient Teaching.	

5 EVALUATE

PATIENT OUTCOME	DATA INDICATING THAT OUTCOME IS REACHED
Airway is patent.	Airways are clear and breathing occurs without obstruction. Breath sounds are clear. Chest x-ray is clear. Cough has subsided. Temperature is normal for patient.
Breathing pattern is effective without pain.	Cough has subsided. Effective, rhythmic, symmetrical breathing pattern without pain.
Nutritional status has improved.	Patient experiences weight gain. Patient is eating a balanced diet with fluid intake of at least 2,500 ml. Albumin = 3.2-4.5 g/dl Lymphocytes = 2100 or 35-40% per ml^3 blood Triceps skinfold = 12.0 mm men; 23.0 mm women Midarm circumference = 32.7 cm men; 29.2 cm women
Performs usual activities without fatigue or dyspnea.	Patient performs self-care activities without fatigue or dyspnea.

→ > >

NURSING DIAGNOSIS	DATA INDICATING THAT OUTCOME IS REACHED
Identifies useful coping strategies.	Patient plans who will be responsible for household duties, for assisting patient with treatments, etc. Patient identifies coping strategies to be used when needed.
Learning is demonstrated.	Patient demonstrates knowledge of home care, disease process and compliance with treatment regimen.

PATIENT TEACHING

1. Teach importance of positioning to facilitate abscess drainage.
2. Teach effective coughing techniques that facilitate expectoration without tiring patient.
3. Teach the importance of deep breathing and coughing to keep the lung aerated and to prevent secondary complications.
4. Instruct about taking prescribed medications, including the name, dosage, action, frequency of administration, and side effects.
5. Provide the patient and family with information regarding lung abscess and the treatment protocol, which may last as long as 6-8 weeks.
6. Teach the importance of frequent oral hygiene, especially as long as there is active lung drainage.
7. Teach methods to reduce the chances of a lung abscess in the future, such as good oral hygiene, avoidance of aspiration, and prompt treatment for potential bacterial infections of the mouth or respiratory tract.

Influenza

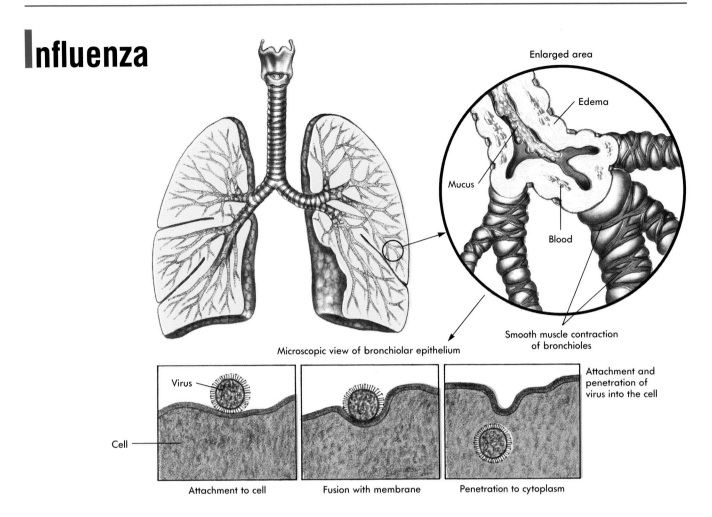

Enlarged area

Edema

Mucus

Blood

Smooth muscle contraction
of bronchioles

Microscopic view of bronchiolar epithelium

Attachment and
penetration of
virus into the cell

Virus

Cell

Attachment to cell

Fusion with membrane

Penetration to cytoplasm

Influenza is a generalized, acute, febrile disease associated with upper and lower respiratory infection: it is characterized by a severe and protracted cough, fever, headache, myalgia, prostration, coryza, and mild sore throat. The disease may be clinically unrecognizable from the common cold.

PATHOPHYSIOLOGY

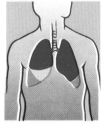

Influenza viruses A, B, or C, each with many mutagenic strains, are inhaled in aerosolized mucus droplets shed from infected persons. The viruses are deposited on and penetrate the surface of upper respiratory tract mucosal cells, producing cell lysis and destruction of the ciliated epithelium. Viral neuraminidase decreases the viscosity of the mucosa, thus facilitating the spread of virus-containing exudate to the lower respiratory tract. An interstitial inflammation and necrosis of the bronchiolar and alveolar epithelium result, filling the alveoli with an exudate containing leukocytes, erythrocytes,

and hyaline membrane.[99] It is difficult to control influenza because surface cell antigens of the virus have a capacity to change.[10] Immunity to influenza A virus is mediated by type specific secretory immunoglobulin A (IgA) in the nasal secretions. Circulating IgG is also highly effective at neutralizing the virus. Stimulation of IgG is the basis of immunization with inactivated influenza A vaccine.[10]

Regeneration of epithelium, following necrosis and desquamation, slowly begins after the fifth day of illness. Regeneration reaches a maximum within 9 to 15 days, at which time mucus production and cilia begin to appear. Before complete regeneration the compromised epithelium is prone to secondary bacterial invasion, resulting in bacterial pneumonia usually caused by S. *aureus*.[99]

The disease is usually self-limiting. Acute symptoms last 2 to 7 days and are followed by a convalescent period of about a week. The disease is important because of its cyclic epidemic and pandemic nature and because of the high mortality associated with pulmonary complications resulting from secondary bacterial pneumonia. This risk is highest in elderly and chronically diseased persons.[99]

See the chain of events in the spread of Influenza in Table 5-3.

COMPLICATIONS

Influenza A—pneumonia
Influenza B—Reye's syndrome

Table 5-3

CHAIN OF EVENTS IN THE SPREAD OF INFLUENZA

Occurrence	Worldwide in pandemics, epidemics, localized outbreaks, and sporadic cases; highest in winter in temperate zones
Etiologic agent	Three types of viruses (A, B, and C), each with many strains
Reservoir	Humans; some mammals suspected as sources of new strains of viruses
Transmission	Direct transmission by inhalation of virus in airborne mucus discharge
Incubation period	24-72 h
Period of communicability	3 days from onset of symptoms
Susceptibility and resistance	Universal; infection produces immunity to a specific strain of virus, but the duration of immunity depends on the antigenic drift in the strain
Report to local health authority	Mandatory case report

From Grimes[99]

DIAGNOSTIC STUDIES AND FINDINGS

Diagnostic Test	Findings
Laboratory tests	
Tissue culture of nasal or pharyngeal secretions	Positive for influenza virus
Sputum culture	Positive for bacteria in secondary infections
Fluorescent antibody staining of secretions	Positive for influenza virus
Hemagglutination inhibition or complement fixation tests	Fourfold increase in antibody titer between acute and convalescent stages
Sedimentation rate elevated	Erythrocyte
Urinalysis	Albuminuria
WBC count	Leukopenia (<5,000 mm^3) or slight leukocytosis (11,000-15,000 mm^3)
Hemoglobin	Elevated
Hematocrit	Elevated

MEDICAL MANAGEMENT

GENERAL MANAGEMENT

Oxygen and IV fluid and electrolytes for complications. Cool mist for congestion.

DRUG THERAPY

Agent-specific antiinfective agents for bacterial complications or for patients with chronic pulmonary disease.

Antipyretics: ASA, 600 mg orally q 4 h for adults; Acetaminophen for children.

Adrenergic agents: Phenylephrine (Neo-Synephrine), 0.25%, 2 drops in each nostril for nasal congestion.

Antitussive agents: Terpin hydrate with codeine, 5-10 ml PO q 3-4 h for adults for cough.

Amantadine (Symmetrel), 100 mg PO bid for duration of epidemic (3-6 weeks) for high-risk persons over the age of 9 years for prevention; 2-4 mg/lb/day (not exceeding 150 mg/day in two or three doses for young children); 100 mg/d PO for persons over the age of 65 years.) (Dosage to be reduced further for persons with impaired renal function.)

Vaccine, 0.5 ml IM for adults; 0.25 ml IM for infants 6-35 months; 0.5 ml IM for children 3-12 years; for infants and children give two doses at 4-week intervals; must be repeated yearly in the fall for viral strain expected in the winter; recommended for elderly individuals, chronically ill adults, children with chronic heart or pulmonary disease, residents of nursing homes and chronic care facilities, and health care providers with contact with high-risk patients.

1   ASSESS

ASSESSMENT	OBSERVATIONS
Head and neck	Conjunctivitis may be present Flushed face Anterior cervical lymphadenopathy may be present Headache, photophobia, and retrobulbar aching
Respiratory	Mild at first: sore throat; substernal burning; nonproductive cough; coryza Later: severe and productive cough; erythema of soft palate, posterior hard palate, tonsillar pillars, and posterior pharynx; increased respiratory rate, rhonchi, crackles
Abdominal	Anorexia
Neurologic	Myalgia, particularly in back and legs
Vital signs	Sudden-onset fever (38° to 39° C <102° to 103° F) that gradually falls and rises again on the third day

→ > >

2 DIAGNOSE

NURSING DIAGNOSIS	SUBJECTIVE FINDINGS	OBJECTIVE FINDINGS
Ineffective airway clearance related to bronchial obstruction		Rhonchi, crackles (rales), tachypnea, cough (non-productive at first, then productive), fever
Fever volume deficit related to hyperthermia and inadequate intake	Complains of thirst and anorexia	Hyperthermia (38° to 39° C; 102° to 103° F), flushed face; warm, dry skin; dry mucous membranes and tongue; decreased urine output, concentrated urine; weight loss
Activity intolerance related to generalized weakness	Reports myalgia, fatigue, headache, and photophobia	Decreased activity level
Hyperthermia related to inflammatory process	Reports feeling hot	Elevated body temperature (38° to 39° C; 102° to 103° F); skin warm and dry

3 PLAN

Patient goals

1. Patient's airway will be patent with clear breath sounds.
2. Patient's fluid volume will be adequate.
3. Patient will be able to perform daily activities without weakness.
4. Patient's body temperature will be within normal limits.
5. Patient will demonstrate understanding of home care and follow-up instructions.

4 IMPLEMENT

NURSING DIAGNOSIS	NURSING INTERVENTIONS	RATIONALE
Ineffective airway clearance related to bronchial obstruction	Auscultate lungs for rhonchi and crackles.	Determines adequacy of gas exchange and extent of airway obstructed with secretions.
	Assess characteristics of secretions: quantity, color, consistency, odor.	Presence of infection is suspected when secretions are thick, yellow and/or foul-smelling.
	Assess patient's hydration status: skin turgor, mucous membranes, tongue, intake and output over 24 h, hematocrit.	Determines need for fluids. Fluids needed if skin turgor is poor, tongue and mucous membranes are dry, intake < output, and/or hematocrit is elevated.
	Monitor sputum Gram stain and culture and sensitivity reports if sputum becomes purulent.	Identifies microorganisms present and appropriate antiinfective agents needed.
	Assist patient with coughing as needed.	Coughing removes secretions.

NURSING DIAGNOSIS	NURSING INTERVENTIONS	RATIONALE
	Position patient in proper body alignment for optimal breathing pattern (head of bed up 45°, if tolerated up to 90°).	Secretions move by gravity as position changes. Elevating head of bed moves abdominal contents away from diaphragm to enhance diaphragmatic contraction.
	Keep environment allergen-free (e.g., dust, feathers, smoke) according to individual needs.	Prevents allergic reactions caused by bronchial irritation.
	Assist patient with ambulation/position changes (turning side to side)	Secretions move by gravity as position changes.
	Increase with cool mist room humidification.	Humidifies and thins secretions to facilitate their expectoration.
	Administer decongestants (Neo-Synephrine) as ordered.	Facilitates breathing through nose and prevents drying of oral mucous membranes.
	Encourage increased fluid intake to 1 1/2 to 2 L/day unless contraindicated.	Liquefies secretions so that they are easier to expectorate.
	Assist patient with oral hygiene as needed.	Removes taste of secretions and moistens oral mucous membranes.
Fluid volume deficit related to hyperthermia and inadequate intake	Weigh patient.	Detects fluid gain or loss.
	Measure intake and output of fluids.	Provides data on fluid balance.
	Assess skin turgor.	Skin remains tented due to inadequate interstitial fluid.
	Observe consistency of sputum.	Thick sputum indicates need for fluid.
	Observe urine concentration.	Concentrated urine may indicate fluid deficit.
	Monitor hemoglobin and hematocrit.	Elevations may indicate hemoconcentration due to fluid deficit.
	Observe tongue and mucous membranes.	Dryness indicates fluid deficit.
	Encourage oral fluids and administer intravenous fluids as ordered.	Replaces fluids lost from sweating associated with fever. Fluids needed to liquefy secretions.
	Assist patient to identify ways to prevent fluid deficit.	May prevent recurrence and involves patient in care.

NURSING DIAGNOSIS	NURSING INTERVENTIONS	RATIONALE
Activity intolerance related to generalized weakness	Observe response to activity.	Determines extent of tolerance.
	Identify factors contributing to activity intolerance, e.g., fever, side effects of drugs.	Eliminating contributing factors may resolve activity intolerance.
	Assess patient's sleep patterns.	Lack of sleep may contribute to weakness.
	Plan rest periods between activities.	Reduces fatigue.
	Perform activities for patient until patient is able to perform them.	Meets patient's need without causing fatigue.
	Provide progressive increase in activity as tolerated.	Gradually increasing activity fosters maximum independence without causing weakness.
	Keep frequently used items within reach.	Provides convenient use of items for patient; decreases oxygen demand.
Hyperthermia related to inflammatory process	Measure body temperature.	Indicates if a fever exists and its extent.
	Assess skin temperature and color.	Warm, dry, flushed skin may indicate a fever.
	Monitor WBC count.	Leukopenia indicates need to protect patient from additional infection. Leukocytosis indicates an inflammatory and/or infectious process are present.
	Measure intake and output.	Determines fluid balance and need to increase intake.
	Encourage fluid intake orally or intravenously as ordered.	Replaces fluids lost by insensible loss and perspiration.
	Administer antipyretics as ordered.	Reduces fever through action on the hypothalamus.
	Provide/encourage frequent oral hygiene.	Maintains moist mucous membranes.
	Increase air circulation in the room with a fan.	Facilitates heat loss by convection.
	Give a tepid sponge bath.	Facilitates heat loss by evaporation.
	Apply an ice bag covered with a towel to the axilla and/or groin.	Facilitates heat loss by conduction.
	Cover the patient with a sheet only.	Prevents chilling; shivering will further increase the metabolic rate.
	Place patient on a hypothermia blanket as ordered.	Facilitates heat loss by conduction.
Knowledge deficit	See Patient Teaching.	

5 EVALUATE

PATIENT OUTCOME	DATA INDICATING THAT OUTCOME IS REACHED
Airway is patent.	Airways are clear and breathing occurs without obstruction. There is no cough. Breath sounds are clear.
Fluid volume is within normal limits.	Fluid intake has increased. Skin is moist. Oral mucous membranes are moist. Hemoglobin = 15.5 ± 1.1 g/dl for men 13.7 ± 1.0 g/dl for women Hematocrit = 42%-50% for men, 35%-47% for women Urine output is normal with normal concentration. No albuminuria.
Usual activities are performed without fatigue or discomfort.	Patient demonstrates ability to perform usual daily activities without fatigue or discomfort. Energy returns.
Temperature is within normal limits.	Normal body temperature 38° C (98.6° F).
Learning is demonstrated.	Demonstrates knowledge of self-care management, disease process, compliance with treatment regimen, and how to prevent recurrence.

PATIENT TEACHING

1. Encourage patient to maintain bed rest for 2-3 days after temperature returns to normal.
2. Teach importance of drinking at least 2 quarts of fluids daily to keep secretions thin so that they can be expectorated.
3. Instruct patient to notify physician of symptoms of secondary infection, including ear pain, purulent or bloody sputum, chest pain, or fever.
4. Teach information about drugs prescribed such as name, dosage, action, frequency of administration, and side effects.
5. Encourage high risk persons to get influenza vaccine before the start of the flu season.

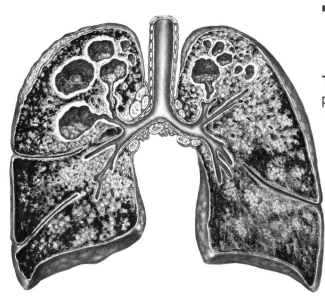

Tuberculosis

Tuberculosis is a chronic pulmonary and extra-pulmonary infectious disease acquired by inhalation into the alveolar structure of the lung of a dried-droplet nucleus containing a tubercle bacillus; it is characterized by stages of early infection (frequently asymptomatic), latency, and a potential for recurrent postprimary disease.

PATHOPHYSIOLOGY

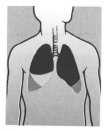

Tuberculosis infection can be differentiated from tuberculosis disease. Tuberculosis infection is characterized by the presence of mycobacteria in the tissue of a host who is free of clinical symptoms and who demonstrates the presence of antibodies against the mycobacteria. Tuberculosis disease is manifested by pathologic and functional symptoms indicating destructive activity of mycobacteria in host tissue. Both infection and disease result from tissue invasion by either *Mycobacterium tuberculosis* or *M. bovis* or a variety of atypical mycobacteria. All are spore formers capable of remaining viable and virulent for long periods inside or outside host tissue. *M. tuberculosis*, the tubercle bacilli, is the most frequent etiologic agent in human tuberculosis. The number of new cases reported annually fell from 27,749 in 1980 to 22,255 in 1984 in the United States. The number of deaths is fairly constant ranging from 1,978 deaths in 1980 to 1,910 deaths in 1983.[94] Transmission is primarily by inhalation of minute dried-droplet nuclei (each containing a single tubercle bacillus) coughed or sneezed into the air by a person whose sputum contains virulent tubercle bacilli. Less commonly, transmission may occur by ingestion or by invasion of the skin or mucous membranes. Repeated exposure usually is necessary for infection. (Refer to Table 5-4 for the chain of

Table 5-4 ⎯⎯⎯⎯⎯⎯⎯⎯⎯⎯⎯⎯⎯⎯ ∿∿

CHAIN OF EVENTS IN THE SPREAD OF TUBERCULOSIS

	Tuberculosis
Occurrence	Worldwide; mortality and prevalence decreasing in many places; highest in males and poor; most active disease arises from a latent infection
Etiologic agent	*Mycobacterium tuberculosis* and *M. bovis*
Reservoir	Humans; *M. bovis* in diseased cattle
Transmission	Inhalation of bacilli in the airborne mucous droplets from sputum of persons with active disease; less frequent: ingestion or skin penetration
Incubation period	4-12 weeks after exposure or anytime when disease is in latent stage
Period of communicability	As long as bacilli are in sputum; some are intermittently communicable for years
Susceptibility and resistance	General; highest in children less than 3 years, those greater than 65 years chronically ill, silicone and asbestos workers, and malnourished and immunosuppressed individuals
Report to local health authority	Mandatory case report

From Grimes, in Thompson.[99]

events in tuberculosis.)

In the initial infection the bacilli inhaled are carried to the peripheral alveoli, usually in the lower lobes. After implantation they multiply with little resistance from the host. The bacilli are engulfed by neutrophils and alveolar macrophages and may continue to multiply within the macrophage. While the cell-mediated immune response is being activated, the bacilli enter the lymphatic system and are carried to the nearest group of lymph nodes, where they also produce an inflammatory response. In addition, hematogenous dissemination of bacilli results in a subclinical bacteremia and the production of inflammatory lesions throughout the body. The sites and the extensiveness of the systemic lesions depend on the numbers of disseminated bacilli and the speed with which the host produces an immune response. These early lesions in the alveoli, in the lymph nodes, and disseminated are referred to as the *primary complex.**

Thus organisms may spread throughout the body before the delayed hypersensitivity response (the cell-mediated response) is available to limit further multiplication and spread of the infection. A delayed hypersensitivity response occurs 4 to 6 weeks after the initial infection and causes a characteristic tissue reaction called an epithelioid cell granuloma. This granuloma (also called epithelioid cell tubercle) develops from fusion of the infiltrating macrophages. The granuloma is surrounded by T-lymphocytes. The central portion of the lesion (called a Ghon tubercle) undergoes necrosis characterized by a cheesy appearance and hence is named caseous necrosis. The lesion also may undergo liquefactive necrosis, with the liquid sloughing into connecting bronchi and producing a cavity. The development of

*References 4, 7, 10, 77, 94, 99.

DIAGNOSTIC STUDIES AND FINDINGS

Diagnostic Test	Findings
Cultures	
Sputum culture	Positive for *M. tuberculosis* within 2-3 wks of active disease; will not be positive during latency
Acid-fast with Ziehl-Neelsen stain smear of sputum (cerebrospinal fluid or blood in extrapulmonary disease)	Positive for acid-fast bacilli
Histologic examination or culture of tissue in extrapulmonary disease	Positive for *M. tuberculosis*
Skin tests	
Intradermal infection of antigen	PPD: 5 tuberculin units of purified protein derivative (PPD)
	Heaf test: old tuberculin (OT) injected with pressure gun
	Mantoux test: PPD or OT injected intradermally
	Tine test: OT pressed into skin with tine unit
	Volmer patch test: OT on gauze strip applied to skin
	Tuberculin reaction begins 3-6 wks after infection; an area of induration greater than 10 mm in 48-72 h indicates past infection and presence of antibodies; does not indicate active disease; nonspecific reactions during first 48 h can be overlooked
	If the reaction is questionable, a second test may be done 1 week later
	If the second test is less than significant, the person is considered to have not been infected
	An increase in size of induration greater than 6 mm to a diameter of 10 mm indicates recent tuberculin infection
Pleural needle biopsy	Positive for granulomas of tuberculosis; giant cells indicating caseation necrosis
Chest x-ray	Findings may show calcification at the original site, enlargement of hilar lymph nodes, parenchymal infiltrate representing extension of the original site of infection, or the appearance of pleural effusion or cavitation
	Not diagnostically definitive of tuberculosis
Laboratory tests	
WBC count	Leukocytosis indicating an inflammatory reaction is occurring
	Elevation of neutrophils initially followed by elevation of monocytes and lymphocytes; indicates inflammatory process

necrosis and cavities destroys the alveoli and connecting bronchi.[81]

The specific immune response results in successful encapsulation of all lesions in 85% to 95% of those persons infected, depending on their age. These people enter the latent stage of the disease, remaining disease free for variable periods of time, depending on their ability to maintain specific and nonspecific resistance. The specific immune response does not preclude reinfection with subsequent exposure.

For 5% to 15% of infected persons, host responses are not adequate to contain the infection, and active disease progresses. Necrosis and cavitation continue in the lesions, forming caseation. The lesions may rupture, spreading necrotic residue and bacilli throughout the tissue and throughout the body. Disseminated bacilli establish new focal lesions that progress through stages of inflammation, noncaseating granulomas, and caseating necrosis.

The disease symptoms vary with the body tissue affected. Extrapulmonary tuberculosis in the meninges, blood vessels, kidneys, bones, joints, larynx, skin, intestines, lymph nodes, peritoneum, or eyes is much less common than pulmonary tuberculosis.

Reactivated disease following latency accounts for most of the active tuberculosis diagnosed today. It occurs most frequently in elderly persons and persons with chronic and debilitating diseases. Although reactivation may occur in any of the focal lesions, it most commonly occurs in those in the upper lobes or at the apex of the lower lobes of the lungs, forming abscesses and tuberculous cavities at those sites. Untreated reactivated disease has a variable course with many exacerbations and remissions. Complications caused by excessive cavitation are common.[77,99]

Healing of the primary lesion usually takes place by resolution, fibrosis, and calcification. The granulation tissue surrounding the lesion may become more fibrous and form a collagenous scar around the tubercle. A Ghon complex is formed, consisting of the Ghon tubercles and regional lymph nodes. Calcified Ghon complexes may be seen on chest roentgenograms.[77]

COMPLICATIONS

Atelectasis	Tuberculosis pericarditis,
Hemoptysis	peritonitis, meningitis,
Pneumothorax	lymphadenitis

MEDICAL MANAGEMENT

SURGERY

Intervention for complications

Resectional procedures for persisting cavitary lesions (less common since antimicrobial therapy). Surgical intervention for massive hemoptysis, spontaneous pneumothorax, abscess drainage, intestinal obstruction, or ureteral stricture.

DRUG THERAPY

A combination of antiinfective agents is recommended: Two primary drugs or primary plus a secondary drug. Initial dosages are higher, followed by prolonged therapy at reduced dosages. The combination of drugs used, the dosage, and duration of administration depend on the stage of the infection or disease, the presence of extrapulmonary disease, and the sensitivity of the patient to certain chemotherapeutic agents.

Antiinfective agents
Primary drugs

Isoniazid (INH), 10-20 mg/kg/day (up to 300 mg/day) PO for 1-2 yr; Ethambutol (Myambutol), 15 mg/kg/day PO for 1-2 yr; Initial dose: 25 mgm/kg/day × 2 mos; Rifampin (Rifomycin, others), 20 mg/kg/day PO for 6 mo to 2 yr; Streptomycin, 30 mg/kg/day IM q 2-3 mo.

7

MEDICAL MANAGEMENT—cont'd

Secondary drugs

Pyrazinamide (Aldinamide), 20-30 mg/kg/day; Ethionamide (Trecator), 10-30 mg/kg/day; Para-amino salicylic acid (PAS), 0.2 mg/kg/day PO for 1-2 yr; Cycloserine (Seromycin), 0.5-1.0 g/day in divided doses PO; Capreomycin (Capastat), 0.75-1.0 g/day IM for 30 days; twice weekly thereafter; Kanamycin (Kantrex), 1 g/day IM; Viomycin (Viocin), 1 g/day IM.

An example of recommended treatment plans:

Primary pulmonary tuberculosis infection—Isoniazid, 300 mg/day PO for 9 mos plus Rifampin, 600 mg/day PO for 9 mos; or Isoniazid, 300 mg/day PO for 18-24 mos plus Ethambutol, 15-18 mg/kd/day PO for 18-24 mos. Chronic pulmonary tuberculosis—Isoniazid, 10-20 mg/kg/day for 18 mo or more; plus Rifampin, 20 mg/kg/day for 18 mo or more; or PAS, 0.2 mg/kg/day for 18 mo or more; or Ethambutol, 15 mg/kg/day for 18 mo or more.

Corticosteroids:　May be used in conjunction with the antiinfective agents for overwhelming and life-threatening disease.

SUPPORTIVE

After stabilization most patients can be effectively managed on an outpatient basis with monitoring for compliance with drug taking, drug side effects, and patient response to the drug therapy.

AFB isolation until antimicrobial therapy is successfully initiated for sputum-positive patients to prevent spread to others.

Secretion precautions until wounds stop draining for patients with external tuberculosis lesions.

Skin testing:　Identify recent converters to tuberculosis skin tests; trace their contacts to identify persons with active disease; isoniazid therapy for 1 yr for recent converters and for close household contacts of persons with active disease (not routine for those over 35 yr old); tuberculosis skin testing is recommended for children at school entry and again at age 14 yr.

BCG vaccine for those persons who are at high risk contact with active cases, who are skin test negative, and who are not immunosuppressed (benefits of BCG vaccine are controversial). Receiving the vaccine results in a positive skin test.

1 ASSESS

ASSESSMENT	OBSERVATIONS
Assessment of extrapulmonary tuberculosis depends on the system involved; the onset of symptoms is generally insidious, as is the onset of pulmonary tuberculosis	
Respiratory	Initially a nonproductive cough; later mucopurulent secretions Advanced: hemoptysis; dyspnea on exertion and at rest; crackles over apex of lung; chest pain with respiratory movement if pleura is involved; hoarseness with involvement of larynx; dysphagia with pharyngeal involvement; sibilant and sonorous rhonchi
Abdominal	Weight loss, anorexia
Vital signs	Tachycardia; slight temperature elevation with chills and night sweats
Respiratory	Miliary tuberculosis; more severe symptoms of respiratory involvement: dyspnea, hyperventilation, and cough; hypoxemia; spontaneous unilateral or bilateral pneumothorax (manifested by sudden chest pain and breathlessness) and fever; painful, nodular cutaneous lesions, which may ulcerate, may be present
Cardiovascular	Tuberculosis pericarditis; precordial chest pain, fever, and pericardial friction rubs; jugular venous distention, hepatic congestion, ascites, and peripheral edema
Abdominal	Tuberculosis peritonitis; abdominal pain simulating that of appendicitis; abdominal distention; anorexia, vomiting, and weight loss; abdominal tenderness when palpated; ascites; tuberculosis of gastrointestinal tract; symptoms depend on the area involved; may have gastrointestinal bleeding, pain, constipation, or diarrhea; partial or complete obstruction; perforation with peritonitis
Genitourinary	Tuberculosis of genitourinary organs; urgency, frequency, dysuria, hematuria, and pyuria; salpingitis with lower abdominal pain and infertility; amenorrhea; abnormal vaginal discharge or bleeding
Neurologic	Tuberculosis meningitis; headache, vomiting, fever, and anorexia; alterations in intellectual function, diminishing levels of consciousness, and neurologic deficits; cerebrospinal fluid leukocytes of 100 to 400 cells/mm^3, and increase in protein
Musculoskeletal	Osteoarticular tuberculosis; pain aggravated by movement, in joints; swelling, minimal erythema, and tenderness to palpation; limitation of motion and gross deformities (most common in vertebral column, hip, and knee joints)
Lymphatic	Tuberculosis lymphadenitis; palpable enlargement of supraclavicular and cervical lymph nodes

2 DIAGNOSE

NURSING DIAGNOSIS	SUBJECTIVE FINDINGS	OBJECTIVE FINDINGS
Ineffective airway clearance related to mucopurulent sputum	Complains of difficulty breathing	Cough (may be productive or nonproductive), crackles and rhonchi, fever, hemoptysis, dyspnea
Ineffective breathing pattern related to inflammatory process and pleuritic pain	Complains of SOB and pain on inspiration	Dyspnea, shallow respirations, cough
Altered nutrition: less than body requirements related to fatigue	Reports inadequate intake and being too tired to eat	Weight loss, inadequate food and fluid intake, fatigue
Fear related to transmitting disease to contacts and to possibility of chronic disease	Expresses fear about contacts developing tuberculosis; expresses fear of developing chronic respiratory disease	
Potential for infection of patient's contacts	Reports living in close contact with patient with active tuberculosis	Positive skin test with no symptoms of tuberculosis

3 PLAN

Patient goals

1. Patient's airways will be patent.
2. Patient will achieve full expansion with adequate ventilation.
3. Patient's nutritional status will be improved.
4. Patient's fears will subside.
5. Patient's contacts will have no pulmonary infections.
6. Patient will demonstrate an understanding of home care and follow-up instructions.

4 IMPLEMENT

NURSING DIAGNOSIS	NURSING INTERVENTIONS	RATIONALE
Ineffective airway clearance related to mucopurulent sputum	Auscultate lungs for rhonchi and crackles.	Determines adequacy of gas exchange and extent to which airway is obstructed with secretions.
	Assess characteristics of secretions: quantity, color, consistency, odor.	Presence of infection is suspected when secretions are thick, yellow, and/or foul-smelling.

NURSING DIAGNOSIS	NURSING INTERVENTIONS	RATIONALE
	Assess patient's hydration status: skin turgor, mucous membranes, tongue, intake and output over 24 h, Hct.	Determines need for fluids. Fluids needed if skin turgor poor, tongue and mucous membranes are dry, intake < output, and/or hematocrit elevated.
	Monitor chest x-rays.	Shows calcification, enlarged hilar lymph nodes, parenchymal infiltrates, and pleural effusion or cavitation.
	Monitor sputum culture and sensitivity reports.	Identifies microorganisms present and the appropriate antiinfective agents needed.
	Assist patient with coughing as needed.	Coughing removes secretions.
	Position patient in proper body alignment for optimal breathing pattern (head of bed up 45°, if tolerated up to 90°).	Secretions move by gravity as position changes. Elevating head of bed moves abdominal contents away from diaphragm to enhance diaphragmatic contraction.
	Administer drug therapy in collaboration with physician.	Primary drugs are bacteriocidal. Secondary drugs are bacteriostatic.
	Avoid suppressing cough reflex unless cough is frequent and nonproductive.	Coughing is needed to mobilize and expectorate secretions, but excessive nonproductive coughing leads to fatigue.
	Encourage increased fluid intake to 1½ to 2 L/day unless contraindicated.	Liquefies secretions so that they are easier to expectorate.
	Assist patient with oral hygiene as needed.	Removes taste of secretions.
	Pace activities to patient tolerance.	Avoids fatigue.
Ineffective breathing patterns related to inflammatory process and pleuritic pain	Observe changes in respiratory rate and depth.	Determines adequacy of breathing pattern.
	Inspect thorax for symmetry of respiratory movement.	Determines adequacy of breathing pattern.
	Observe breathing pattern for SOB.	Identifies increased work of breathing.
	Assess for pain on inspiration.	Pain may limit inhalation.
	Position patient in optimal body alignment in semi-Fowler's position for breathing or turn side to side.	Optimizes diaphragmatic contraction.
	Medicate with analgesic as ordered without depressing respirations.	Reduces pain that may be interfering with breathing.

NURSING DIAGNOSIS	NURSING INTERVENTIONS	RATIONALE
Altered nutrition: less than body requirements related to fatigue	Assess dietary habits and needs.	Helps to individualize the diet.
	Weigh patient weekly.	Improved nutrition will result in weight gain.
	Auscultate bowel sounds.	Documents GI peristalsis needed for digestion.
	Assess psychologic factors, e.g., depression, that might decrease food and fluid intake.	Identifies effect of psychologic factors on food intake.
	Monitor albumin and lymphocytes.	These values indicate adequate visceral proteins, which are low when nutrition is inadequate. Protein needed to promote healing and support immune system.
	Encourage oral care before meals.	Removes taste of sputum that may reduce appetite.
	Provide frequent small feedings.	Lessens fatigue.
	Provide foods in appropriate consistency for eating. Soft or liquid foods may be preferred.	Requires less energy to eat soft foods and liquids, thereby reducing oxygen requirement.
	Provide high-protein diet.	Supports immune system.
	Provide a high-carbohydrate diet.	Metabolism of carbohydrates needed for calories during an inflammatory process.
	Assist patient by cutting food and feeding patient if needed.	Lessens fatigue.
	Administer vitamins as ordered.	Supplements diet and promotes healing.
Fear related to transmitting disease and to possibility of chronic disease	Validate source of fear with patient.	Ensures congruence between nurse and patient in trying to resolve fears.
	Assess vital signs.	Determines effects of fear on heart and respiratory rates.
	Encourage patient to discuss contributing factors to fear and actions to allay fear.	Facilitates problem solving; reviews coping skills used in the past.
	Explain tuberculosis; provide information related to fear when possible. Encourage patient to ask questions.	Knowledge can decrease fear.
	Promote patient's control of situation when possible.	Provides some power and control.
	Accept patient's fears.	Facilitates problem solving, supports therapeutic relationship.

→ ❯ ❯

NURSING DIAGNOSIS	NURSING INTERVENTIONS	RATIONALE
Potential for infection of patient's contacts	Employ AFB isolation until antimicrobial therapy is successfully started for sputum-positive contacts.	Prevents inhalation of droplet nuclei by people around the patient.
	Employ secretion precautions until wounds stop draining for patients with tuberculosis lesions.	Wound secretions may contain tubercle bacilli that can spread to others.
	Skin test all contacts.	Determines if contacts have been infected.
	Collect sputum specimens from contacts.	Determines if sputum contains tubercle bacilli.
Knowledge deficit	See Patient Teaching.	

5 EVALUATE

PATIENT OUTCOME	DATA INDICATING THAT OUTCOME IS REACHED
Airways are patent.	Breath sounds are clear. Chest x-rays show reduction in size of cavities and decrease in the thickness of cavity walls. Sputum cultures are consistently negative.
Respiratory pattern is effective.	No dyspnea or cough. No pain on inspiration. Respiratory pattern symmetric with regular rate. Breath sounds are clear.
Nutritional status has improved.	Patient experiences weight gain. Patient is eating a balanced diet. Fluid intake is at least 2,500 ml daily.
Fear is relieved.	Patient reports lessened fear with the return of adequate breathing pattern and with knowledge about how to prevent recurrence of tuberculosis.
There is no infection of contacts.	Contacts' temperature remains within normal limits. Contacts do not convert to positive skin tests or develop symptoms of TB.
Learning is demonstrated.	Patient demonstrates knowledge of self-care management, disease process, compliance with treatment regimen and how to prevent the spread and recurrence.

PATIENT TEACHING

1. Teach patient that if sputum cultures are positive at discharge, he or she needs to handle sputum carefully. Cover nose and mouth with paper tissue *every* time patient coughs, sneezes, or coughs up sputum. The tissues should be flushed down the toilet or discarded in a paper bag that is burned or disposed with the trash. After handling sputum or soiled tissues the patient must wash hands thoroughly.
2. Teach importance of reporting symptoms to the physician, including hemotypsis, chest pain, difficulty breathing, hearing loss, or vertigo.
3. Instruct about taking prescribed medications including the name, dosage, action, frequency of administration, and side effects.
4. Teach importance of eating a balanced diet to build up resistance to further infections.
5. Teach importance of drinking at least 2 quarts of fluid daily to keep secretions thin so they can be expectorated.
6. Emphasize the need for periodic reculturing of sputum during period of therapy; monthly until cultures are negative; then every 3 months for duration of therapy.

CHAPTER 6

Surgical and Therapeutic Interventions

Breathing Techniques

Breathing techniques are useful and specific measures to increase the volume of air entering the lungs as well as being expelled from the lungs.

ABDOMINAL OR DIAPHRAGMATIC BREATHING

Patients with chronic and acute respiratory dysfunction may be taught to use the abdominal muscles and diaphragm as the primary structures for breathing rather than as accessory muscles.

Procedural Guidelines

1. Ensure that nasal passage and trachea are free of secretions and congestion. If necessary, suction, use aerosol, encourage coughing, or perform postural drainage before teaching diaphragmatic breathing.
2. Assist patient to attain position of comfort, either lying down or in semi-Fowler's position in bed. Abdominal muscles should be relaxed and knees and hips flexed. The patient places one hand on his chest and the other on his abdomen.
3. Instruct patient to inhale deeply though nose (keep mouth shut). As patient inhales, the focus should be to pull the diaphragm down and to force the abdominal wall outward. The hand on the patient's abdomen should rise.
4. Instruct patient to pause slightly after a deep and even inspiration and then, using a pursed-lip technique, to exhale quietly and naturally.
5. Encourage patient to use the abdominal muscles during expiration to remove all air from the lungs.
6. Explain that expiration should last two to three times longer than inspiration.
7. After the technique is mastered, place a 5-pound (2.25 kg) weight on the patient's abdomen to further strengthen the abdominal muscles.
8. Have patient practice the diaphragmatic breathing technique 10 to 20 minutes at least every 4 hours until ability and willingness to implement the technique are demonstrated.

PURSED-LIP BREATHING

This technique is used to control expiration and to facilitate maximum emptying of the alveoli. It functions to maintain a positive pressure in the airways and thus keep them open longer. In this way more air may be exhaled.

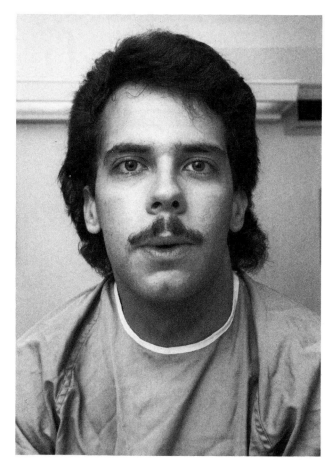

FIGURE 6-1
Pursed-lip breathing.

DEEP BREATHING, COUGHING, AND SPLINTING

This technique is most frequently used during the first 48 hours after surgery to loosen secretions and force them to be expelled. The deep breathing dilates the airways, stimulates surfactant production, and expands the lung tissue surface, thereby increasing the area for respiratory gas exchange. Coughing is used to force collected and consolidated secretions to be expelled. Splinting of the chest wall is used to produce stabilization, which in turn decreases discomfort.

Procedural Guidelines

1. Position patient to facilitate deep inspiration and coughing.
2. The incisional area may be splinted with a pillow and hand pressure. As the patient coughs, firmly assist the patient to stabilize the incisional area.
3. Instruct patient to take a slow, deep inspiration. If patient is postoperative, pain medications may need to be administered 20 to 30 minutes before initiating procedure.
4. Instruct patient to quickly close glottis and forcefully expel an explosive current of air.
5. Provide patient with tissues to collect expelled sputum.

INCENTIVE SPIROMETERS

The incentive spirometer may be used postoperatively to encourage deep breathing. While it may provide assistive deep breathing exercises, it should not replace other deep breathing and coughing interventions.

Procedural Guidelines

1. Position patient in seated or semi-Fowler's position.
2. Instruct patient to seal mouth around mouthpiece and to inhale or exhale so as to activate the spirometer (Figure 6-2). Each brand of spirometer functions slightly differently. Some are operated by exhalation into the system; others are activated by inspiration. In either case the deeper the ventilatory effort, the more successful the use of the spirometer. Carefully inspect the operation of a specific unit before instructing the patient.
3. Instruct the patient to hold a deep breath for a few seconds before exhaling. This will help prevent pulmonary complications.
4. After the spirometer is used, wash the mouthpiece and tubing. They should not be used for any other patient.

Procedural Guidelines

1. Assist patient to a position of comfort.
2. Instruct patient to inhale deeply through the nose (with mouth shut) and to pause slightly at end of inspiration.
3. Instruct patient to exhale slowly through pursed lips so a blowing effect occurs (Figure 6-1).
4. Explain that exhalation should be slow and purposeful.
5. As the technique is practiced and used on a continual basis, patient anxiety and anxiety-related dyspnea should decrease.

5. The incentive spirometer should be used at least every 3 or 4 hours during the postoperative period until the patient is ambulatory and initiates effective deep breathing and coughing on his own.

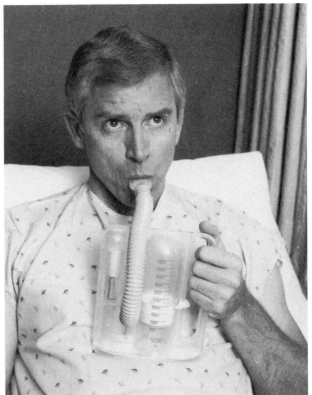

FIGURE 6-2
Patient using incentive spirometer.

Chest Physiotherapy and Postural Drainage

The components of **chest physiotherapy** include percussion (cupping and clapping), vibration, coughing, and deep breathing. Together postural drainage and chest physiotherapy provide effective methods of loosening and moving secretions into the large airways where they can be coughed up.

Postural drainage may be performed alone or in combination with percussion and vibration.

INDICATIONS

Postoperative patients with secretions related to decreased cough or pain

Patients with pneumonia

Patients with diseases in which secretions would predispose to infection, e.g., cystic fibrosis

Patients with tenacious secretions or bronchospasm that make it difficult to raise secretions

Comatose patients without voluntary cough

Very obese patients or very inactive patients

Patients with neuromuscular reasons for an ineffective cough, e.g., quadriplegia, myasthenia gravis, Guillain-Barré syndrome.

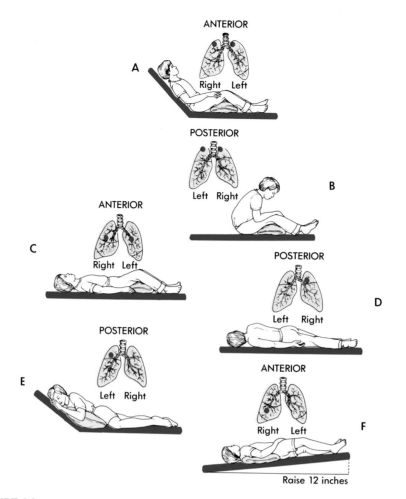

FIGURE 6-3
Positions for postural drainage. **A,** Anterior apical segment (sitting). **B,** Posterior apical segment (sitting). **C,** Anterior segment (lying flat on back). **D,** Right posterior segment (lying on left side). **E,** Left posterior segment (lying on right side). **F,** Right middle lobe (lying on left side).

CONTRAINDICATIONS

Cyanosis or dyspnea caused by chest physiotherapy and postural drainage

Increased pain or discomfort with chest physiotherapy and postural drainage

Patients with prolonged bleeding and clotting times

Extremely obese patients

Patients with history of predisposition to pathologic fractures

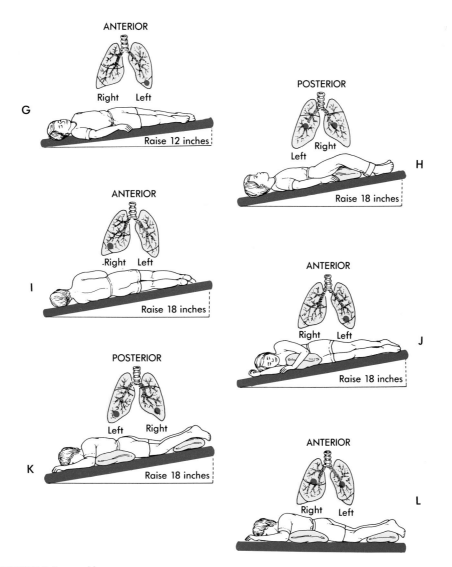

FIGURE 6-3—cont'd.
G, Left lingula (lying on right side). **H,** Anterior segments (lying on back). **I,** Right lateral segment (lying on left side). **J,** Left lateral segment (lying on right side). **K,** Posterior segments (lying on stomach). **L,** Superior segments (lying on stomach).
(From Hirsch).[56]

Procedural Guidelines

Postural drainage consists of positioning the patient in specific and controlled positions to drain and remove secretions from particular segments of the lungs. The positions used are those needed to drain the specific lobes where secretions have accumulated (Figure 6-3). The upper lobes are drained first.

The patient should maintain each postural drainage position for at least 5 minutes. At the end of each positioned period the patient should cough and deep breathe before moving to the next position. Should one position cause the patient dyspnea or discomfort, move on to the next position. Do not terminate the techniques completely.

Chest percussion and vibration are performed after postural drainage. Place a towel over the chest area to be percussed. Each indicated lung lobe area may be percussed and vibrated as indicated in Figure 6-4.

To **percuss,** cup hands and lightly and rhythmically strike the chest wall. A hollow, deep sound indicates that the technique is being performed correctly. Each area should be percussed for 1 to 2 minutes. Do not percuss over soft tissue or areas where the technique causes increased pain. **To vibrate** the area, gently but firmly vibrate hand against the thoracic wall directly over the area that was percussed. This technique should be done at least 5 to 7 times during the patient's expiration.

Chest physiotherapy and postural drainage techniques should be performed systematically and routinely as ordered by the physician. The therapy most frequently involves the following:

1. Patient assumes a specific postural drainage position for 5 minutes. Upper lobes are drained first.
2. The area is percussed for 1 to 2 minutes.
3. The area is vibrated.
4. Patient is encouraged to cough up and spit out sputum.
5. A different postural drainage position is attained, and the percussion and vibration techniques are repeated.

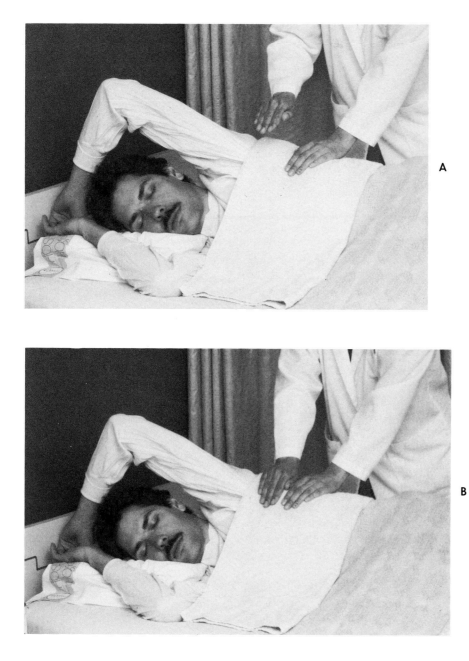

FIGURE 6-4
Chest percussion **(A)** and vibration **(B).**

PATIENT TEACHING

1. Teach patient to perform postural drainage at home; a specific routine should be encouraged.
2. Although it is impossible for patient to perform chest physiotherapy on self, teach patient to perform tapping movements on the chest wall by using the fingertips of both hands. This may loosen secretions.
3. Teach family members vibratory and percussion techniques.

4. Encourage patient to perform oral hygiene after the procedure.
5. Complete procedure at least 30 minutes before meals or at least 2 hours after the last meal.
6. Encourage patient to use tissues during coughing and to inspect characteristics of sputum.

Oxygen Therapy

The goal of **oxygen therapy** is to provide sufficient amounts of oxygen to the tissues so that normal metabolism can occur.

Clinically this means to provide oxygen at the lowest fractional inspired oxygen (FiO_2) to maintain a PaO_2 of at least 55 mm Hg. Therapy is indicated when a patient is unable to maintain an adequate PaO_2 by his own ventilatory efforts, known as hypoxemia. Hypoxemia may be caused by a variety of factors:

Reduced alveolar oxygen: results from either low ambient PaO_2 or hypoventilation

Impaired alveolar-capillary diffusion: occurs secondary to pathologic changes such as fibrosis, increased connective tissue, interstitial edema, or tumors

Hemoglobin deficiencies: may be either absolute owing to anemia or relative as in patients with carbon monoxide inhalation

Ventilation/perfusion ratio imbalance: anatomic shunting that occurs secondary to congenital defects, disease or trauma, or physiologic shunting

Circulatory failure: occurs secondary to decreased cardiac output of hypovolemia

EQUIPMENT

Oxygen therapy equipment may be divided into two major types: low-flow and high-flow systems.

Low-flow systems do not apply to all of the inspired gases that the patient breathes. This means that the patient breathes some room air along with the oxygen. For the system to be effective, the patient must be able to maintain a normal tidal volume, have a regular ven-

tilatory pattern, and be able to cooperate. As the patient's ventilatory pattern changes, so does the concentration of inspired oxygen. Examples of low-flow systems include nasal cannula, simple oxygen mask, partial rebreathing mask with reservoir bag, and nonrebreathing mask with reservoir bag (Figure 6-5).

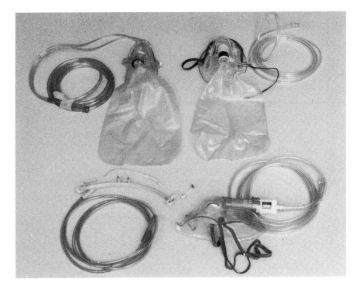

FIGURE 6-5
Low-flow oxygen therapy systems: nasal cannula (lower left); simple oxygen mask (lower right); partial re-breathing mask with reservoir bag (top right); nonrebreathing mask with reservoir bag (top left).

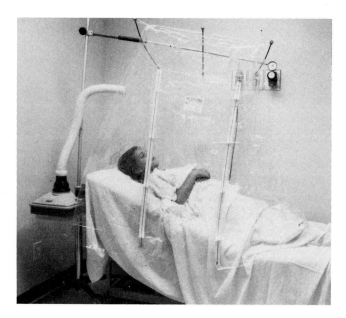

FIGURE 6-6
Patient in oxygen tent.

High-flow systems supply all gases at a preset Fio_2. These systems are generally not affected by changes in ventilatory pattern. The Venturi mask is the most common example of the high-flow system.

In addition to these two main systems there are blended-type systems that may use either high-flow or low-flow techniques. Examples of this type include oxygen hoods, Isolettes, T-tubes, and oxygen tents (Figure 6-6). Table 6-1 summarizes the major types of oxygen therapy systems, their benefits, problems, and nursing care.

CAUTION

Patients with arterial carbon dioxide tension > 50 mm Hg are at risk for oxygen-induced hypoventilation. Therefore maintain oxygen therapy so the arterial oxygen tension remains at about 50 to 60 mm Hg. Be especially cautious with patients who have chronic lung diseases. These patients experience such prolonged hypercarbia that the medulla oblongata loses its sensitivity to increased $Paco_2$ as a stimulus for breathing. Instead, receptors in the carotid bodies and aortic arch use low Pao_2 as the stimulus to breathe. Thus if high flow rates of oxygen are administered to such patients, their stimulus to breathe is eliminated.

COMPLICATIONS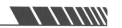

Atelectasis. The collapse of alveoli may occur secondary to high concentrations of oxygen in inspired air, which causes malfunctioning pulmonary surfactant. To prevent this complication, if possible limit the duration of 100% inspired oxygen to no more than 20 minutes; maintain patent airway; provide the patient with a deep breath by using the sigh function of the ventilator; and provide high tidal volumes.

Oxygen toxicity. The lungs can normally handle oxygen concentrations of 21%. Although it is not clear exactly what fractional inspired oxygen (Fio_2) percent causes oxygen toxicity, it is most probable that an Fio_2 of over 50% administered for longer than 24 hours increases the risk. Oxygen toxicity is thought to be caused by end products of oxygen formed during biochemical reactions. These end products, called free radicals, include hydrogen peroxide, superoxide radical, and hydroxyl radical. Prolonged exposure to high concentrations of oxygen may form free radicals that damage tissue. Recognition of oxygen toxicity may be difficult because the symptoms are similar to the respiratory diseases for which oxygen is given, e.g., cough, dyspnea at rest, and substernal pain. Other symptoms are vague, such as nausea, vomiting, orthostatic hypotension, headache, anorexia, sore throat, and paresthesia. To further impair data collection to substantiate oxygen toxicity, the patient usually is critically ill, intubated and unable to verbally communicate the above mentioned symptoms. Clinical signs after 6 hours of 100% oxygen therapy would include sharp chest pain and dry cough; after 18 hours decreased pulmonary function; and after 24 to 48 hours, ARDS occurs.

Arterial blood gases are the best source of data to prevent oxygen toxicity. The goal is to try to keep the Pao_2 between 60 and 90 mm Hg. If the patient's Pao_2 > 90 mm Hg and the Fio_2 >40%, then he may be needlessly at risk for oxygen toxicity.

Guidelines to prevent oxygen toxicity:

1. Limit use of 100% oxygen to brief periods.
2. As early as possible reduce Fio_2 to lowest possible level to maintain oxygenation.
3. Up to 70% oxygen may be used safely for 24 hours.
4. Up to 50% oxygen may be used safely for 2 days.
5. After 2 days an Fio_2 about 40% is potentially toxic.
6. Prolonged use of Fio_2 below 40% rarely causes oxygen toxicity.

Table 6-1

OXYGEN THERAPY SYSTEMS

Type of System	Description	Flow Rate (L/min)*	Approximate Oxygen Concentration Delivered (%)	Benefits	Problems	Nursing Care
Low-flow systems						
Nasal cannula	Two short hollow prongs direct oxygen into the nostrils. Prongs attach to tubing that connects to an oxygen source, a humidifier, and a flow meter	2 3 4 5 6	24-28 28-30 32-36 36-40 40-44	Comfortable, convenient method of delivering concentration of oxygen ranging from 44% If minute ventilation is relatively low and constant, Fio_2 delivered approaches the percentages presented Major advantages of this method are low cost of equipment, allowance for patient mobility, ability to deliver oxygen and still permit patient to eat and talk, and lack of necessity for humidification of inspired gas Practical system for long-term therapy mixture Mouth breathing will not affect concentration of delivered oxygen	Unable to deliver oxygen concentration over 44% Assumes an adequate breathing pattern Equipment may not be used if patient has nasal problem or if unable to tolerate nasal prongs Patient must be able to cooperate to keep prongs in place	Clean equipment daily Evaluate for pressure sores over ears and cheek areas Lubricate nasal prongs before inserting into nose Liter flow > 6 L/min will *not* increase the Fio_2 Avoid kinking or twisting tubing, which impedes oxygen flow
Nasal catheter	Oxygen catheter with several holes at the distal end for delivering oxygen. Catheter is inserted into one nostril and advanced to the oropharynx.	Same as nasal cannula		Same as nasal cannula, but not as comfortable	Same as nasal cannula Even when properly placed in the oropharnyx, gas flow can be misdirected into the stomach causing gastric distention. Do not operate at flow < 5 L/min (will not flush out accumulated CO_2)	Remove catheter every 8 hrs to prevent drying of the oropharynx mucosa Lubricate catheter with water-soluble lubricant before inserting. Avoid kinking or twisting tubing, which impedes oxygen flow.

*Normal breathing patterns are assumed.

Continued.

Table 6-1

OXYGEN THERAPY SYSTEMS—cont'd

Type of System	Description	Flow Rate (L/min)*	Approximate Oxygen Concentration Delivered (%)	Benefits	Problems	Nursing Care
Simple face mask	The mask fits over the nose and mouth and is held in place by elastic around the head. The mask is attached to oxygen tubing, a humidifier, and a flow meter	5 6 8	40 45-50 55-60	If patient's ventilatory needs exceed flow of gas, holes on sides of mask allow for entry of room air Permits higher oxygen delivery than nasal cannula System does not tend to dry out mucous membranes of nose or mouth	Mask must be removed prior to patient's eating May not be operated at flow < 5 L/min A tight face mask seal may cause facial irritation Face mask may increase anxiety in some patients, especially children Not practical for long-term therapy May feel hot and confining for some patients Fio_2 is variable	Do not operate at flow < 5 L/min (will not flush out accumulated CO_2) If Fio_2 above 60% is desired, patient must be switched to rebreathing mask with reservoir bag Should not be used for patients with chronic lung diseases Powdering may be necessary along bony prominence of face Equipment should be removed and cleaned several times each day.
Partial rebreathing mask with reservoir bag	Mask similar to simple face mask with addition of a reservoir oxygen bag; the purpose of the rebreathing mask is to conserve oxygen by permitting it to be rebreathed from the reservoir bag	8 10-12	40-50 60	The bag makes possible delivery of oxygen concentration between 40% and 60% provided that the reservoir is kept full by a continuous flow of oxygen	Requires tight face seal Impractical for long-term therapy Must be removed for eating and talking May lead to signs of oxygen toxicity	Apply mask as patient exhales Arterial blood gases should be monitored Check mask for leaks around face; Fio_2 may decrease if mask is not tight fitting The reservoir bag should remain full on expiration and partially deflate at peak inspiration All other functions as with simple mask
Nonrebreathing mask with reservoir bag	Similar to rebreathing bag, but this mask has a one-way expiratory valve that prevents rebreathing of expired gases	6 8 10 12-15	55-60 60-80 80-90 90	Effective as short-term therapy May provide oxygen concentration up to 90%	Requires tight face seal Impractical for long-term therapy Must be removed for eating and talking May lead to signs of oxygen toxicity If oxygen tubing is kinked the one-way valves give only a small hole to breathe through	Arterial blood gases should be monitored Check mask for leaks around face; Fio_2 may decrease if mask is not tight fitting; ensure that all rubber flaps stay in place All other functions as with simple mask

*Normal breathing patterns are assumed.

Table 6-1

OXYGEN THERAPY SYSTEMS—cont'd

Type of System	Description	Flow Rate (L/min)*	Approximate Oxygen Concentration Delivered (%)	Benefits	Problems	Nursing Care
Oxygen hood	Most convenient method to provide oxygen therapy to infants Hood covers head only, leaving rest of body available for patient care	10-12	Oxygen analyzer should be used to determine level of concentration	May be used in conjuction with high-flow Venturi system May be used in conjuction with Isolettes, which provide temperature and humidity regulation	Oxygen between 10 and 12 L/min may be necessary to keep oxygen concentrations steady (dependent on size of oxygen hood)	Make sure oxygen is warmed and humidified Active infants must be carefully observed; they may dislodge hood Pad edges of hood with towels or foam Condensation in tubing will build and must be emptied frequently Heat nebulizer should be maintained between 34.4° (94° C) and 35.6° C (96° F)
Oxygen tent	Tent covers entire bed and provides oxygen through an inlet port	10 12 15	30-40 40-50 50	Provides convenient method to provide oxygen to children while sleeping	High liter flows are necessary to fill tent. Humidity in tent dampens child's hair, which may contribute to chilling. Child cannot see well through tent when condensation forms.	Make sure oxygen is warmed and humidified Condensation in tubing will build up and require emptying frequently Heated nebulized should be maintained between 34.4° C (94° F) and 35.6° C (96° F)
High-flow systems						
Venturi mask	Works on Bernoulli principle of air entrainment: for each liter of oxygen that passes through a fixed orifice, a fixed proportion of room air will be entrained; by varying size of orifice and flow of oxygen, precise Fio_2 is maintained The system operates by actually setting Fio_2	4 4 6 8 8	24 - blue† 28 - yellow† 31 - white† 35 - green† 40 - pink†	Delivers exact concentration Fio_2 remains constant regardless of the patient's ventilatory pattern Fio_2 may be measured directly by an oxygen analyzer Fio_2 adaptor may be changed and set to deliver a calculated oxygen concentration	May irritate facial skin Interferes with eating and drinking Tight face seal must be maintained Condensation may collect within system	Arterial blood gases should be monitored Check mask for leaks around face; Fio_2 may be altered if system not properly fitting All other functions as with simple face mask

*Normal breathing patterns are assumed.
†Color of adaptor.

OXYGEN THERAPY AT HOME

Oxygen is available for home use in three forms—liquid oxygen, oxygen concentrator, and oxygen cylinder (Figures 6-7 to 6-9).

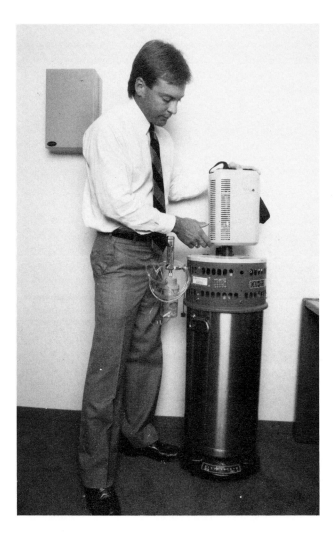

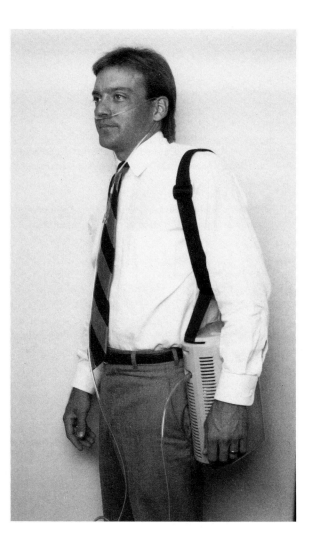

FIGURE 6-7
A, Liquid oxygen used with the Linde Oxygen Walker System is used by patients who use oxygen 16 to 24 hours a day and will be active outside of the home. **B,** The Linde Walker is filled from the larger liquid oxygen container and carried by the shoulder strap.

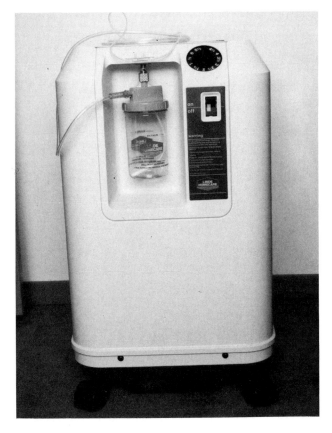

FIGURE 6-8
The oxygen concentrator is used for individuals who will be using oxygen 12 to 24 hours a day and *only* inside the home. It concentrates oxygen out of room air making it economical for the high volume user.

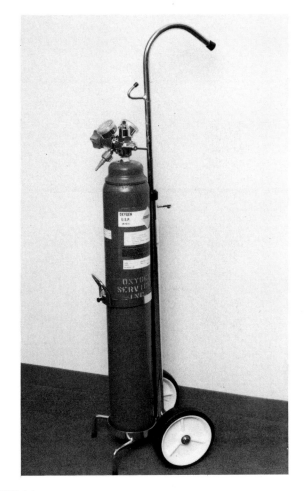

FIGURE 6-9
The oxygen cylinder provides compressed gaseous oxygen and is used by patients who need oxygen only on an "as needed" basis. The E cylinder is shown here; other sizes are available. **Caution:** Traveling with an oxygen cylinder, such as an E cylinder, can be dangerous because the oxygen gas is compressed within the cylinder. If the oxygen gauge is knocked off, the oxygen will discharge at a rapid rate because the gas is under very high pressure. The cylinder may act as a torpedo as the gas discharges.

1 ASSESS

ASSESSMENT	OBSERVATIONS
Respiratory	Hypoxia, tachypnea, cyanosis, dyspnea, shallow respirations Anxiety, nausea, restlessness, irritability Disorientation, confusion $Pa_{O_2} < 55$ mm Hg $Pa_{CO_2} > 42$ mm Hg Airway obstruction, nasal flaring, retractions, atelectasis CNS depression, muscle weakness
Cardiovascular	Hypotension, sudden hypertension, tachycardia, cardiac dysrhythmia
Skin and mucous membranes	Dry nasal or oral mucous membranes Red or broken skin when in contact with oxygen delivery equipment

2 DIAGNOSE

NURSING DIAGNOSIS	SUBJECTIVE FINDINGS	OBJECTIVE FINDINGS
Impaired gas exchange related to altered oxygen supply and alveolar-capillary membrane changes	Complains of not getting enough air	Rapid and shallow respirations, use of accessory muscles, restless, irritable, disoriented, confused, $Pa_{O_2} < 55$ mm Hg
Ineffective airway clearance related to fatigue, tracheobronchial obstruction or secretions	Complains of congestion	Tachypnea, dyspnea, cyanosis, crackles, rhonchi
Altered oral mucous membranes related to dehydration	Reports lips and mouth being dry	Dry mucous membranes in nostrils and/or mouth, decreased salivation
Altered nutrition: less than body requirements related to need for oxygen by mask	Complains of oxygen mask interfering with eating; reports continuous need for oxygen	Oxygen mask ordered to provide needed oxygen Difficulty eating with mask in place, but need for oxygen delivery
Anxiety related to need for oxygen therapy	Expresses concern about need for oxygen therapy and about breathlessness without therapy	Worried facial expression, restlessness, insomnia, anxiousness

3 PLAN

Patient goals

1. Patient will have adequate gas exchange.
2. Patient's airways will be clear.
3. Patient will have intact, moist mucous membranes.
4. Patient's nutritional status will be maintained to meet body's needs.
5. Patient's anxiety will be reduced.
6. Patient will demonstrate understanding of the purpose for and the maintenance of oxygen therapy.

4 IMPLEMENT

NURSING DIAGNOSIS	NURSING INTERVENTIONS	RATIONALE
Impaired gas exchange related to altered oxygen supply and alveolar-capillary membrane changes	Assess patient for signs of confusion, irritability, disorientation.	These signs may indicate hypoxia.
	Monitor arterial blood gases. Administer oxygen as ordered.	Indicates oxygen present in arterial blood and need to adjust oxygen flow rate.
Ineffective airway clearance related to fatigue, tracheobronchial obstruction or secretions	Auscultate breath sounds for crackles and rhonchi.	These sounds indicate secretions in the airways that impede flow of oxygen to alveoli.
	Assist patient to semi-Fowler's position for optimal lung expansion.	This position moves the abdominal contents away from the diaphragm to optimize lung expansion.
	Encourage patient to cough or assist patient by suctioning airways.	Coughing and suctioning remove secretions that narrow airways.
	Encourage patient to increase fluid intake at least to 2,500 ml daily unless contraindicated.	Fluids thin secretions so they are easier to expectorate or suction.
Altereded oral mucous membranes related to dehydration	Assess mucous membranes of the mouth and nose.	Determines if they are intact and moist.
	Encourage fluid intake to at least 2,500 ml unless contraindicated.	Adequate fluid intake prevents dry mucous membranes.
	Provide oral hygiene several times daily.	Cleanses and moistens the mucous membranes of the mouth.
	Apply water soluble ointment or hand lotion to lips and around nares if they are dry.	Moistens mucous membranes and skin when these areas are dried by oxygen. Oil-based ointments are combustible.
Altered nutrition: less than body requirements related to need for oxygen mask	Consult with physician about patient using a nasal cannula for oxygen therapy during mealtime.	Nasal cannula provides oxygen without covering the mouth, whereas an oxygen mask interferes with intake of food and fluid.
Anxiety related to need for oxygen therapy	Assess patient's level of anxiety as related to air hunger and need for oxygen therapy.	Determines presence and cause of anxiety so that nursing interventions can be implemented.
	Provide accurate information about oxygen therapy.	Knowledge can relieve anxiety.
	Encourage patient to verbalize feelings and fears.	Helps patient put thoughts into perspective, identifies misconceptions that can be clarified by the nurse.
Knowledge deficit	See Patient Teaching.	

5 EVALUATE

PATIENT OUTCOME	DATA INDICATING THAT OUTCOME IS REACHED
Gas exchange is adequate.	Arterial blood gases are within acceptable range. There is no dyspnea.
Airways are patent.	Breath sounds are clear. Arterial blood gases are within acceptable range.
Oral mucous membranes are intact.	Mucous membranes are warm, moist, and intact.
Maintains adequate nutritional status.	Weight remains stable and within normal range for patient.
Anxiety is reduced.	Patient has a relaxed facial expression and verbalizes feelings of less anxiety.
Knowledge is demonstrated.	Patient and family have sufficient information to comply with oxygen therapy plan.

PATIENT TEACHING

1. Assess the patient's knowledge and skills regarding the use of oxygen equipment.
2. Teach the patient the purpose and process of the selected type of oxgyen equipment.
3. Teach importance of not smoking (and not permitting others in the area to smoke) during administration of oxygen.
4. Provide the patient and family with information regarding the care, cleaning, and maintenance of oxygen equipment being used in the hospital or to be used at home.

   Refer to Patient Teaching Guide on Using Oxygen at Home.

Airway Maintenance

Airway maintenance may occur in many forms, including: coughing, orotracheal or nasotracheal suctioning, oropharyngeal or nasopharyngeal airway insertion, endotracheal intubation, and endotracheal or tracheostomy tube suctioning.

The purpose of airway maintenance is to permit ventilation. Certain airway maintenance methods, such as endotracheal intubation, usually are initiated along with oxygen therapy and/or mechanical ventilators.

COUGHING

Coughing is the body's defense mechanism for maintaining clear airways. It can be an effective intervention, but may require patient teaching.

INDICATIONS

Secretions in the large airways of any patient
Postoperative patient
Patient who is on bed rest

PROCEDURAL TECHNIQUES AND ASSOCIATED CARE

1. Assess patient's ability to cough, e.g., ability for deep inhalation, glottic closure, contraction of expiratory muscles, and forced expulsion of air.
2. Facilitate loosening of secretions by encouraging fluid intake if not contraindicated or by using a nebulizer (Figure 6-10).
3. Instruct the patient regarding:
   a. The ideal position for coughing is sitting with head slightly flexed, shoulders relaxed, and knees flexed.
   b. Huff cough: The patient inhales deeply, bends forward slightly and then performs a series of 3 or 4 small coughs ("huffs") in a forced expiratory technique. This maneuver may stimulate the natural cough reflex.
   c. Splinting the thorax or abdomen with a towel or pillow may be necessary to achieve a maximum cough.
   d. End-expiratory cough: The patient takes a deep breath, exhales to below the normal tidal volume, and then coughs. The maneuver is repeated 2 or 3 times. This cough technique is effective with patients with bronchiectasis.

COMPLICATIONS

Rupture of rectus abdominus muscles
Rib fractures
Pneumothorax
Rupture of subconjunctival, nasal, or anal veins
Bradycardia

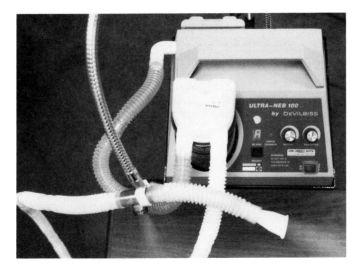

FIGURE 6-10
Ultrasonic nebulizer.

OROTRACHEAL OR NASOTRACHEAL SUCTIONING

When the patient is unable to cough up secretions, the nurse can use orotracheal or nasotracheal suctioning to remove secretions from the airways.

INDICATIONS

Signs of respiratory distress
Noisy, wet breathing
Tight wheeze with bronchospasm or croup

PROCEDURAL TECHNIQUES AND ASSOCIATED CARE

1. If possible, position patient in semi-Fowler's position.
2. Use sterile, gloved technique.
3. Select smallest catheter size possible to remove secretions.
4. Lubricate catheter tip with sterile saline or water or water-soluble gel.
5. Ask patient to take several deep breaths while on prescribed oxygen.
6. Ask patient to stick out the tongue as the catheter is passed through the nasal cavity.
7. Advance the catheter with a smooth motion directing it medially along the floor of the nasal cavity.
8. Encourage patient to breathe slowly during procedure.
9. If any difficulty is found advancing the catheter, rotate it gently. If resistance is met, attempt insertion of the other side.
10. The sound of air moving out with each expiration can be heard. If no air movement is heard, the catheter is in the esophagus.
11. Once the catheter is in the trachea, attach catheter to suction.
    a. One method of practice is to apply suction intermittently for 5- to 10-second intervals and then slowly removing catheter, waiting at least 3 minutes before catheter insertion is attempted again if additional suctioning is required.
    b. Another method of practice is to apply suction intermittently, but not to withdraw the catheter if additional suction is required. Instead the catheter is disconnected from suction, the patient receives oxygen followed by additional suctioning if needed.

12. Note and record amount and characteristics of sputum.
13. Note and record patient's response to suctioning procedure.
14. Discard catheter after each treatment.
15. Change vacuum container and tubing every day.

COMPLICATIONS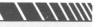

Wheezing or crowing respiratory sounds after or during procedure indicating potential bronchospasm or laryngospasm (if noted, administer oxygen and contact physician)

Bloody drainage owing to trauma or respiratory secretions

Prolonged spasmodic coughing

Traumatic ulceration of the airways

Infection

Atelectasis if catheter greater than two thirds the size of bronchus is used

Hypoxemia

Cardiac rhythm and rate disturbance

ENDOTRACHEAL INTUBATION AND EXTUBATION

The patient who requires assistance with ventilation may be intubated so that a mechanical ventilator can be used to maintain ventilation. An orotracheal or nasotracheal tube is used for short term therapy. When long-term therapy is required, the endotracheal tube is replaced with a tracheostomy tube (Figures 6-11 and 6-12).

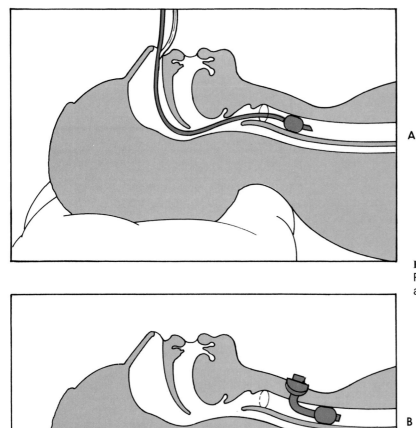

FIGURE 6-11
Placement of endotracheal tube **(A)** and tracheostomy tube **(B).**

INDICATIONS

Airway obstruction that occurs despite the use of an oral airway

To prevent possible aspiration in an unconscious patient

To remove secretions from the tracheobronchial tree

To provide controlled ventilation, which may or may not be accomplished by face masks

To provide high concentrations of oxygen

PROCEDURAL TECHNIQUES AND ASSOCIATED CARE

1. Assemble all equipment before attempting intubation procedure.
2. Check the cuff on endotracheal tubes for leakage.
3. Assist to position patient so the neck is flexed and the head is extended; this should bring the mouth, larynx, and trachea in line.
4. Before intubation, explain the procedure and ensure that any false teeth or bridges have been removed.
5. If patient is awake or combative, succinylocholine may be given to block voluntary ventilation; before administration of this drug, ventilatory assistance equipment must be available for immediate use.
6. Before intubation, hyperventilate patient using a manual resusciator bag (e.g., Ambu bag) with supplemental 100% oxygen (Figure 6-13).
7. If intubation is prolonged, interrupt the procedure and oxygenate the patient.
8. Once the endotracheal tube is in place, assist to determine proper endotracheal tube placement; this is done by considering the following:
   a. Correct placement: bilateral lung inflation, breath sounds heard equally throughout all lobes.
   b. Note the position at the patient's lips in reference to the centimeter (cm) markers on the tube. Document the proper placement in centimeters.
   c. Incorrect placement:
      Esophagus: absence of breath sounds, respiratory distress and cyanosis; if these are noted, the endotracheal tube should be removed and reinserted.
      Right mainstem bronchus or carina: the endotracheal tube has been inserted too far; clinical signs include unilateral breath sounds, lung inflation, and coughing; if this is noted and confirmed by x-ray examination, the endotracheal tube should be retracted slightly and resecured; reassessment should indicate proper placement.

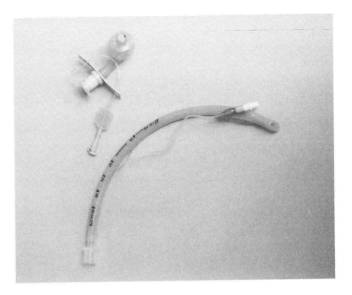

FIGURE 6-12
Cuffed tracheostomy tube (top) and cuffed endotracheal tube.

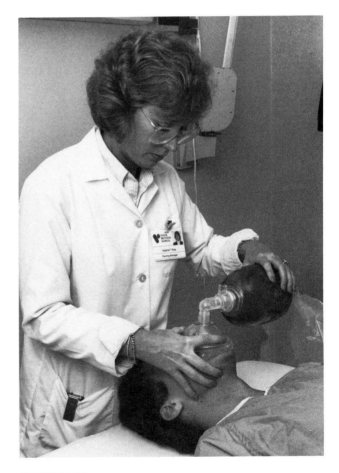

FIGURE 6-13
Using manual resuscitator bag to hyperoxygenate patient prior to intubation.

d. After repositioning tube
  1. Note the tube position at the lips in reference to the cm markers on the tube to insure the tube has not slipped down or been pulled outward by the repositioning, and
  2. Check bilateral breath sounds after repositioning tube.
9. Once the endotracheal tube is in correct position, tape it securely so movement of tube is impossible.
10. If tube has a cuff, use minimal occlusion volume (MOV) or minimal leak technique (MLT) for inflation.
  a. MOV is accomplished by injecting air slowly into the cuff pilot during the inspiratory phase of ventilation until the patient receives the prescribed tidal volume on the ventilator, or until no air can be heard leaking when auscultating the trachea. This represents just enough air to seal the area between the trachea and the tube. MOV does not prevent tracheal injury, but does reduce the potential for aspiration.
  b. MLT is accomplished using the same steps as MOV, but then withdrawing 0.1 ml of air to allow a small leak. MLT may produce less injury to the tracheal mucosa, but does not reduce the potential of aspiration.
11. Check the cuff pressure to ensure it is in a safe range. Normal tracheal capillary perfusion pressure is 30 mm Hg. The MOV should not exceed 20 mm Hg or 25 cm H_2O. Excessive air causes pressure against the trachea and restricts blood supply to the tracheal mucosa.
12. To deflate cuff a second person is needed.
  a. Suction the trachea using sterile technique.
  b. Deflate the cuff by inserting the syringe into the end of the stopcock, turning the stopcock arm to close the open port, and pulling back on the syringe. Meanwhile the second person delivers positive pressure either by compressing the manual resuscitation bag or using the ventilator to force the secretions into the mouth where they are suctioned. If positive pressure is not applied, the secretions from atop the cuff fall into the trachea.
13. Monitor tube placement and patency at least every hour. This assessment should include:
  a. Tube position
  b. Tube patency
  c. Lung inflation
  d. Absence of respiratory distress
  e. Generalized respiratory response
  f. Monitoring of arterial blood gases

14. Provide ongoing care for patients with endotracheal tube in place:
  a. Provide mouth care every 2 hours.
  b. Clean nares and around endotracheal tube at least every 6-8 hours.
  c. Reposition and retape endotracheal tube at least every 6-8 hours.
15. Use bite block or oral airway if the patient bites the endotracheal tube.
16. Perform chest physiotherapy at least every 4 hours.
17. If patient is awake, provide writing materials for communication.
18. Extubation:
  a. Assess patient's ability to breathe on own before extubation.
  b. Determine that patient is able to maintain spontaneous respiratory rate sufficient to maintain stable blood gas values.
  c. Carefully suction endotracheal tube and mouth before extubation; then deflate cuff and remove.
  d. Immediately after extubation, assess for signs of respiratory distress or laryngeal spasm e.g., dyspnea, noisy breathing, use of abdominal or accessory muscles, restlessness, irritability, tachycardia, tachypnea, decreased Pao_2, increased $Paco_2$. If these are noted, consult physician immediately and prepare for reinsertion of endotracheal tube.

COMPLICATIONS

Delay of oxygenation or ventilation during intubation procedure

Placement of endotracheal tube into right mainstem bronchus, resulting in unilateral and thus diminished lung aeration

Ulceration of trachea or tracheoesophageal fistula resulting from endotracheal tube cuff inflated for more than 8 hours

Mucus plugs or other blockage of endotracheal tube may lead to hypoxia and respiratory distress

Unplanned extubation by combative patient or secondary to poor securement of tube will require immediate airway and ventilatory assessment by the nurse as well as potential need for oral airway, patient positioning, and ventilation by Ambu bag with supplemental oxygen

Aspiration of secretions secondary to poorly inflated cuff, inadequate suctioning before cuff deflation, or too small noncuffed endotracheal tube used

Potential laryngospasm or edema follwing intubation

ENDOTRACHEAL OR TRACHEOSTOMY TUBE SUCTIONING

INDICATIONS

Rhonchi heard over large airways
Diminished breath sounds
Difficulty breathing
Cyanosis
Restlessness
Crowing (ineffective cough)

PROCEDURAL TECHNIQUES AND ASSOCIATED CARE

1. Auscultate breath sounds to determine the need for suctioning. Assess heart rate and rhythm as a baseline. Unless contraindicated, elevate the head of the bed to facilitate deep breathing and effective coughing.

2. Wash hands, use sterile gloves, catheter, and solution. The wearing of gown, mask, and/or wearing goggles because of the risk of AIDS is controversial. This procedure is altered somewhat when a 24-hour catheter is used. This is a suction catheter enclosed in a sterile sheath and attached to the endotracheal tube. The catheter sterility is maintained in the sheath so that the same catheter is used for a 24-hour period. Steps 5, 7, 9, and 13 described below are not necessary with this type of suction catheter.

3. Explain procedure to the patient including why it is necessary, summarizing explanations each time suctioning is repeated. Perform the explanation even if the patient is unconscious, because he may be able to hear.

4. Be sure the connecting tubing is attached to the suction collection bottle and that you have enough tubing to maneuver comfortably.

5. Choose a catheter that is at least 4 inches (10.2 cm) longer than the endotracheal tube with a diameter no larger than half the inside of the tube.

General guide

Adult:	12 to 18 French
Child:	6 to 12 French
Infant:	5 to 6 French

6. Pinch the catheter to check the vacuum pressure just high enough to remove secretions.

Usually above	120-150 mm Hg for adult
	100-120 mm Hg for child
	60-100 mm Hg for infant

7. Dip tip of catheter in sterile saline to lubricate it and apply suction to check the catheter patency.

8. Second person uses a manual resuscitator bag attached to 100% oxygen to hyperinflate and hyperoxygenate the patient's lungs four to five times.

   An alternate approach is to change the ventilator oxygen setting to 100% and use the "sigh" mode to hyperventilate and hyperoxygenate. Care must be taken after suctioning is complete to return the ventilator oxygen setting to the prescribed percentage.

9. First person inserts the suction catheter into tracheostomy or endotracheal tube and advances the catheter until resistance is met.

10. Withdraw the catheter back 1 cm and apply intermittent suction as the catheter is withdrawn with a gentle rotating motion. Suction should not be applied longer than 10 seconds. From catheter insertion to withdrawal should take no longer than 15 seconds.

11. Immediately after first person withdraws catheter, the second person gives 4-5 more hyperinflations with 100% oxygen.

12. Suctioning is repeated until the airway is clear.

13. If secretions are tenacious, 3 to 5 ml of sterile normal saline can be instilled into tube followed by hyperinflation to disperse the saline. The usefulness of this procedure is controversial. The use of heat and humidity has also been used to liquefy tenacious secretions.

14. When suctioning is completed, reconnect the ventilator tubing to the endotracheal tube. Suction the patient's mouth to remove excess saliva produced during the procedure.

15. Auscultate the patient's breath sounds and check the heart rate and rhythm; compare these with the baseline and document accordingly.

COMPLICATIONS

Hypoxemia
Dysrhythmias (atrioventricular (AV) heart block, premature ventricular contractions (PVCS), cardiac arrest)
Infection
Atelectasis
Hypotension
Bradycardia

1 ASSESS

ASSESSMENT	OBSERVATIONS
Respiratory	Restlessness, wheezing, noisy respirations, dyspnea, tachypnea, rhonchi over large airways, decreased breath sounds, retractions (intercostal, suprasternal, supraclavicular), nasal flaring, stridor, low tidal volumne, respiratory depth changes, cyanosis, hypoxia
Cardiovascular	Tachycardia
Oral mucous membrane	Airway in mouth, mouth breathing, dry mucous membranes
Psychosocial	Worried facial expression, restlessness, inability to speak due to intubation, confusion

2 DIAGNOSE

NURSING DIAGNOSIS	SUBJECTIVE FINDINGS	OBJECTIVE FINDINGS
Ineffective airway clearance related to tracheobronchial secretions	Complains of chest congestion; reports increased frequency of nonproductive cough	Decreased breath sounds, rhonchi over large airways, dyspnea, tachypnea
Anxiety related to difficulty breathing	Reports concern about meaning of chest congestion and its treatment	Tachypnea, restlessness, worried facial expressions, tachycardia
Ineffective breathing pattern related to pain, decreased lung expansion, or inflammatory process	Complains of pain on inspiration; reports reluctance to breathe deeply	Dyspnea, cyanosis, respiratory depth changes, altered chest excursion, nasal flaring, cough
Potential for aspiration related to excessive secretions and compromised respiratory system		Artifical airway in use; in supine or side-lying position, altered gag reflex, fatigue
Altered oral mucous membranes related to dehydration, ineffective oral hygiene, or malnutrition	Complains of a dry mouth	Airway in mouth, little to no oral intake, mouth breathing
Impaired verbal communication related to artificial airway		Patient unable to talk
Potential for infection related to inadequate primary defense mechanisms		Artificial airway bypassing upper airway, malnutrition, stress from disease process, invasive procedure

3 PLAN

Patient goals

1. Patient's airways will be clear to auscultation.
2. Patient's anxiety will be reduced.
3. Patient will have an effective breathing pattern.
4. Patient will not aspirate secretions or gastric contents.
5. Patient's oral cavity will be clean, moist, and odor-free.

6. Patient will be able to communicate.
7. Patient will not develop an infection.
8. Patient and family will understand purpose of airway maintenance procedures.

4 IMPLEMENT

NURSING DIAGNOSIS	NURSING INTERVENTIONS	RATIONALE
Ineffective airway clearance related to tracheobronchial secretions	Auscultate breath sounds for rhonchi.	Indicates need for coughing or suctioning.
	Position patient in semi-Fowler's position.	This position maximizes airway clearance.
	Assist patient to cough or suction airway as needed.	Coughing/suctioning removes secretions from large airways.
	If secretions are thick, increase humidification and fluid intake if not contraindicated.	Helps to liquefy secretions so they are easier to remove.
	Provide oxygen as needed.	Prevents hypoxemia; replaces oxygen removed by suctioning.
Anxiety related to difficulty breathing	Use a calm, reassuring voice.	This type of voice may help patient relax so he will take slower, deeper breaths.
	Explain procedures to be used to ease breathing difficulties.	Telling the patient the plans to help make him breathe easier may reduce anxiety.
	Remain with the patient.	Provides support; patient will not feel alone.
	Encourage patient to express feelings and thoughts, if possible.	Expressing feelings may reduce anxiety.
Ineffective breathing pattern related to pain, decreased lung expansion, or inflammatory process	Observe chest for equal excursion.	Determines symmetry and fullness of breathing pattern.
	Measure tidal volume and vital capacity.	Determines amount of air moving in and out of airways.
	Administer supportive ventilation as ordered.	Maintains ventilation.
	Administer analgesics as ordered.	Reduces pain that may cause altered breathing.

→ ❯ ❯

NURSING DIAGNOSIS	NURSING INTERVENTIONS	RATIONALE
Potential for aspiration related to excessive secretions and compromised respiratory system	Assess patient's ability to swallow secretions and patient's level of consciousness.	Patients who have difficulty swallowing or have decreased level of consciousness are more likely to aspirate.
	If patient has a cuffed endotracheal or tracheal tube, ensure the cuff is inflated at the proper pressure.	Cuff may prevent aspiration of fluid into the trachea.
	Elevate head of bed when performing mouth care and administering gastric feedings.	Gravity helps prevent fluids from entering trachea.
	Suction secretions as needed.	Maintains a patent airway.
Altered oral mucous membranes related to dehydration, ineffective oral hygiene, or malnutrition	Assess integrity of oral mucous membranes.	Determines if mucous membranes are intact.
	Provide oral care at least q 2 h for patients with an artificial airway. Change oral airway daily.	Cleans and moistens oral mucous membrane.
	Move orotracheal tube to the other side of the mouth daily.	Prevents continuous pressure of the tube on oral mucous membranes.
	Avoid lemon-glycerine swabs.	Lemon and glycerine dry mucous membranes and cause cracking.
Impaired verbal communication related to artificial airway	Assess psychologic response to impaired communication, e.g., anxious, angry, hostile.	Determines the patient's response to altered communication so the nurse can intervene appropriately.
	Maintain eye contact.	Shows interest in communicating.
	Explore alternate means of communication aids, e.g., paper and pencil, magic slate, picture board, letter board. Allow adequate time for communication.	Provides alternate forms of communication, for addressing patient's needs and relieving anxiety.
	Administer oxygen as ordered.	Decreases dyspnea that interferes with communication.
	Anticipate patient needs. Keep call bell within patient's reach.	Prevents patient from having to communicate needs.
	Ask questions that require a "yes" or "no" answer.	Allows patient to communicate nonverbally.
Potential for infection related to inadequate primary defense mechanisms	Monitor temperature.	Detects fever indicating actual infection.
	Auscultate lungs for rhonchi and crackles.	These sounds indicate increased secretions which may lead to pulmonary infection.

NURSING DIAGNOSIS	NURSING INTERVENTIONS	RATIONALE
	Monitor leukocytes.	Indicates adequacy of secondary defense and immune system. An increase in leukocytes indicates infection.
	Use sterile technique when suctioning airway.	Prevents exposure of patient to microorganisms.
	Encourage coughing and deep breathing if possible.	Maintains clear airways; prevents atelectasis.
	Administer prophylactic antibiotics as ordered.	Interrupts growth of microorganisms.
Knowledge deficit	See Patient Teaching.	

5 EVALUATE

PATIENT OUTCOME	DATA INDICATING THAT OUTCOME IS REACHED
Airway is patent.	Breath sounds are clear and bilaterally equal. There are no adventitious sounds. Lung fields are clear on chest x-ray.
Anxiety is reduced.	Patient verbalizes feeling less anxious. Patient appears more calm, relaxed.
Breathing pattern is effective.	Breathing occurs easily and seems adequate for patient's attempts.
Aspiration did not occur.	Temperature and respiratory rate are within normal limits. Lung fields are clear on chest x-ray.
Oral mucous membranes are intact.	Oral mucous membranes appear moist, clean, and odor-free.
Patient is able to communicate.	Patient is able to communicate verbally or nonverbally.
No infection is present.	Temperature is within normal limits. Leukocytes are normal.
Knowledge deficit is resolved.	Patient and/or family verbalize understanding of procedure.

PATIENT TEACHING ■

Because of the patient's situation requiring airway maintenance procedures, preprocedural teaching may seem inappropriate. The care provider is still required to anticipate teaching opportunities and to provide the following information as appropriate (see specific teaching guidelines under Procedural Techniques and Associated Care):

1. Explain procedure to patient and family members.
2. Discuss with patient and family what procedure will be like for the patient.
3. Demonstrate equipment and its purpose.

Mechanical Ventilation

Mechanical ventilation allows administration of 100% oxygen and control of breathing pattern for patients who are unable to maintain adequate ventilation on their own. The ventilator does not cure pulmonary disease, but is a temporary support that "buys time" for correction of the underlying pathologic process.

There are two categories of ventilators: positive pressure and negative pressure. Positive pressure ventilators include the volume-cycled and pressure-cycled ventilators (Figure 6-14). These ventilators use positive pressure to push air into the lungs. Positive pressure ventilators require the patient to use a mouthpiece or have an endotracheal tube or tracheostomy tube in place. In contrast, the negative pressure ventilators use negative pressure to raise the rib cage and lower the diaphragm to create negative pressure within the lungs so that air flows into the lungs. Although not used as frequently, this latter type approximates normal respiration. This type of ventilator includes the iron lung and cuirass ventilators.

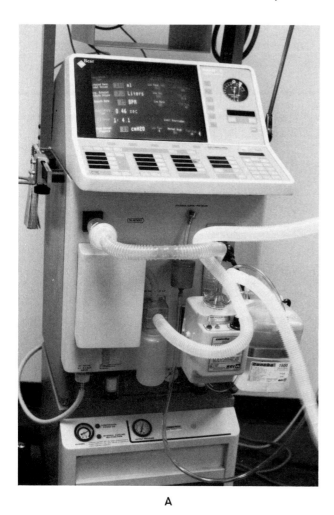

A

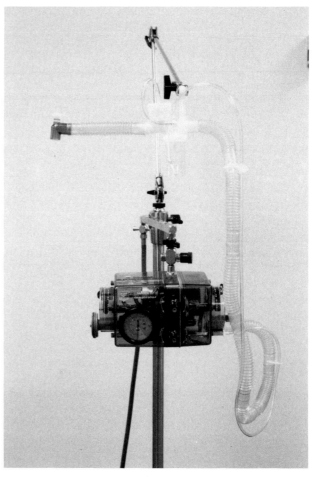

B

FIGURE 6-14
Positive pressure ventilators. **A,** Volume-cycled ventilator. **B,** Pressure-cycled ventilator.

POSITIVE PRESSURE VENTILATORS
Volume-Cycled Ventilators

Volume-cycled (volume-preset) ventilators terminate inspiration after delivering a preset volume of gas (Figure 6-14, A). A piston or bellows pushes a predetermined volume (VT) into the patient's lungs at a set respiratory rate. The desired volume of gas is delivered regardless of the required pressure to do so. The ventilator continues to deliver a constant tidal volume regardless of the changes in the airway resistance or in the compliance of the lungs and thorax. The volume remains the same unless excessively high peak airway pressures are reached, in which case safety release valves stop the flow. The safety release pressure is usually set at about 10 cm H_2O above the inspiratory pressure.*

*Some examples include the Bennett MA-3, Ohio 560, Servo 900, Emerson, Bourns Bear 1 and 2, and the Engstrom.

Pressure-Cycled Ventilators

Pressure-cycled (pressure-preset) ventilators terminate inspiration when a preset pressure is achieved (Figure 6-14,B). When the pressure is reached, the gas flow stops and the patient passively exhales. The largest patient variable is that varying degrees of resistance interfere with gas flow. Thus the delivered volume may vary as the degree of resistance varies. These ventilators are most commonly used for patients whose ventilatory resistance has not changed (e.g., drug overdose). They are not appropriately used for patients whose resistance may have changed (e.g., postoperative status or patients with severe respiratory infections). These respirators have only a low peak pressure capability (30 to 40 cm).†

†Some examples include Bird Mark 7 and 8, Bennett PR-1 and PR-2, and Monaghan 300.

POSITIVE PRESSURE VENTILATOR SETTINGS

Tidal volume (V_t) sets the number of milliliters of air to be delivered with each breath. This volume is dialed in on volume ventilators. For pressure ventilators the inspiratory time flow-rate control is manipulated to determine the magnitude of inspiration.

Pressure limit or *inspiratory pressure limit* is the highest pressure allowed in the ventilatory circuit. If the pressure limit is reached, inspiration is terminated. The high pressure alarm will sound if the pressure limit is reached. When this alarm sounds the patient is not receiving the desired tidal volume. The cause of the high pressure alarm may be coughing, accumulation of secretions, kinked ventilator tubing, pneumothorax, decreased compliance, or simple pressure limits set too low.

Respiratory rate is the number of breaths per minute delivered to the patient. The rate is dialed in for volume ventilators. For pressure ventilators, the inspiratory time flow-rate control determines the duration of inspiration by regulating the velocity of gas flow.

Sigh volume delivers a larger volume of air than the tidal volume. The specific volume and rate per hour can be selected. The sigh is incorporated to provide a deep breath to help to prevent atelectasis.

Peak flow is the velocity or speed of air flow per unit of time and is expressed as liters per minute. For volume ventilators this is a separate knob that is set (more rapid the flow, shorter the inspiratory time; slower the flow, longer the inspiratory time). For pressure ventilators this is manipulated by the inspiratory time flow-rate control.

Sensitivity is the amount of effort the patient must exert (negative inspiratory pull) to initiate an inspiration. *Fraction of inspired oxygen* (Fio_2) is the percentage of oxygen delivered to the patient. Concentrations vary from 21 to 100%.

Positive End Expiratory Pressure (PEEP) maintains positive pressure in the patient's alveoli at all times, even during exhalation. PEEP minimizes alveolar collapse, increases mean airway pressure, increases the functional reserve capacity, increases compliance, decreases shunting, and promotes clearing of lung fields. In the cardiovascular system PEEP decreases venous return and increases pulmonary vascular resistance. The goal of PEEP is to improve oxygenation with subsequent decrease in inspired oxygen concentration needed to correct life-threatening hypoxemia. Complications of PEEP include peripheral vasoconstriction, hypotension, increased pulmonary capillary wedge pressures (>15 mmHg), and increased incidence of pneumothorax and barotrauma. Continuous positive airway pressure (CPAP) is similar to PEEP but is intended for patients who can breathe spontaneously.

VENTILATORY MODES

Volume-cycled ventilators are able to deliver four modes of ventilation. The **control** mode delivers a predetermined volume at a fixed rate. The ventilator breaths are not synchronized with the patient's own respiratory effort. When this mode is used, the patient usually receives sedation such as morphine or paralyzing agents such as pancuronium to diminish or eliminate his respiratory effort so that the patient will not fight against the ventilator.

The **assist** mode augments the patient's own breaths with an additional preset volume of air. Each time the patient inhales, he creates a negative pressure in the airways. When this negative pressure equals or exceeds the preset pressure level, the ventilator responds by giving the patient an assisted breath.

The **assist-control** mode is a combination of the last two modes described. This mode works in the assist mode unless the patient stops breathing. Then the ventilator automatically responds with a predetermined respiratory rate and volume, as it would in the control mode.

The **synchronized intermittent mandatory ventilation** mode (SIMV) or (IMV) is a combination of the patient's own respiratory rate and the assist-control mode. The ventilator is set at a predetermined rate and volume of air, which is delivered to the patient who may breath in between the ventilator breaths. However, unlike the assist-control mode, any breaths the patient takes above the set rate are spontaneous at his own rate and tidal volume. This mode is used when weaning a patient from a ventilator. The goal is to gradually decrease the rate on the ventilator while the patient breaths increasingly on his own.

NEGATIVE PRESSURE VENTILATORS

Negative pressure ventilators have settings for respiratory rate and the pressure of the negative force exerted. These two settings are adjusted based on the patient's tidal volume. These ventilators are used for patients who have neuromuscular diseases, which impair the intercostal and/or diaphragmatic muscles from contracting to maintain ventilation. Many of these patients have healthy lungs but lack the muscular ability to inhale. As a result, they need assistance with ventilation, but breathe room air. Supplemental oxygen can be added with the usual oxygen therapy devices. Some examples include the Emerson and Monoghan.

INDICATIONS

$Paco_2$ > 55 mm Hg
Pao_2 < 50 mm Hg on a Fio_2 > 0.60 or Pao_2 > 50 mm

Hg with pH < 7.25
Dead space to tidal volume ratio (V_D/V_T) > 0.60
Inspiratory force (IF) < 25 cm H_2O
Tidal volume (V_T), 5 ml/kg
Vital capacity (VC) < 10 ml/kg
Expiratory force < 60 cm H_2O
Respiratory rate > 35/min

COMPLICATIONS

Complications of positive pressure ventilation include respiratory arrest from disconnection from ventilator, respiratory infection, acid-base imbalances, oxygen toxicity, pneumothorax, gastrointestinal bleeding, barotrauma, and decreased cardiac output.

PROCEDURAL PROBLEMS

Pao_2 >110 mm Hg

1. Determine Fio_2; report Fio_2 setting and Pao_2 to physician (make sure Fio_2 was not left on 100% oxygen)
2. Note patient's position; diaphragm movement and blood flow and ventilation (V/Q) relationships are affected by gravity and position

Pao_2 < 50 to 90 mm Hg, depending on patient's underlying disease

1. If patient shows signs of cyanosis, tachycardia, arrhythmias, restlessness, or decreased sensorium, remove patient from ventilator and bag breathe patient with 100% oxygen until physician's help and further assessment are possible
2. Assessment of problem should include:
   Machine or tubing malfunction
   Patient's need for suctioning
   Diminished patient lung functioning owing to pneumothorax or atelectasis
   Malplaced endotracheal tube

STANDARD INITIAL VENTILATOR SETTINGS

Fraction of inspired oxygen $(Fio_2)\approx100\%$	
Tidal volume (V_T)	10-15 ml/kg body weight
Respiratory rate	10-15 breaths/min
Inspiratory flow	40-60 liters/sec
Sensitivity	12 cm H_2O
Sigh rate (optional)	1-2/min, V_T 20 ml/kg

$Paco_2 > 45$ mm Hg or patient's baseline if the patient has COPD

1. Verify that patient is connected to ventilator and that ventilator tubing is clear of obstruction or water accumulation
2. Suction airway if necessary and determine position and patency of endotracheal tube
3. Evaluate patient for metabolic acidosis
4. If patient is on low, intermittent mandatory ventilation, determine whether patient has recently received respiratory depressing sedation, which would affect respiratory status

$Paco_2 < 35$ mm Hg (unless desired control of cerebral blood flow)

1. Assess patient's respiratory rate and depth
2. Assess for metabolic acidosis

WEANING FROM THE VENTILATOR

The following criteria can be used to determine when the patient is ready for weaning:

1. Vital capacity at least 10-15 ml/kg body weight.
2. Tidal volume greater than 5 ml/kg.
3. Maximum inspiratory force greater than 20 cm H_2O.
4. Resting minute volume greater than 100 per minute.
5. $Paco_2$ in stable range for patient.
6. Pao_2 greater than 70-80 mm Hg on 0.5 Fio_2.

One strategy for weaning patient is first to reduce the Fio_2 to 30%, then to decrease the PEEP if it has been used, and finally to use intermittent mandatory ventilation (IMV). IMV allows the patient's own reasonable breathing pattern to be maintained with positive pressure breaths intermittently delivered by the ventilator as needed. IMV also allows for the gradual conditioning of the diaphragm, which becomes weak from disuse during mechanical ventilation. Before mechanical ventilation is disconnected, explain the weaning process to the patient. The longer the patient uses mechanical ventilation, the longer the weaning process takes due to psychologic and physical dependence on the machine. Prior to disconnection the airways should be suctioned and the patient positioned in a 60- to 90-degree angle to move the abdominal contents away from the diaphragm. A T-tube may be used to provide oxygen while the patient breathes without assistance.

1   ASSESS

ASSESSMENT	OBSERVATIONS
Respiratory	Decreased tidal volume, dyspnea, tachypnea, $Pao_2 < 50$ mm Hg, $Paco_2 > 50$ mm Hg, rhonchi, crackles, decreased or absent breath sounds
Gastrointestinal	Decreased food and fluid intake

2   DIAGNOSE

NURSING DIAGNOSIS	SUBJECTIVE FINDINGS	OBJECTIVE FINDINGS
neffective breathing pattern related to neuromuscular impairment, inflammatory process, or decreased lung expansion	*Since the patient cannot verbally communicate, there are usually no subjective findings.*	Decreased tidal volume, dyspnea, tachypnea, $Pao_2 < 50$ mm Hg, $Paco_2 > 50$ mm Hg
Impaired gas exchange related to alveolar-capillary membrane changes		$Pao_2 < 50$ mm Hg, $Pao_2 > 50$ mm Hg, decreased or absent breath sounds, inability to move secretions

→ › ›

NURSING DIAGNOSIS	SUBJECTIVE FINDINGS	OBJECTIVE FINDINGS
Potential altered nutrition: less than body requirements related to NPO status		Unable to take food or fluids by mouth
Potential for infection related to loss of respiratory defense mechanisms, decreased ciliary action, and stasis of secretions		Crackles, rhonchi, fever, increased secretions

3   PLAN

Patient goals

1. Patient will have effective breathing pattern.
2. Patient will have adequate gas exchange.
3. Patient's nutritional status will be maintained to meet body needs.
4. Patient will not develop a pulmonary infection.
5. Patient and/or family will indicate understanding of the purpose for mechanical ventilation.

4   IMPLEMENT

NURSING DIAGNOSIS	NURSING INTERVENTIONS	RATIONALE
Ineffective breathing pattern related to neuromuscular impairment, inflammatory process, or decreased lung expansion	Observe changes in respiratory rate and depth; observe for SOB and use of accessory muscles.	An increase in the work of breathing will add to fatigue; may indicate patient fighting ventilator.
	Inspect thorax for symmetry of movement.	Determines adequacy of breathing pattern; asymmetry may indicate hemothorax or pneumothorax.
	Measure tidal volume and vital capacity.	Indicates volume of air moving in and out of lungs.
	Assess for pain.	Pain may prevent patient from coughing and deep breathing.
	Monitor chest x-rays.	Shows extent and location of fluid or infiltrates in lungs.
	Maintain ventilator settings as ordered.	Ventilator provides adequate ventilatory pattern for the patient.
	Elevate head of bed 60°-90°.	This position moves the abdominal contents away from the diaphragm, which facilitates its contraction.
Impaired gas exchange related to alveolar-capillary membrane changes	Monitor ABGs.	Determines acid-base balance and need for oxygen.
	Assess level of consciousness, listlessness, and irritability.	These signs may indicate hypoxia.

NURSING DIAGNOSIS	NURSING INTERVENTIONS	RATIONALE
	Observe skin color and capillary refill.	Determines adequacy of blood flow needed to carry oxygen to tissues.
	Monitor CBC.	Indicates the oxygen-carrying capability available.
	Administer oxygen as ordered.	Decreases work of breathing and supplies supplemental oxygen.
	Reposition patient q 1-2 h.	Repositioning helps all lobes of the lung to be adequately perfused and ventilated.
Potential altered nutrition: less than body requirements related to NPO status	Monitor lymphocytes and albumin.	Indicates adequate visceral protein.
	Measure mid-arm circumference and triceps skin fold.	The former indicates protein stores, the latter fat stores.
	Provide nutrition as ordered, e.g., total parenteral nutrition or continuous tube feedings and serum lipids.	Calories, minerals, vitamins, and protein are needed for energy and tissue repair.

5 EVALUATE

PATIENT OUTCOME	DATE INDICATING THAT OUTCOME IS REACHED
Breathing pattern is effective without dyspnea.	Respiratory rate and rhythm are adequate; absence of dyspnea.
Gas exchange is adequate.	ABGs within acceptable range, no dyspnea.
Maintains adequate nutritional status.	Weight remaining stable and within normal range for patient; albumin and lymphocytes are in normal range.
Patient/family understand purpose of mechanical ventilation.	Patient breathes in synchrony with ventilator, does not appear anxious when alarm sounds. Family explains purpose of the mechanical ventilation.

PATIENT TEACHING

1. Explain to the patient and family the purpose for mechanical ventilation and respiratory mode (e.g., assist-control,)
2. Encourage the patient to relax and not to fight against the breathing (mode) pattern of the ventilator.
3. Explain that alarms may sound periodically, indicating the ventilator may need to be checked. Encourage patient to take a deep breath and relax when the alarm sounds and that a nurse or respiratory therapist will check on the patient and the ventilator.
4. Teach patient the importance of periodic deep breathing.
5. Inform the patient that although he is not able to communicate verbally there are alternate methods for expressing his needs and his fears (e.g., magic slate or similar writing material, picture board). Let the patient know that a call bell is within his reach.

Chest Tubes and Chest Drainage Systems

A **chest tube** (also called thoracostomy tube or thoracic catheter) is generally a firm plastic drain with several eyelets in the proximal end that is inserted into the pleural space, sutured to the skin, and taped securely.

The purpose of this tube is to drain fluid, blood, or air from the pleural cavity and to reestablish a negative pressure that will facilitate the reexpansion of the lung.

To drain air from an adult a no. 16 or no. 24-gauge French tube is used and to drain liquid a no. 28 to no. 36-gauge tube is used. Smaller size tubes are used with children.

The underwater seal drainage to which the chest tube is connected prevents backflow into the pleural space. Chest tubes may be inserted postoperatively, as an emergency procedure following chest trauma, or therapeutically as a disease treatment modality.

Chest tubes may be terminated when x-ray examination determines that the lung is reexpanded and when the drainage has slowed to less than 75 ml/day.

CAUTIONS

Cautions specific to chest tubes and drainage systems include the following:

Sterility must be maintained so as not to introduce infection into pleural cavity.

The system must remain patent: the tubing must not become blocked; if this occurs, a tension pneumothorax may result.

If the drainage tubing becomes dislodged from the patient or a drainage bottle breaks, cross-clamps should be quickly applied to the tube(s) nearest the patient until the system's integrity can be reestablished.

If the chest tube becomes dislodged from the patient's chest, the patient should exhale forcefully, and the chest wall incision should be quickly covered with a petrolatum jelly gauze.

INDICATIONS

Postoperative patient after surgical procedure requiring a surgical incision of the chest wall (thoracotomy)
Patient with a pneumothorax or hemothorax
Patient with pleural effusion or empyema

PROCEDURAL TECHNIQUES AND ASSOCIATED CARE

Carefully assess patient's preprocedural condition including respiratory rate and quality. Note evidence of dyspnea, labored breathing, tachypnea, tachycardia, quality and distribution of breath sounds, mediastinal shift, subcutaneous emphysema, and crepitus.

Set up drainage equipment appropriately for the type of system being used.

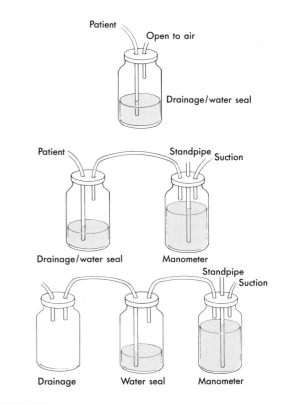

FIGURE 6-15
Bottle chest drainage systems. **A,** Single-bottle system. **B,** Double-bottom system. **C,** Triple-bottle system. (From Thompson.)[99]

One-bottle System (Figure 6-15, *A*)

1. Unwrap bottle and tubing; maintain sterility.
2. Fill bottle with sterile water until the long glass tubing is submerged 2 cm. This bottle is called the water-seal bottle. The depth of the rod in the water determines the degree of negative pressure in the bottle.
3. The short glass tubing (air vent) should never be covered with water.
4. The long glass tubing is connected to the patient's chest tube, and the short tubing (air vent) allows air to escape.
5. The force of the patient's exhalation pushes air out through the bottom of the long glass tube. The air may be absorbed in the fluid or bubble to the surface. The amount of force necessary for the patient to push air through the water seal depends on how deeply the long tube is submerged in the solution. Drainage from the patient's chest raises the fluid level in the collection bottle. If the fluid level in a one-bottle system gets too high, a new collection bottle is needed. Otherwise the patient will not be able to push air from the pleural space through the water seal. If the amount of drainage is large, a two-bottle system is needed.

Two-bottle System (Figure 6-15, *B*)

1. Prepare the second bottle as described for the single-bottle system. This bottle acts as a water-seal bottle with one long tube submerged 2 cm under water and a short tube open to air.
2. The bottle closest to the patient is a collection bottle for drainage. It has one short tube that allows drainage to collect and a second short tube that is connected to the second bottle by a rubber tubing.
3. Drainage falls into the first collection bottle and air flows beyond into the water seal bottle.
4. Bubbling from an air leak and fluctuations in the water-seal tube will occur in the same way as they do in the one-bottle system.

CHEST TUBE INSERTION SITES

For pneumothorax: usually in second and third intercostal space (anterior)
For hemothorax: usually in seventh, eighth, or ninth intercostal space (posterior)
For thoracotomy: one tube generally inserted in second or third intercostal space (anterior) and another in lower posterior axillary line

---

CHECKING CHEST TUBES AND CHEST DRAINAGE

Chest tubes

1. Inspect all tubing connections for leaks and kinks. Make sure the extra tubing is coiled and lying on top of the bed.
2. Maintain chest tubes at a level below the patient's chest. This prevents fluid and air from reentering the pleural space.
3. Keep two clamps at the bedside to temporarily clamp a chest tube if a break or disconnection occurs.
4. Keep petrolatum jelly gauze at the bedside to cover the insertion site after the chest tubes are removed.

Chest drainage

1. Check water level in water seal drainage system.
2. Observe amount, color, and consistency of drainage from lung.
3. Observe fluctuations in the water seal bottle. Fluid level rises during inhalation and falls during exhalation when the patient is breathing spontaneously. Fluctuations are reversed when the patient is on mechanical ventilation due to the positive pressure. If the patient has a pleural air leak and there is no suction applied, there is bubbling in the water seal bottle when the patient exhales or coughs; if suction is applied, the bubbling is continuous.

Three-bottle System (Figure 6-15, *C*)

1. Prepare the first two bottles as described in the two-bottle system.
2. A third bottle, used as a suction control bottle, is placed between the water seal bottle and the suction source. The bottle has a long tube with the lower end submerged in sterile water or saline and the upper end open to atmosphere pressure. The maximal level of suction that can be exerted on the drainage system is determined by how deeply the control tube is submerged, usually 20 cm of water.
3. Suction may be added to the drainage system if the air leaking into the pleural space accumulates faster than the gravity system can remove it.

Commercial Disposable Three-chamber System (Figure 6-16)

Disposable plastic units include Atrium Compact, ConMed Pleura-Gard, Deknatel Pleurevac, Emerson 550, and Sherwood Medical Thora-Seal. These systems function like the three-bottle systems. Setup and operation directions are provided with the sterile units.

REMOVAL OF CHEST TUBES

Chest tubes may be removed after the lung has been reinflated for 24 hours to several days. Indications for removal are usually confirmed by chest x-ray examination. Removal procedures include the following:

1. Place patient in semi-Fowler's position or on side.
2. Physician instructs patient to take a deep breath and hold it.
3. The chest tube suture is clipped and the tube is quickly removed.
4. A pressure dressing with antibiotic ointment or petrolatum jelly gauze is placed over chest wall wound.
5. Patient is instructed to breathe normally, and the pressure dressing is taped securely.

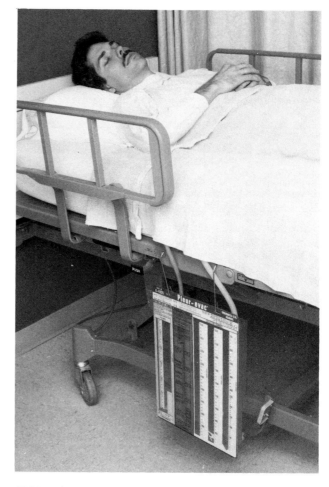

FIGURE 6-16
Pleur-Evac commercial three-chamber system used to drain the pleural cavity.

6. Careful patient assessment should follow on a continuing basis, including rate of respirations, quality of breath sounds, any drainage from the pressure dressing, sudden chest pains, or shortness of breath.

---

1   ASSESS

ASSESSMENT	OBSERVATIONS
Respiratory	Dyspnea, labored breathing, tachypnea, tachycardia, non-symmetrical chest expansion Breath sounds on affected side: absent, decreased, crackles, rhonchi Anxiety, restlessness

2 DIAGNOSE

NURSING DIAGNOSIS	SUBJECTIVE FINDINGS	OBJECTIVE FINDINGS
Ineffective breathing pattern related to pain and decreased lung expansion	Complains of SOB, difficult and/or painful breathing	Dyspnea, labored breathing, tachypnea, non-symmetric chest expansion Absent or decreased breath sounds on affected side Crackles, rhonchi
Impaired physical mobility related to pain and discomfort	Reports pain when breathing and moving	Reluctant to move; limited range of motion in arm adjacent to chest tube
Potential for infection related to inadequate primary defenses and invasive procedure		Broken skin at chest tube insertion site; traumatized tissue

3 PLAN

Patient goals

1. Patient will have an adequate breathing pattern.
2. Patient will resume physical mobility.
3. Patient will not develop an infection.

4. Patient will demonstrate an understanding of the need for chest tubes.

4 IMPLEMENT

NURSING DIAGNOSIS	NURSING INTERVENTIONS	RATIONALE
Ineffective breathing pattern related to pain and decreased lung expansion	Auscultate breath sounds.	Determines gas exchange.
	Observe chest excursions.	Symmetrical excursions indicate adequate breathing pattern.
	Assist patient to change position, cough and deep breathe, splinting chest as necessary.	Helps reexpand lung; prevents atelectasis or stasis of secretions.
Impaired physical mobility related to pain and discomfort	Assess range of motion in affected upper extremity.	Determines whether a contracture has developed.
	Encourage active or passive range of motion exercises for arm and shoulder of affected side.	Prevents stiffness and contractures from disuse.
	Encourage patient to exercise lower legs. Assist patient with ambulation as ordered.	Prevents venous stasis and muscle weakness.

→ > >

NURSING DIAGNOSIS	NURSING INTERVENTIONS	RATIONALE
Potential for infection related to inadequate primary defenses and invasive procedure	Monitor temperature.	Fever may indicate an infection.
	Auscultate lungs for crackles and rhonchi.	Adventitious sounds indicate secretions in airways.
	Monitor leukocytes.	Indicates adequacy of immune system; an increase indicates an infection.
	Observe drainage from chest tube for foul odor and purulent drainage.	Indicates an infection in pleural space.
	Encourage coughing and deep breathing.	Helps to reexpand lungs; prevents stasis of secretions.
	Encourage an increase in fluid intake unless contraindicated.	Helps to liquefy secretions.
	Administer antiinfective agents as ordered.	Prevents or interrupts growth of microorganisms.
	Encourage optimum nutrition.	Maintains nutritional status; supports immune system.
Knowledge deficit	See Patient Teaching	

5 EVALUATE

PATIENT OUTCOME	DATA INDICATING THAT OUTCOME IS REACHED
Breathing pattern is adequate.	Breath sounds are clear bilaterally. Patient is able to breathe deeply without pain. Chest x-rays indicate lungs are reexpanded.
There is no infection.	Temperature is within normal limits. Leukocytes are within normal limits.
Physical mobility is restored.	Patient has full range of motion of affected arm and shoulder.
Knowledge deficit is resolved.	Patient expresses an understanding of the need for chest tubes and chest drainage.

PATIENT TEACHING ■

1. Explain the purpose for chest tubes and the drainage system.
2. Encourage patient to maintain good body alignment.
3. Encourage patient to change position frequently when possible.
4. Teach patient to move arm and shoulder of the affected side through range of motion exercises several times each day.
5. Teach patient importance of deep breathing and coughing.
6. Instruct patient to request pain medication when coughing is painful.

Thoracic Surgery

Thoracic surgery refers to surgical incision of the chest wall for the purpose of obtaining a biopsy, controlling a source of bleeding, removing lung tissue, or transplanting one or both lungs.

Thoracotomy refers to a surgical incision of the chest wall. Many times an exploratory thoracotomy is performed to obtain a biopsy specimen or locate a source of bleeding. During the procedure the ribs are spread and the pleura is opened. Closed chest drainage is generally required postoperatively.

Pneumonectomy refers to surgical removal of an entire lung. The surgeon severs and sutures off the main arteries, veins, and the mainstem bronchus at the bifurcation. The major indication for pneumonectomy is lung cancer. Closed chest drainage is generally not done postoperatively. It is desirable for the thoracic cavity on the affected side to fill with serous exudate. The exudate eventually consolidates. The phrenic nerve on the affected side may be severed by the surgeon. This permits the diaphragm to assume an elevated position, which also assists to fill the empty thoracic space.

Lobectomy refers to removal of a lobe of the lung. Major indications for this procedure include isolated tumors, cysts, tuberculosis, abscess, or localized injury. Closed chest drainage is used following a lobectomy.

Segmental resection refers to the removal of one or more segments of the lung lobe. Indications for the procedure include tuberculosis, bleb, localized abscess, or bronchiectasis. Closed chest drainage is used following this procedure.

Wedge resection refers to the removal of a small, wedge-shaped localized area near the lung surface. Indications for the procedure include biopsy and removal of a small area of tuberculosis. The resected area is sutured off before removal. There is generally little disruption of overall lung function. Closed chest drainage is used after the procedure.

Decortication refers to the stripping off of a thick fibrous membrane that may develop over the visceral pleura secondary to empyema or the prolonged presence of blood or fluid in the pleural space. Closed chest drainage is required postoperatively.

Thoracoplasty refers to a surgical procedure intended to remove select portions of the ribs with the intent of reducing the overall size of the thoracic cavity.

Lung transplantation is the removal of the recipient lung and replacement of a donor lung from a cadaver. Surgical procedures have been developed to transplant a single lung, both lungs, and both heart and lungs. Indications for single lung transplants are patients who have end-stage irreversible acute or chronic lung disease without serious infection such as pulmonary fibrosis, interstitial fibrosis, emphysema, and cystic fibrosis. Single lung as well as heart-lung transplants have been successful for patients with end-stage primary pulmonary hypertension. Three anastomoses are involved for a *single* lung transplant—bronchial, pulmonary artery, and pulmonary vein. The bronchial anastomosis is accomplished by telescoping the donor bronchus within the recipient bronchus. The anatomosis is then wrapped with a pedicle flap of intercostal muscle to provide structural reinforcement and early neovascularity. The pulmonary artery anastomosis is constructed to prevent stenosis. The pulmonary venous anastomosis is done by transplanting a cuff of left atrium containing the ostia of the pulmonary veins, rather than performing direct pulmonary venous anastomoses.

COMPLICATIONS

Respiratory insufficiency
Tension pneumothorax
Cardiac failure or myocardial infarction
Thrombosis or pulmonary embolism
Atelectasis
Bronchopleural fistula
Pulmonary edema
Subcutaneous emphysema
Infection

CRITERIA FOR SINGLE LUNG TRANSPLANT

Criteria for recipient

6-12 month prognosis
Under 55 years of age (selected patients over 55 years of age)
Absence of infection, diabetes, malignancy, and renal disease
Adequate cardiac function

Criteria for donor

ABO match between donor and recipient
Age 12-50 years
No active or histologic pulmonary disease
Absence of thoracic trauma or chest tubes
Arterial Pao_2 >250 mm Hg on 100% Fio_2
Chest x-ray free of infiltrates or edema
Compatible side of hilar and bronchial structures
Absence of purulent tracheobronchial secretions

PREPROCEDURAL NURSING CARE

Carefully determine preoperative status of patient including the following:

Baseline pulmonary function studies
Electrocardiogram
Arterial blood gases
Electrolytes
Other existing medical problems
Current respiratory status: amount and extent of dyspnea, cough, and respiratory distress
General nutrition and hydration state

Provide preoperative teaching to include the following:

1. Emphasize the need to stop smoking preoperatively.
2. Teach coughing and deep breathing techniques.
3. Discuss need for and technique of suctioning and closed chest drainage postoperatively.
4. Present an overview of equipment and procedures that will most likely occur postoperatively.
5. Listen preoperatively to patient and family questions and concerns; provide information and clarification when indicated.
6. Assure patient that pain medication will be available postoperatively to assist with discomfort.
7. Teach patient the need for postoperative range of motion and leg exercises.

1 ASSESS

ASSESSMENT	OBSERVATIONS
Respiratory	Dyspnea, tachypnea, shallow respirations, crackles, rhonchi, decreased tidal volume, Pao_2 < 55 mmHg, $Paco_2$ > 50 mm Hg cough, chest tubes Pain on coughing and deep breathing
Skin	Thoracic incision covered with dressing; stab wounds at chest tube insertion sites; skin warm and dry
Nutrition	Inadequate intake of fluids and food

2 DIAGNOSE

NURSING DIAGNOSIS	SUBJECTIVE FINDINGS	OBJECTIVE FINDINGS
Ineffective breathing pattern related to pain, fatigue, and chest tubes	Complains of fatigue; complains of pain when breathing; expresses need for oxygen	Dyspnea, tachypnea, shallow respirations, decreased tidal volume $Pa_{O_2} < 55$ mm Hg $Pa_{CO_2} > 50$ mm Hg
Ineffective airway clearance related to tracheobronchial secretions	Complains of painful coughing	Crackles, rhonchi, tachypnea, dyspnea, cough
Pain related to surgical procedure	Complains of incisional pain on moving, deep breathing, and coughing	Hesitant to turn, move, deep breathe, or cough due to pain; facial grimace
Impaired physical mobility related to incisional pain and chest tubes	Requests assistance in moving	Limited range of motion in affected arm; reluctant to move
Impaired verbal communication related to intubation for mechanical ventilation		Unable to speak
Potential for infection related to incision, stasis of secretions, or immunosuppression		Thoracic incision, crackles, rhonchi, fever, leukocytosis, receiving immunosuppressants

3 PLAN

Patient goals

1. Patient's respiratory pattern will be effective without pain and fatigue.
2. Patient's airways will be patent.
3. Patient will be free of pain.
4. Patient will regain full range of motion.
5. Patient will be able to communicate adequately.
6. Patient will not develop an infection.
7. Patient and family will demonstrate knowledge of home care and follow up instructions.

4 IMPLEMENT

NURSING DIAGNOSIS	NURSING INTERVENTIONS	RATIONALE
Ineffective breathing pattern related to pain, fatigue, and chest tubes	Observe changes in respiratory rate and depth. Observe for SOB and use of accessory muscles.	An increase in the work of breathing will add to fatigue.
	Inspect thorax for symmetry of movement.	Determines adequacy of breathing pattern; asymmetry may indicate hemothorax or pneumothorax.

NURSING DIAGNOSIS	NURSING INTERVENTIONS	RATIONALE
	Monitor ABGs.	Determines acid-base balance and need for oxygen.
	Measure tidal volume and vital capacity.	Indicates volume of air moving in and out of lungs.
	Assess for pain.	Pain may prevent patient from coughing and deep breathing.
	Assess function of chest tubes.	Ensures that chest tubes remove fluids and air from pleura so that lungs can reexpand.
	Monitor chest x-rays.	Shows extent and location of fluid or infiltrates in lungs.
	Administer oxygen as ordered.	Decreases work of breathing and supplies supplemental oxygen.
	Elevate head of bed 60°-90°.	This position moves the abdominal contents away from the diaphragm, which facilitates its contraction.
	Administer pain medication as ordered.	Altering pain perception will make deep breathing and coughing easier.
	Encourage use of incentive spirometer.	Facilitates deep breathing to improve gas exchange.
Ineffective airway clearance related to tracheobronchial secretions	Auscultate lungs for crackles and rhonchi.	These adventitious sounds indicate secretions in alveoli and airways.
	Assess characteristics of secretions: quantity, color, consistency, and odor.	Suspect infection if secretions increase in quantity and are thick, yellow, or green, and/or foul smelling.
	Assess patient's hydration status: skin turgor, mucous membranes, tongue, intake and output, and Hct.	Fluids needed if turgor is poor, mucous membranes and tongue are dry, intake and output, and/or hematocrit is elevated.
	Assist patient with coughing, after pain medication is given.	Coughing clears airways and prevents atelectasis. Pain medication reduces discomfort of this painful surgery.
	Splint incision while coughing.	Splinting applies gentle pressure, which makes coughing less painful.
	Suction airway when patient is unable to cough.	Suctioning removes secretions from large airways.
	Assist patient to turn (be sure chest tube is not occluded).	Turning allows secretions to drain by gravity so they can be expectorated.
	Encourage fluid intake up to 2,500 ml daily if not contraindicated.	Fluids thin secretions so they are easier to remove.

NURSING DIAGNOSIS	NURSING INTERVENTIONS	RATIONALE
Pain related to surgical procedure	Assess patient for pain.	Pain will interfere with deep breathing, coughing, and turning.
	Administer pain medication as ordered, especially before asking patient to cough.	This drug alters pain perception, which will facilitate coughing and deep breathing.
	Assist patient to use alternate pain relief measures, e.g., relaxation, imagery.	May produce comfort without drugs.
Impaired physical mobility related to incisional pain and chest tubes	Assess range of motion in arm on the same side as chest tube.	Mobility in this arm is limited due to incision and chest tube.
	Encourage patient to rotate shoulder 360° as ordered. (Begin with passive ROM if patient unable to do active.)	Rotation prevents contracture of the joint.
	Encourage ambulation as ordered.	Prevents complications of bed rest.
Impaired verbal communication related to intubation for mechanical ventilation	If patient is unable to talk because of mechanical ventilation, endotracheal tube, or tracheostomy, provide a magic slate or similar writing material and use a picture board. Make sure a call bell is within reach.	Facilitates communication of patient's needs and concerns.
Potential for infection related to incision, stasis of secretions, or immunosuppression	Monitor leukocytes and albumin.	Leukocytosis indicates an infection; low albumin indicates inadequate immunity.
	Monitor temperature.	Fever may indicate infection.
	Encourage coughing and deep breathing.	These actions remove secretions and prevent atelectasis.
	Inspect chest tube insertion sites and incision for infection.	Red, edematous skin with purulent drainage indicates infection.
	If patient is receiving immunosuppressants, isolate patient from others with infections.	Immunosuppressants are necessary to prevent rejection of transplant graft, but reduce one's immunity.
	Administer antiinfective agents as ordered.	These drugs interrupt growth of microorganisms.
	Use sterile technique when changing dressings.	Protects patient from microorganisms.
Knowledge deficit	See Patient Teaching.	

5 EVALUATE

PATIENT OUTCOME	DATE INDICATING THAT OUTCOME IS REACHED
Breathing pattern is effective without pain or fatigue.	Arterial blood gases are within acceptable range.
Airways are patent.	Breath sounds are clear. Arterial blood gases are within acceptable range.
Patient is free of pain.	Patient is able to breathe effectively and move around without pain.
Full range of motion evident in affected shoulder.	Patient is able to rotate affected shoulder 360° without difficulty.
Communicates verbally.	Patient is able to talk without difficulty.
There is no infection.	Temperature is within normal limits. WBCs are within normal limits. Breath sounds are clear. Incision is intact with no redness, swelling, or drainage.
Knowledge is demonstrated.	Patient and family demonstrate knowledge of home care and follow up instructions.

PATIENT TEACHING

1. Explain the need to continue coughing and deep breathing at least four times each day at home.
2. Explain the importance of not smoking.
3. Explain the importance of exercising to tolerance daily, increasing the amount of exercises gradually.
4. Explain that numbness, heaviness, or pain in the operative site is normal.
5. Explain need to avoid persons with upper respiratory infections.
6. Explain the need to report any of the following symptoms to physician: persistent dyspnea, cough, elevated temperature, upper respiratory infection, and redness, swelling, pain, or drainage from incision.
7. Discuss the following about medications: name, purpose, action, frequency of administration, and side effects.

CHAPTER 7

Patient Teaching Guides

PATIENT TEACHING GUIDES	Acute bronchitis	Asthma	COPD (chronic bronchitis, emphysema)	Cystic fibrosis	Occupational lung diseases	Pulmonary embolism	Respiratory infection	TB
Preventing respiratory infections			√	√	√	√		
Smoking and your lungs	√	√	√		√	√	√	√
Quitting smoking	√	√	√		√	√	√	√
Chronic obstructive pulmonary disease			√					
Asthma		√						
What to do about an asthma attack		√						
Pulmonary embolism						√		
Pneumonia							√	
Tuberculosis								√
Chest physiotherapy			√	√			√	
Breathing exercises		√	√	√			√	
Using oxygen at home			√	√				
Traveling around town with oxygen			√					
Vacationing with oxygen			√					

PREVENTING RESPIRATORY INFECTIONS

Respiratory infections can be a serious complication for anyone with a chronic lung disease. Unfortunately, people with chronic lung diseases are more susceptible to respiratory infections; even an ordinary cold that causes only sniffles in someone else can turn into pneumonia. Because of this, you must make every effort to prevent infection. You must also learn the early danger signs and see your doctor at once when any symptoms appear.

Preventing Infection

Follow your doctor's orders. Take your medications exactly as ordered. Perform chest physiotherapy as directed. If oxygen therapy is prescribed, take it as ordered.

Take care of yourself every day. Drink at least six glasses of water daily (unless your doctor tells you differently). Eat a nutritious, well-balanced diet. Sleep 7 or 8 hours every night. Take several short rests during the day. Learn to conserve your energy and avoid getting too tired.

Stay away from people who have colds and flu, if at all possible. If this can't be avoided, wear a disposable mask (available at medical supply companies and many grocery stores) when around people with colds or flu.

Avoid air pollution, including tobacco smoke, wood or oil smoke, car exhaust, and industrial pollution.

Take special precautions with your personal hygiene. Wash your hands before taking your medication or handling your oxygen equipment. Wash your hands after handling soiled tissues and before and after using the bathroom. Always rinse your oral inhaler after each use.

Ask your doctor about flu vaccines.

Detecting Infections

Symptoms of respiratory infections can appear suddenly and worsen quickly. When an infection develops, it's important to start treatment right away. Your doctor may decide to prescribe antibiotics or other drugs to get the infection under control before it becomes serious. (**Don't try to treat yourself.** Over-the-counter cold remedies may worsen the problem, so don't use them unless your doctor tells you it's okay.) Call your doctor immediately if any of these signs occur:

Fever

Increased coughing, wheezing, or trouble breathing

Mucus changes in any of these ways: the mucus is thicker; the amount is either more or less than usual; it has a foul odor; or the color is green, yellow, brown, pink, or red

Stuffy nose, sneezing, or sore throat

Increased fatigue or weakness

Weight gain or loss of more than 5 pounds within a week

Swollen ankles or feet

Confusion, memory loss, or persistent drowsiness

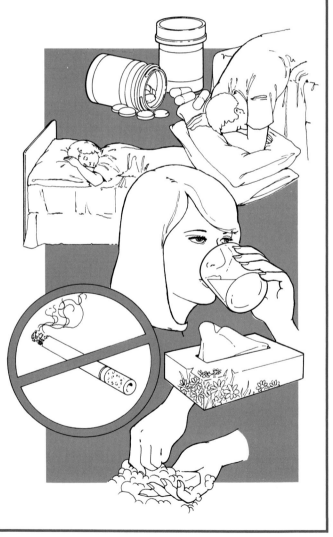

Mosby's
Clinical Nursing
Series

SMOKING AND YOUR LUNGS

Chances are, you started smoking because it was cool, sophisticated, glamorous. Or your friends smoked and you were curious about what smoking was like.

Now you know smoking is anything but cool. It makes you cough, cuts your "wind," gives you bad breath, and stains your teeth. It's also expensive; in one year, a heavy smoker may spend $1,000 or more on cigarettes.

More important, smoking causes emphysema, chronic bronchitis, lung cancer, heart disease, and gum disease. It increases your chances of having a stroke, diseases of the blood vessels, and stomach ulcers. Women who smoke during pregnancy may have premature babies. And smoke in the air harms nonsmokers.

Your and Your Defense System

The insides of your lungs are exposed to the environment every time you breathe. To protect them from foreign particles that could enter the body through this route, the lungs have several defense mechanisms.

Tiny hairlike cilia line your bronchial tubes. Normally they are in constant movement, sweeping germs, dirt, and mucus out of your lungs. But tobacco smoke slows down and actually paralyzes the cilia. Dirt particles and germs that enter the lungs are not removed. And the mucus that collects in the lungs provides a fertile environment for germs to multiply. This is the reason smokers suffer more respiratory infections.

Mucus lining the airways serves two purposes: it helps remove dirt and germs and it moistens the air you breathe. Smoking dries out the mucus, further hampering the defensive action of removing foreign matter. Smokers often experience dry, scratchy throat because the normal moisture is absent.

The Chemicals in Tobacco

Tar is a cancer-causing substance that clings to the inside of your lungs, forming a brown, sticky coat. All tobacco contains tar. Many people switched to low-tar cigarettes in the belief that these brands were less damaging. But the fact is, even small amounts of tar can still cause cancer. In addition, many smokers who switch to low-tar brands take deeper draws and smoke more cigarettes.

Nicotine causes the blood vessels to constrict, raising your blood pressure and forcing your heart to work harder than it should. Smokers suffer from cold hands and feet caused by poor circulation. In time, this can cause vascular diseases.

Burning tobacco produces carbon monoxide. Each time you inhale the hot smoke, you are taking carbon monoxide into your lungs. The tiny blood vessels in your lungs pick up this carbon monoxide instead of oxygen. Tests on smokers have found that carbon monoxide levels in their blood are 15 times higher than in the blood of nonsmokers. As a smoker, your entire body is chronically oxygen-deficient.

It's Not Too Late to Quit

Even if you have been smoking for years—even if you already have a lung disease—quitting smoking now will greatly improve your health. The cilia will begin working again and help keep your lungs swept clean. Your blood vessels will relax, allowing the blood to flow normally, so your heart will no longer work so hard. Your lung tissue will become healthier and you will breathe easier.

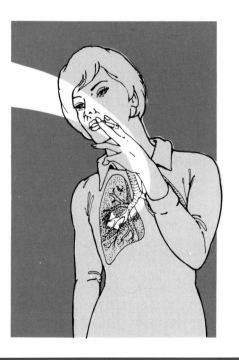

QUITTING SMOKING

Your doctor has told you to quit smoking. You want to, but you aren't sure of the best way. Perhaps you've tried before. Or you're afraid you'll gain weight.

"What's the Best Way to Quit?"

There are many ways to quit smoking, but you need only one thing—*the desire to quit.* Once you have that all-important ingredient, you will succeed.

You can quit "cold turkey," or you can set a quit date and taper off gradually over a 2-week period. Some people find it helpful to have support from others who are quitting at the same time. Your local chapter of the American Lung Association, the American Cancer Society, the American Heart Association, or a hospital in your community can help you locate a smoking cessation class. Or, you can use the "buddy system" — make a pact with a friend who wants to quit and provide support for each other.

Many people find nicotine chewing gum helpful for the first few weeks. Talk to your doctor about prescribing this for you.

Adopt as many techniques that you think will work for you and use them all.

"What about Withdrawal Symptoms?"

Keep in mind that most smokers actually have a double addiction: physical and psychological. You will need to deal with both aspects.

Physical withdrawal can be a problem for heavy smokers (over one pack a day). The symptoms vary from one person to another, but common complaints are headache, constipation, irritability, nervousness, trouble concentrating, and insomnia. You may even cough more for the first week after quitting as your cilia become active again. This is actually a sign that your body is healing itself.

But there are several things you can do to ease the withdrawal symptoms. Although you may fear that you'll be craving a smoke all the time, each urge actually lasts only 2 or 3 minutes. When it hits, do a minute or two of deep breathing exercises to calm the urge; close your eyes, take a deep breath, and slowly let it out. If you still feel a craving, change your activity—walk around or do something that requires both hands, or do something that you especially enjoy.

Drink lots of water to help flush the toxins from your body. Eat a healthy, well-balanced diet. Many authorities say that eating less meat and more fresh vegetables and fruits helps reduce withdrawal symptoms. To combat after-meal cravings, leave the table immediately and brush your teeth. Sugarless gum or hard candy, a toothpick, or unsalted, shelled sunflower seeds satisfy the oral craving without adding calories.

Daily exercise (unless your doctor advises you not to) will help relax you and hasten recovery from the effects of nicotine.

Try to avoid situations that you associate with smoking, such as a morning cup of coffee or a before-dinner drink. You may need to modify your habits for a while until the withdrawal period is over. This also means avoiding spending much time around other smokers.

Write down all your reasons for quitting smoking to remind yourself whenever you're discouraged or tempted to smoke. Keep the list handy and look at it often. And feel proud of yourself for quitting.

"Won't I Gain Weight?"

According to recent studies, only about one third of exsmokers gains some weight, one third loses weight, and one third stays the same. The key to not gaining weight is to not eat every time you crave a smoke. As long as you maintain a well-balanced diet, don't snack between meals, and exercise, you shouldn't experience any weight problems.

"What if I Fail?"

Many people who have successfully quit smoking failed the first time they tried. Often they describe these "failures" as valuable learning experiences that helped them succeed the next time. Whatever you do, don't give up. Over 36 million Americans have already quit. You can, too.

CHRONIC OBSTRUCTIVE PULMONARY DISEASE

What is it?

Chronic obstructive pulmonary disease (COPD) describes conditions of chronic bronchitis, asthma, or emphysema that cause persistent obstruction to bronchial and bronchiolar airflow.

The symptoms include difficulty breathing (dyspnea), shortness of breath, wheezing, thick mucus in the lungs, and susceptibility to lung infection.

How Normal Airways Work

The lungs contain millions of tiny air passages, called bronchioles, that end in clusters of even smaller air sacs. These smaller air sacs, called alveoli, are lined with capillaries, which are tiny blood vessels. When you breathe in, air travels through the large airways (the trachea and bronchi) and bronchioles into the alveoli. Here oxygen passes through the thin walls of the alveoli and enters the blood through the capillaries. The arteries of the circulatory system deliver oxygen to all parts of the body, where it is used to nourish the cells. As the blood returns to the heart through the veins, it picks up carbon dioxide from the cells. The heart routes this carbon dioxide-laden blood back through the lungs' capillaries. The carbon dioxide passes through the alveoli walls, travels through the bronchi, and is breathed out when you exhale.

What happens in COPD

Chronic irritation of the lungs causes inflammation, which prompts the lungs to produce more mucus. The mucus partially or completely blocks the bronchioles so that only very small amounts of air can get to the alveoli. Eventually, the bronchioles become permanently narrowed, and many of the alveoli walls are destroyed, enlarging the air spaces. Air becomes trapped in these enlarged alveoli.

COPD begins gradually and gets progressively worse over the years. The earliest symptom is usually a mild "smoker's cough." Later, physical exertion causes difficulty breathing, or dyspnea. Wheezing, susceptibility to respiratory infections, sputum production, and sometimes weight loss and weakness occur. It becomes more difficult to breathe out. After several years, a person with COPD has a "barrel chest" appearance from over-inflation of the lungs. And as less oxygen gets into the blood stream, COPD causes cyanosis (bluish lips, nails, and skin). Swelling of the lower legs and eventually heart failure can occur.

What Causes COPD?

Smoking is the most common cause of COPD. Some people develop emphysema in early adulthood because of a deficiency of alpha-1 antitrypsin, a substance that gives the lungs their elasticity. This deficiency is rare, however, and accounts for only about 10% of the cases. Other causes of COPD are long-term exposure to industrial pollutants and scarred lung tissue.

How is COPD Treated?

Although there is no cure for COPD, treatment can slow down the progression and minimize the discomfort. Your doctor will decide the best treatment in your case, depending on how severe the symptoms are and the underlying disease (remember that COPD has different causes). Medications often used to treat COPD include bronchodilators (to open the airways and make breathing easier) and antibiotics to prevent or treat respiratory infections. Oxygen therapy is often prescribed.

You must learn chest physiotherapy to help loosen and remove the mucus in your lungs. The special techniques of pursed lip breathing and abdominal breathing are helpful.

Finally, you must take very good care of yourself by eating well-balanced meals, drinking fluids, getting plenty of rest, learning to conserve your energy, and avoiding respiratory infection.

ASTHMA

Asthma is a condition involving repeated attacks of shortness of breath, wheezing, and coughing. These attacks occur when the airways contract, swell, and clog up with mucus. An attack may last a few minutes or a few hours. In mild cases the attacks occur only occasionally, but people with severe asthma may have several attacks in a week (or even in a single day). Although it's a chronic disease, people with asthma can learn how to manage these attacks and lead normal, active lives.

What Causes Asthma?

There are two types of asthma: **atopic (extrinsic) asthma** and **nonatopic (intrinsic) asthma.**

The term *atopic,* which means *external,* gives a clue to the cause of this type of asthma. Atopic asthma is a type of allergic reaction. Many people with atopic asthma have other allergies, and there is often a family history of allergies. Common causes are dust, pollen, mold spores, insecticides, animals, and certain food. Atopic asthma usually, but not always, begins in childhood.

Nonatopic asthma typically begins after age 35 years, and the attacks are more frequent as time goes by. The cause is unknown, but it is believed to be an over-response of the immune system. Attacks are sometimes triggered by viruses (such as the common cold), exercise, emotional stress, or exposure to cold air, dust, or fumes.

How is Asthma Diagnosed?

Unfortunately, no single test can diagnose asthma, and several tests must be performed. Lung function tests involve breathing into a special machine to evaluate breathing performance. Blood tests are made, which often include checking the amount of oxygen in the blood. This is done by drawing a small amount of blood from an artery. Sputum is examined under the microscope, and a chest x-ray is made. Skin tests are usually performed (if they have not been in the past) to identify allergies to common foods or other substances.

How is Asthma Treated?

Bronchodilators are prescribed to relax the airways and are the main type of medication used for treating asthma. Daily doses in pill form (either theophylline or aminophylline) or aerosol inhalers are prescribed to help prevent attacks. Oral aerosols are also used when an asthma attack begins to keep the airways open.

When asthma is severe, corticosteroids (oral or aerosols) are prescribed to suppress the body's reaction. Because steroids can have serious side effects, these drugs usually are prescribed only for a short period of time.

How can Attacks be Avoided?

People who have asthma are wise to learn what triggers an attack and to avoid that item or situation. The following are common triggering agents:

Foods—chocolate, nuts, eggs, shellfish, milk, oranges, wine, beer

Pollen, mold spores

Tobacco smoke

Animals—cats, dogs, rabbits, hamsters, gerbils, chickens, insects

Dust—dirty filters on heating and air conditioning systems; brooms and dusters; upholstered furniture, carpets, and curtains that might harbor dust

Smog, automobile fumes

Feathers

Wool

Personal care products—sprays, cosmetics, powder

Aerosol sprays of any kind

Cold or hot air, high humidity or very dry air

Emotion—anger, frustration, fear, crying, laughing too hard

Exercise

Common cold, flu

WHAT TO DO ABOUT AN ASTHMA ATTACK

Asthma attacks usually give you warning signs before they start. This gives you time to "short circuit" the attack, but you must take immediate action. Go into action as soon as any of the following warning signs appear: tightness in your chest, coughing, wheezing, dyspnea, (difficulty breathing), or shortness of breath. Here's what you do:

Use the Oral Inhaler

1. Take the mouthpiece and cap off. Fit the metal stem of the inhaler into the hole in the mouthpiece. Shake the inhaler 5 times.
2. Purse your lips and breathe out completely. Put the mouthpiece in your mouth, forming a seal with your lips and teeth. (Make sure the inhaler is upside down.)
3. With your head tilted back slightly, take a slow, deep breath and press the inhaler down once. Keep breathing in until your lungs feel as if they are full of air. (Press the inhaler only one time. One press equals one dose.)
4. Remove the mouthpiece from your mouth. Hold your breath for 5 seconds. (Silently count one 100, two 100, three 100, four 100, five 100.) Purse your lips and breathe out slowly.
5. If your doctor has prescribed a second dose, wait 2 minutes before taking the second dose.

Relax and Breathe Slowly

It takes a few minutes for the medication to completely open your airways. In the meantime, it's important that you try to relax, because fear and anxiety add to the shortness of breath. Do your pursed lip breathing until you no longer feel breathless. (Don't gasp for air! That only makes it worse.) Here are two relaxation techniques to help you keep calm and slow your breathing:

1. *Tension-relaxation exercise.* Sit in a chair with your eyes closed, doing your pursed lip breathing for a minute or so. Now tighten the muscles in your forehead (frown as if you're furious!), hold it for 3 seconds, and relax those muscles. Next tighten the muscles in your lower face (clench your jaw in determination), hold it for 3 seconds, and relax. Now

you're ready to tighten-relax your arms and hands, then your buttocks, then your legs and feet. After that, let your entire body go limp and feel how relaxed your muscles are.

2. *Visualization.* Sit in a chair with your eyes closed, doing your pursed lip breathing for a minute or so. Now imagine the most peaceful scene you can think of—perhaps a calm lake, mountaintop at sunset, floating clouds, or whatever especially appeals to you. Visualize the scene, with you in it, in as much detail as possible. Repeat to yourself how relaxing it is to be in that place and how easily you can breathe there. For example, you might tell yourself, "The air is so sweet and fresh here. Every time I breathe, the air cleanses my lungs and I can breathe more easily."

Coughing

Asthma attacks sometimes trigger a coughing spell. This is actually good, because it brings up mucus and helps clear your airways. But you need to be sure the coughing is effective. To do this, keep your feet on the floor and lean forward slightly. Breathe in deeply and hold it for 2 or 3 seconds. Cough to loosen the mucus. Cough again to bring the mucus up, spitting it into a tissue. (Don't swallow mucus because this can cause nausea.)

When to Call Your Doctor

If the asthma attack gets worse—in spite of doing everything you were supposed to—call your doctor immediately.

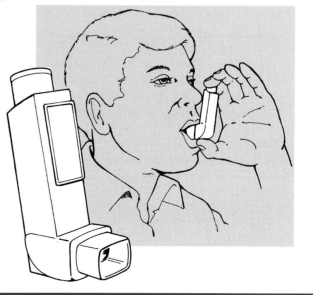

PULMONARY EMBOLISM

Pulmonary embolism is a condition in which a blood clot has lodged in a blood vessel inside the lungs. This clot interferes with the ability of that section of the lung to carry oxygen to the tissues of the body.

Most blood clots start in the leg veins, break loose, and travel to the lungs. Clots form when blood in the legs stagnates from poor circulation, long periods of sitting, prolonged bed rest, or leg injuries.

Anticoagulants (medications that slow down clotting) are given to prevent new clots. If you have a blood clot, it will dissolve in 7 to 10 days without any treatment. The anticoagulant heparin is usually given in a vein for about a week. After you leave the hospital, the oral anticoagulant warfarin sodium (Coumadin) is prescribed for several months.

Improving your circulation is also important to help prevent new clots. Your doctor may recommend an exercise program, such as daily walking. Avoid sitting for long periods of time, and be sure that stockings and other clothing are not too tight. If you smoke, you must quit. Smoking constricts the blood vessels and increases the chances of another clot forming.

Taking your Coumadin

It is important to take the medication exactly as ordered because too much can cause bleeding and too little can cause clotting. Regular blood tests are necessary to be certain your blood is clotting the way it should. If it is not, your doctor will change the dosage. Here are important guidelines for taking your medication:

1. Take the warfarin at the same time of the day. If you are supposed to take it on alternate days, marking a calendar will help you keep track of when your next dose is due.
2. If you skip a dose, don't double up next time; just take your next dose as scheduled. If you miss two doses, call your doctor.
3. Keep your appointments for blood tests.
4. Refill your prescription one week ahead of time so you won't run out.
5. Store warfarin away from heat and cold.

Helping the Medication Work

Too much vitamin K increases clotting, so don't eat excessive amounts of green leafy vegetables (such as spinach and broccoli) and don't take vitamin supplements that contain vitamin K.

If you drink alcohol, limit the amount to one drink per day. Excessive amounts of alcohol can affect blood clotting.

The liver produces many blood clotting factors. Alcohol is broken down (metabolized) by the liver. An excessive intake of alcohol can alter liver function so that it cannot produce enough clotting factors to maintain the normal blood clotting mechanism. Many drugs can interact with coumadin. Don't take aspirin or any drugs containing aspirin. Aspirin interferes with the platelets that normally form blood clots. Check with your doctor or pharmacist before taking over-the-counter drugs to be sure they don't contain aspirin or other substances that might affect blood clotting. Take prescription drugs only as prescribed by your doctor.

Safety First

Warfarin causes your blood to clot more slowly, so you must take steps to prevent injuries that could cause bleeding.
Use a toothbrush with soft bristles.

Don't use toothpicks or other sharp objects in your mouth.

Don't walk barefoot and don't trim corns or calluses. Use corn or callus removers.

Don't use cutting tools or sharp objects.

Don't engage in rough sports.

Protect yourself from falling—put a nonskid mat in your bathtub or shower, remove hazardous throw rugs, and wear low-heeled shoes with nonslip soles.

If you cut yourself, keep pressure on the injury for 10 minutes.

Remember to tell the dentist that you are taking warfarin.

CALL YOUR DOCTOR IF:
A cut doesn't stop bleeding in 10 minutes.
A bruise gets larger.
You see blood in your urine, or your stools are black and tarry.
You have a nosebleed, bleeding gums, purplish or reddish spots on your skin, unusual vaginal bleeding or excessive menstrual flow, or bleeding hemorrhoids.

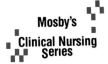
PNEUMONIA

Pneumonia is an infection of the lungs that can be caused by many different organisms. The symptoms can vary considerably, depending on the cause.

Viral Pneumonia

Upper respiratory viral infections and influenza sometimes spread to the lungs. In addition to influenza-type symptoms (fever, headache, general aching, and loss of appetite), viral pneumonia is marked by an irritating cough that may produce sputum, shortness of breath, and chest pain. The so-called walking pneumonia can cause very mild symptoms.

Viral pneumonia is usually treated at home with bed rest, plenty of liquids, and cough medicine that contains an expectorant to clear the lungs of mucus. A humidifier to add moisture to the air also helps loosen the mucus. Antibiotics or other drugs are not effective in treating viral pneumonia.

Most otherwise healthy people recover within a week or so. However, viral pneumonia can lead to bacterial infection in certain people. For this reason, doctors may prescribe antibiotics for people with chronic lung diseases or other chronic illnesses to prevent this complication.

Bacterial Pneumonia

Bacterial pneumonia is usually caused by either *Streptococcus, Staphylococcus,* or *Haemophilus.* The infection can start from an upper respiratory infection such as "strep" throat, from inhaling fluid or other foreign substance into the lungs, or from viral pneumonia. The symptoms include fever, shortness of breath, chest pain, coughing, and sputum that is yellowish or greenish and often has a foul odor.

It is a serious infection that often requires hospitalization. Treatment consists of antibiotics, bed rest, fluids, humidified air, and an expectorant cough medication. Oxygen and chest physiotherapy may be necessary for hospitalized patients.

Legionnaires' disease is a serious type of bacterial pneumonia that occurs in older people and people who smoke or who have chronic diseases such as emphysema, chronic bronchitis, diabetes, renal disease, and cancer. It is treated with erythromycin.

Other Types of Pneumonia

Mycoplasma pneumonia is caused by one of the *Mycoplasma* bacteria. It most often infects children and young adults, and it is a common cause of "walking pneumonia." *Mycoplasma pneumonia* is treated with the antibiotic erythromycin.

Pneumocystis pneumonia is caused by the protozoa *Pneumocystis carinii.* This serious infection occurs in patients with AIDS and those whose immune systems are deficient.

A chronic fungus infection of the lungs can lead to pneumonia. *Histoplasma, Blastomyces, Cryptococcus, Aspergillus,* and *Candida* are fungi that can establish themselves in the lungs. This type of pneumonia is rare and occurs mainly in patients whose immune systems are deficient.

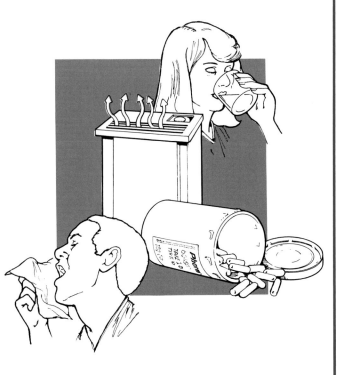

TUBERCULOSIS

What is Tuberculosis?

Tuberculosis (TB) is a serious lung infection caused by the bacteria *Mycobacterium tuberculosis*. If it is not treated, these bacteria multiply in the lungs, causing permanent damage, and can even spread to other parts of the body. TB is transmitted by sneezing and coughing, but it is not highly contagious. Infection usually results only after close or prolonged exposure to someone who is infected.

Today, the majority of TB cases occur in people who are in poor health and in elderly persons. In most cases these people were infected years ago, but the bacteria stayed dormant until age or illness depleted their immune systems and the bacteria reactivated.

At one time, TB was a serious health problem in the United States. It required a long period of hospitalization and often surgery. During this century, improved sanitation and public health measures help to prevent its spread. However, TB remains a serious problem in many parts of the world.

How is it Diagnosed?

A doctor may suspect TB because of a chest x-ray, recent exposure to someone with active TB, or symptoms. The symptoms of TB are a chronic cough that produces blood-streaked sputum, weight loss, fatigue, fever, and night sweats. Although the person will usually have a positive reaction to a tuberculin skin test, this can also mean past exposure to TB or a similar bacteria. The only way to confirm the diagnosis is to examine the sputum under a microscope to detect the bacteria.

How is it Treated?

Antibiotic drugs must be taken for several months to completely kill all the bacteria. Most people can be treated at home. However, you must take the prescribed drugs every day, exactly as your doctor orders. If you take them irregularly or stop taking them, it will cause the TB to worsen and may spread the infection to others.

Several combinations of antibiotics are used to treat TB. Usually both isoniazid and rifampin are prescribed for a 9-month period. They must be taken once a day, 1 hour before or 2 hours after a meal. Sometimes other drugs are prescribed in addition to these two antibiotics.

While you are being treated for TB, your doctor will need to monitor you every month to be sure the drugs are working and are not causing side effects. Although it's not common, hepatitis is a very serious complication of treatment. Call your doctor immediately if any of these symptoms develop: increased fatigue, weakness, appetite loss, nausea, vomiting, or jaundice.

Bed rest is not necessary, unless you are seriously ill from other diseases. Eat a nutritious, well-balanced diet to avoid fatigue.

How to Prevent the Spread of TB

If you have TB, it is important that you take steps to protect those around you from infection. Taking your prescribed medication will help wall off the bacteria so they cannot spread. Always cover your nose and mouth when coughing and sneezing. Throw away used tissues promptly and wash your hands frequently. Good ventilation is important to keep fresh air circulating through the house.

Your close contacts (family members or friends) should be tested to see if they are infected, even if they do not have symptoms. It may be necessary for them to take a daily dose of isoniazid for 6 to 12 months to prevent illness.

Call your Doctor if:

You notice blood in your sputum.

You feel pain in your chest or have difficulty breathing.

You feel dizzy or hear ringing in your ears. These symptoms are side effects of some medications for TB.

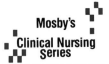
CHEST PHYSIOTHERAPY

In some lung conditions, such as chronic bronchitis, emphysema, and cystic fibrosis, thick mucus collects in the lungs. This makes breathing more difficult and increases the chance of getting pneumonia or other infections. To help loosen the mucus and move it out of the lungs, your doctor has suggested that you perform chest physiotherapy. This consists of postural drainage, chest percussion, and coughing.

You should do chest physiotherapy twice a day (unless your doctor tells you otherwise)—once when you first get up in the morning and once in the evening before you go to bed. Whenever you have more mucus than usual, you should do chest physiotherapy more often.

Remember that drinking a lot of fluids (at least 2 quarts daily) will also help thin the mucus.

You can do the postural drainage and coughing by yourself. Someone will need to help you with chest percussion.

Postural Drainage

1. Place pillows on the floor beside the bed and a box of tissues close by.
2. Lie on the bed with your trunk over the side, head and arms resting on the pillows. You will lie on your stomach and on each side. Stay in each position 10-20 minutes.

Chest Percussion

Here's where a friend or family member will have to help you. You will stay in the postural drainage position for percussion.
1. The helper should make a cup with his or her hands. This is done by keeping fingers together, flexing the fingers, and tucking the thumb tightly against the index finger.
2. The helper firmly pats your back rhythmically, alternating the cupped hands, for 3 to 5 minutes. When done correctly, this will make a sound like a galloping horse. (With just a little practice, this technique is easy to master.)

Coughing

Stay in the postural drainage position.
1. Take a slow, deep breath through your nose. Hold your breath for 3 seconds. (Counting one 100, two 100, three 100 will help you hold your breath long enough.)
2. Open your mouth slightly, coughing three times as you breathe out. A good cough that helps bring up mucus sounds hollow, deep, and low. (A high-pitched cough is not effective.)
3. Take a slow, deep breath through your nose and breathe normally for a few minutes. Then repeat the coughing procedure several more times.
4. Be sure you spit the mucus into a tissue. (Do not swallow it, since this can cause nausea.)

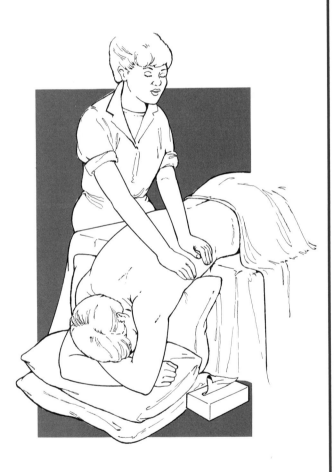

BREATHING EXERCISES

The feeling of not being able to get enough air into your lungs is frightening. Shortness of breath or difficulty breathing—called dyspnea—is a problem for people with chronic lung diseases. However, there are several things you can do to help you breathe more easily.

Avoiding Trouble

Breathing pollutants can aggravate dyspnea. Avoid heavy traffic and smog as much as possible. Don't use aerosol sprays. Stay away from products that produce fumes, such as paint, kerosene, and cleaning agents.

Cold weather can trigger dyspnea. If you must go outside when it's cold, cover your mouth with a scarf or mask.

Very dry air increases dyspnea and thickens the mucus in your lungs. A portable room humidifier is helpful, especially in the winter.

Physical exertion brings on dyspnea. Learn to conserve your energy by resting frequently, alternating light and heavy tasks, and minimizing movement. Instead of standing, sit. Instead of pushing or lifting objects, pull. Be creative in managing tasks—for example, a cart or child's wagon can be used to haul groceries, and wheels can be installed on furniture that is frequently moved.

Breathing Exercises

There are two simple exercises that can help you breathe more easily. You can do pursed lip breathing anywhere. With abdominal breathing, you will need to lie down. Practice them daily so when you are having problems with dyspnea, you will immediately know what to do.

Pursed Lip Breathing

Pursed lip breathing will help get rid of the stale air trapped inside the lungs. It will slow down your breathing so it is more efficient. (Breathing fast only makes the dyspnea worse.)
1. Breathe in slowly through your nose. Hold your breath for three seconds (count to yourself by saying one 100, two 100, three 100). Be sure to breathe through your nose to avoid gulping air.
2. Purse your lips as if you were going to whistle or give someone a kiss.
3. Breathe out slowly through your pursed lips for six seconds (count one 100, two 100, three 100, four 100, five 100, six 100.) The sound you make breathing out will be like a soft whistle.

Abdominal Breathing

Abdominal breathing will also slow down your breathing to make it more effective. It also helps relax your entire body and is a wonderful technique to use before you go to sleep.
1. Lie on your back in a comfortable position with a pillow under your head. Place another pillow under your knees to help relax your abdomen.
2. Rest one hand on your abdomen just below your rib cage. Rest the other hand on your chest.
3. Slowly breathe in and out through your nose using your abdominal muscles. The hand resting on your abdomen will rise when you breathe in, and it will fall when you breathe out. The hand on your chest should be almost still.

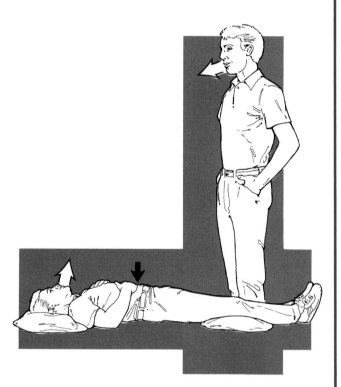

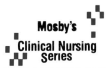

Mosby's
Clinical Nursing Series

USING OXYGEN AT HOME

Your doctor has prescribed extra oxygen at a flow rate of _____ liters per minute for _____ hours every day. The medical supply company will show you how to set the flow rate and how to care for the equipment. Keep the supplier's phone number handy so you can call if the system doesn't work properly.

You will be using a liquid oxygen unit, an oxygen tank, or an oxygen concentrator. You will breathe the oxygen through either a mask or a nasal cannulae (two short prongs that fit just inside your nostrils). The system will also have a humidifier to warm and moisturize the oxygen.

It's a good idea to also have a small portable oxygen tank for an emergency backup system in case of power failure.

Here are some general guidelines and safety tips for using oxygen equipment.

General Guidelines

Always keep your oxygen flow rate where your doctor prescribes.

Sometimes it's hard to tell whether oxygen is flowing through the tubes. If you have doubts, check to be sure that the system is turned on and there are no kinks in the tubing. If you still aren't sure, place the nasal cannulae in a glass of water with the prongs up and watch for bubbles. (Always shake the water off before inserting the cannulae into your nostrils.) If no bubbles appear, oxygen is not flowing through the tubes and you need to call your supplier.

Each time before using your oxygen, check the humidifier bottle. If it's near the fill line, empty the bottle and refill it with sterile or bottled water.

Even with the humidifier, oxygen can dry the inside of your nose. A water-soluble lubricant (such as K-Y Jelly) helps ease dryness and cracking. Don't use petroleum-based products like Vaseline because this will make the dryness worse.

To avoid running out of oxygen, reorder your new supply when the register reads ¼ full—2 or 3 days before you need a new tank.

Safety First

Oxygen is very combustible. By following these rules, you can be confident that your oxygen system is not posing a serious fire hazard.

Keep your oxygen unit away from open flames and heat. This includes smoking—don't smoke and don't allow others to smoke around you. If you have a gas stove, gas space heater, or kerosene heater or lamp, stay out of the room while it's on.

To prevent leakage, always keep your oxygen system upright, and make sure the system is turned off when not in use. Don't place carpets, bed clothes, or furniture over the tubing, since this may cause a leak.

Keep an all-purpose fire extinguisher close by.

If a fire should occur, turn off the oxygen and leave the house at once.

Notify your local fire department that you have oxygen in the house. In most areas, the fire department offers free safety inspections, which can help make your home even safer for using oxygen.

Call your Doctor Immediately if:

Your breathing is difficult, irregular, shallow, or slow.

You become restless or anxious.

You are tired, drowsy, or have trouble waking up.

You have a persistent headache.

Your speech becomes slurred, you can't concentrate, or you feel confused.

Your fingernails or lips are bluish.

These symptoms may arise when you are not getting enough oxygen or when you are getting too much oxygen. Only your doctor can determine how much oxygen you need. Therefore you must never change the flow rate without instructions from your doctor.

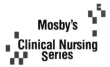
TRAVELING AROUND TOWN WITH OXYGEN

Having oxygen equipment doesn't mean you must stay at home. By carefully planning ahead, you can continue to lead an active life. The following guidelines will help you make arrangements to travel safely and comfortably, whether you just want to travel around town or take short trips.

Plan Ahead

1. First, consult your doctor. Ask if it's all right for you to travel around town.
2. Your oxygen supply company will recommend the equipment you need and help determine the time you can safely travel between refills. This time will depend on your prescribed flow rate. Always allow for a 20% to 25% safety margin to cover any unexpected delays. Use the equipment they recommend at home first, so you can get familiar with how to operate it.
3. Always plan your time. Know what time you leave home and what time you need to return (a watch with an alarm function is a helpful reminder). Don't be tempted to "cut it too close" because unexpected delays—a traffic tie-up or a flat tire—can happen. For example, an E cylinder will last 4-5 hours with a flow rate of 2-3 liters per minute.
4. You will encounter people who do not understand the safety precautions of oxygen equipment. Do not hesitate to tell people around you "Do not smoke." From Linde HomeCare Medical Systems, Inc., Grand Prairie, Texas, 1989.

Traveling by Automobile

1. Secure your walker unit with a seatbelt and shoulder harness. If you can't use a shoulder belt, set the walker on the floor and belt the shoulder strap through the inside door handle. (Be sure you lock the door to prevent accidental opening!)
2. Keep the oxygen container upright at all times. Laying a liquid oxygen container on its side will cause rapid release of oxygen through the pressure relief valve. (This means you cannot store extra tanks in the trunk of your car, since most tanks are too large to stand upright.) However, slight tipping of liquid oxygen tanks during loading and unloading is not dangerous.
3. Always keep a window partially open while you are using oxygen. All liquid oxygen containers release a small amount of gas periodically, so good ventilation is essential—regardless of weather.
4. Campers and motor homes offer a lot of flexibility. With the help of your oxygen supply company, a liquid oxygen reservoir can be installed. However, ventilation is still important, and a window or overhead vent should be left open. Cooking appliances that have an open flame are fire hazards and should not be used in a vehicle carrying oxygen.

Local Public Transportation

Most cities have no restrictions about oxygen equipment on local transportation systems, as long as you have no trouble getting your equipment on and off buses, subways, or trains. Call your city's transportation department to be sure there are no restrictions. The first time you use public transportation, take a companion along to be sure you can manage by yourself. Since smoking is prohibited on public transportation in most areas, this will not present a problem.

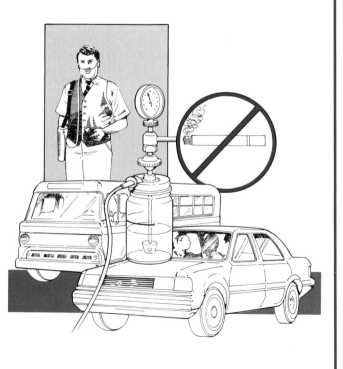

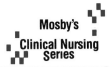

VACATIONING WITH OXYGEN

First, discuss your travel plans with your doctor to be sure it's all right for you to travel and for how long. If you are going to higher or lower elevations (mountains or sea level), your doctor may need to change the flow rate.

Contact your oxygen supply company about your travel plans. They will recommend the equipment you need and help determine the time you can safely travel between refills. Obtain the oxygen equipment you will travel with ahead of time so you can get familiar with how to operate it. Your supplier can also help arrange to have oxygen supplied to you at your destination.

Check with your insurance company. You may have to pay in advance for equipment and submit the insurance claims after you return home. Be sure to keep all receipts.

Contact the airline, busline, rail line, or cruise line and hotels or motels about your medical needs well in advance.

Always keep your prescription with you throughout the trip.

Traveling by Bus

Travel with oxygen equipment is permitted on buslines. However, check in advance to prevent any unexpected problems. Greyhound, Trailways, and some tourlines permit you to take one E cylinder onto the bus, but extra tanks are not allowed in the baggage compartment. You must be able to put your tank on and take it off by yourself. You must sit up front in the "No Smoking" section.

Traveling by Train

Make reservations with Amtrak at least 4 days in advance, even for short distances. You may bring only two cylinders, either size E or F, and the oxygen unit must be self-contained and cannot be on wheels. On overnight trips, you must have a sleeper, where you are required to stay while using oxygen. You can have meals sent to your sleeper.

Traveling by Ship

Cruise line regulations differ and are subject to change, so you must contact the company re-garding current rules. Some cruise lines permit you to travel only with oxygen cylinders and limit the number you may bring on board. Be prepared to supply the following information from your doctor: a prescription stating the quantity of oxygen and flow rate, a letter describing your diagnosis, and a statement that you are approved for travel.

Traveling by Plane

Regulations vary from one airline to another and are subject to change. Always call ahead of time to inquire about current rules. Some airlines will not permit passengers to use oxygen. Others are willing to provide oxygen if you make advance arrangements, but you must use their oxygen supply. They do not allow passengers to bring oxygen on board the plane. Always bring your own nasal prongs, because some airlines use only simple oxygen masks, which allow carbon dioxide build-up. Also bring a nipple adaptor that fits all tubing.

You must make reservations 2 to 5 days in advance, depending on the individual airline's rules. Be sure to ask what documents you will need to supply. Airline document requirements are similar to those of cruise lines, and some airlines also have special forms that must be filled out by your doctor. You may have to sign a liability statement. In a few cases, you are required to bring a companion with you on the flight. Additional charges vary, but expect to pay about $50 extra.

Allow at least 1 hour between connecting flights. Remember that you must arrange for oxygen during the time between flights. Local oxygen suppliers will provide this service for layovers between flights. Whenever possible, use small airports because they usually have fewer delays and their boarding gates are closer together.

Lodging

Hotels and motels are usually very accommodating about special needs. Someone is usually available to transport your oxygen tank. Contact your oxygen supply company about arranging for a local supply company to set up the equipment in the room before you arrive.

CHAPTER 8

Respiratory Drugs

BRONCHODILATORS

SYMPATHOMIMETIC DRUGS

Sympathomimetic drugs are classified as *nonselective adrenergic, nonselective beta adrenergic,* or *selective beta-2 receptor* drugs based on their activity at adrenergic receptor sites.

Nonselective Adrenergic Drugs

Epinephrine (Adrenalin, Bronkaid Mist, Primatene Mist)

Epinephrine bitartrate inhalation (AsthmaHaler, Bronkaid Mist Suspension, Medihaler-Epi, Primatene Mist Suspension)

Racepinephrine inhalation solution (AsthmaNefrin, microNEFRIN, S-2 Inhalant, Vaponefrin)

Ethylnorepinephrine (Bronkephrine)

Ephedrine (Ectasule, Ephedsol, Vatronol)

Nonselective adrenergic drugs exert their effects on blood vessels (alpha activity), the heart (beta-1 activity), and bronchial smooth muscle (beta-2 activity). Alpha activity (or stimulation) may reduce mucosal edema by causing vasoconstriction. Beta-1 activity accounts for most of the undesirable cardiac effects, including increased heart rate and contractility. Beta-2 activity increases the level of cyclic AMP, which in turn relaxes bronchial and vascular smooth muscle, producing bronchodilation and vasodilation. Adverse effects of beta-2 stimulation include muscle tremors. Sympathomimetic drugs may also produce undesirable CNS stimulation.

Indications: Acute and temporary relief of bronchial asthma and reversible bronchospasm.

Usual dosage: *Epinephrine*—SC: 0.3-0.5 ml of 1:1,000 solution (0.3-0.5 mg); **inhaled:** As microaerosol from metered dose inhaler (0.16-0.25 mg/spray) repeated once if necessary, or through nebulizer. *Ethylnorepinephrine*—SC or IM 0.5-1 ml (1-2 mg). *Ephedrine*—SC, IM, or IV: Parenteral 25-50 mg, **oral:** 25-50 mg q 3-4 h as needed.

Precautions/contraindications: Use with extreme caution in the presence of hypertension, history of seizures, advanced age, diabetes, unstable vasomotor systems, hyperthyroidism, or prostatic hypertrophy. Contraindicated in cardiogenic or hypovolemic shock, narrow-angle glaucoma, cerebral or coronary artery disease.

Side effects/adverse reactions: CNS: Stimulation, including nervousness, tremors, and seizures; **CV:** Tachycardia, dysrhythmias, angina pectoris, hypertension, cerebral hemorrhage; **GI:** Dry mouth (following inhalation) nausea, vomiting, anorexia; **GU:** Urinary retention or difficult urination. Severe paradoxic airway resistance and bronchospasm have been reported in patients following excessive use of inhalation preparations.

Pharmacokinetics: Onset of action: Maximal bronchodilation generally occurs within 5 min of inhalation of aerosols or within 20 min following SC or IM injection. **Duration of action:** 1-3 h for inhalation and 1-4 h for SC or IM. **Route of elimination:** Locally at sympathetic nerve endings, systemic metabolism in the liver with renal excretion of metabolites.

Interactions: Combination therapy with other sympathomimetic agents may lead to an increase in cardiovascular and CNS effects. The effects of sympathomimetics are potentiated by tricyclic antidepressants and some antihistamines. Sympathomimetics may decrease the effects of antihypertensive agents. Alpha-and beta-blocking agents will antagonize some or all of the effects of the sympathomimetic drugs.

Nursing considerations: Inhalation: 80%-90% of aerosol dose is generally deposited in the mouth or pharynx. Deposition depends on particle size, pattern of breathing, and condition of the airways. Pressurized inhalation should be administered during the second half of inhalation for best distribution when the airways are open the widest. Breath holding following inhalation may increase deposition in the lower airways. Wait at least 1 min between inhalations to allow first dose to take effect. This will allow the second dose to be better distributed in the lower airways. Instruct patient in proper use for each product and inhaler based on manufacturer's instructions, to notify physician if dizziness or chest pain develops or if there is a lack of response to usual dose, and to not exceed recommended dosage. (See Patient Teaching Guide, page 281.) Dryness of pharyngeal membranes may be prevented by rinsing the mouth with water immediately after use. **Parenteral:** Take care to avoid inadvertant IV administration.

Monitor closely for signs of adverse effects and for response to therapy. Treatment of toxicity or overdosage usually involves supportive care. Beta-adrenergic-blocking drugs may precipitate bronchospasm if used to treat toxicity.

Nonselective Beta-adrenergic Drugs

Isoproterenol (Isuprel, Isuprel Mistometer)

Nonselective beta adrenergic drugs do not stimulate alpha-adrenergic receptors. Their primary action is on the heart and bronchial smooth muscle, with little or no effect on BP. However, they still may cause many of the undesirable beta-2 cardiac effects, such as tachycardia, increased conduction velocity, and increased automaticity.

Indications: Acute and temporary relief of bronchial asthma and reversible bronchospasm.

Usual dosage: Metered dose inhaler 1-2 inhalations (80-160 μg/inhalation), not more than 6 inhalations/h 4-6 times daily or 5-15 deep inhalations of a nebulized 1:200 solution.

Precautions/contraindications: Use with extreme caution in hypertension, coronary artery disease, history of seizures, advanced age, and hyperthyroidism.

Side effects/adverse reactions: CNS: Stimulation, including nervousness, tremors, and seizures; **CV:**

Tachycardia, dysrhythmias, angina pectoris; **GI:** Nausea, vomiting, anorexia, dry mouth.

Pharmacokinetics: Onset of action: 2-5 min. **Duration of action:** ½-2 h. Metabolized in sympathetic nerve endings, gastrointestinal tract, and other tissues, excreted in kidneys.

Interactions: May potentiate other sympathomimetic drugs.

Nursing considerations: Pressurized inhalation should be administered during the second half of inhalation for best distribution when the airways are open the widest. Wait at least 1 min between inhalations to allow first dose to take effect. This will allow the second dose to be better distributed in the lower airways. Instruct patient in proper use for each product and inhaler based on manufacturer's instructions, to notify physician if dizziness or chest pain develops or if there is a lack of response to usual dose, and to not exceed recommended dosage. Dryness of pharyngeal membranes may be prevented by rinsing the mouth with water immediately after use.

Monitor closely for signs of adverse effects and for response to therapy. Treatment of toxicity or overdosage usually involves supportive care. Beta-adrenergic-blocking drugs may precipitate bronchospasm if used to treat toxicity.

Selective Beta-2 Adrenergic Drugs

Albuterol (Proventil, Ventolin)
Bitolterol (Tornalate)
Isoetharine inhalation (Bronkometer, Bronkosol)
Metaproterenol sulfate (Alupent, Metaprel)
Terbutaline sulfate (Brethaire, Brethine, Bricanyl)

Selective beta-2 adrenergic drugs are used to avoid the undesirable cardiac effects caused by beta-1 stimulation. Because of their relative specificity for beta-2 adrenergic receptors, these drugs exert their effects primarily on bronchial smooth muscle and vasculature, with little cardiac stimulation. However, these drugs are not pure beta-2 agonists, and some beta-1 stimulatory effects may occur.

Indications: Acute and temporary relief of bronchial asthma and reversible bronchospasm; prevention of bronchospasm.

Usual dosage: *Albuterol*—aerosol: 1-2 inhalations (90-180 μg) repeated q 4-6 h as needed; **oral:** 2-4 mg, 3-4 times/day, maximum total daily dose of 32 mg. *Bitolterol*—aerosol: Metered dose inhaler, 2-3 inhalations (370 μg/inhalation), not to exceed 3 doses/6 h. *Isoetharine*—metered aerosol: 1-2 inhalations (340-680μg) q 4 h as needed; **Hand-held nebulizer:** 3-7 inhalations of 0.5-1% solution; **IPPB or oxygen aerosolization:** 0.5-1 ml of 5% or 0.5 ml of 1% solution diluted 1:3 with diluent. *Metaproterenol*—**aerosol:** metered dose inhaler, 2-3 inhalations (650 μg/inhalation), up to 12 inhalations/day; **nebulizer,** 5-15 inhalations or 0.3 ml of 5% solution, 3-4 times/day; **oral:** 20 mg, 3-4 times/day. *Terbutaline*— **aerosol:** metered dose inhaler, 2 inhalations (200 μg/inhalation) q 4-6 h; **oral:** 2.5-5 mg 3 times/day; **subcutaneously:** 0.25 mg, may be repeated 15-30 min, not to exceed 0.5 mg in 4 h.

Precautions/contraindications: See Nonselective Beta-adrenergic Drugs, page 291.

Side effects/adverse reactions: See Nonselective Beta-adrenergic Drugs, page 291.

Pharmacokinetics: Onset of action: rapid onset following inhalation, maximal bronchodilation by 30 min with 3-4 h duration. Following oral administration (metaproterenol, terbutaline), onset within 30 min with 4-8 h duration. Following SC administration (terbutaline) onset within 15 min, peak effect 30-90 min with a duration of 90 min to 4 h. **Route of elimination:** Metabolized by liver with GI or renal excretion.

Interactions: see Nonselective Beta-adrenergic Drugs, page 291.

Nursing considerations: see Nonselective Beta-adrenergic Drugs, page 291.

XANTHINE DERIVATIVES

Theophylline (Bronkodyl, Elixophyllin, Somophyllin-T, Aerolate, Slo-Phyllin Gyrocaps, Theo-Dur, Theo-24)
Aminophylline (Aminophyllin, Somophyllin)
Oxtriphylline (Choledyl)
Dyphylline (Dilor, Lufyllin)

Xanthine drugs include **caffeine, theobromine,** and **theophylline.** Food sources containing these substances include tea, cocoa, and coffee. Since drugs used in this category are methylated forms of xanthine, they are often referred to as **methylxanthines.** The effectiveness of these drugs depends on their conversion into theophylline, the most active of the xanthine derivatives. Aminophylline and oxtriphylline are soluble salts of theophylline. Aminophylline contains about 86% theophylline, and oxtriphylline contains about 64% theophylline. Dyphylline is a synthetic analog of theophylline that is less potent.

Theophylline works in two ways. The primary action is to increase the level of cyclic AMP, which relaxes bronchial and vascular smooth muscle, producing bronchodilation and vasodilation. Theophylline appears also to be effective in inhibiting the release of bronchoconstricting substances, including histamine, from lung tissues.

Indications: Relief or prevention of bronchial asthma and reversible bronchospasm.

Usual dosage: *Theophylline*—**IV:** Loading dose 5 mg/kg, maintenance 0.5-0.7 mg/kg/h intravenous infusion; **oral:** loading 3 mg/kg q 6 h × 2 doses, maintenance 3 mg/kg q 6-8 h. Sustained release: 3-6 mg/kg q 12-24 h. *Aminophylline*—**IV:** Loading dose 6 mg/kg, maintenance 0.5-0.7 mg/kg/h intravenous infusion; **oral:** loading 3 mg/kg q 6 h × 2 doses, maintenance 3 mg/kg q 6-8 h. *Oxtriphylline*—**oral:** 200 mg, 4 times/day. *Dyphylline*—**oral:** Up to 15 mg/kg, 4 times/day.

Doses must be individualized based on patient condition and preparation used. Doses are generally higher in smokers and children and decreased in the presence of congestive heart failure or liver disease and in the elderly. Oral doses differ between sustained and immediate-release forms.

Precautions/contraindications: Use caution in patients with myocardial infarction, angina, severe hypoxemia, renal or hepatic disease, severe hypertension, congestive heart failure, or alcoholism and in elderly patients. Contraindicated in patients with hypersensitivity to any xanthine or who have peptic ulcer or active gastritis.

Side effects/adverse reactions: Reactions are rare with serum levels <20 μg/ml; at levels >20-25 μg/ml, nausea, vomiting, diarrhea, headache, CNS excitement, insomnia, and irritability may occur; at levels > 30-35 μg/ml, hyperglycemia, hypotension, dysrhythmias, tachycardia, seizures, and death may occur. Side effects may not occur in any specific order or may not appear until life-threatening reaction occurs.

Pharmacokinetics: Onset of action: Varies with route and preparation. **Plasma half-life:** 7-9 h in adult nonsmokers and 4-5 h in smokers. **Therapeutic blood levels:** 10-20 μg/ml. **Route of elimination:** Renal excretion. Decreased serum clearance may occur in patients with heart failure, liver dysfunction, alcoholism, respiratory infections, COPD, or high fever.

Interactions: Decreased effects with cigarette and marijuana smoking, phenobarbital; increased effects with cimetidine, erythromycin, oral contraceptives, troleandomycin, influenza virus vaccine, clindamycin, lincomycin. Theophylline increases the effects of sympathomimetics and enhances sensitivity to or toxicity of digitalis and may increase excretion of lithium carbonate.

Nursing considerations: Oral administration: Food may alter the absorption and bioavailability of some sustained release preparations. For predictable results, the sustained release forms of theophylline should consistently be taken on an empty stomach. Changes in doses result in new steady-state serum levels in about 2 days. **Intravenous administration:** The drug should be administered slowly to avoid toxic serum levels (no more than 25 mg/min infusion rate). Loading doses should be given over at least 30 min. Monitor the patient closely, especially while administering the loading dose, for adverse effects and signs of toxicity. Plasma clearance varies significantly even between healthy patients. Serum theophylline levels should be monitored 24 h after institution of IV therapy and later after oral therapy is begun. During long-term therapy, serum levels tend to remain constant; serum levels may be rechecked at 6-12 month intervals, following dosage adjustments, or at any sign of toxicity. Obtain serum sample at time of peak absorption (1-2 h after administration of immediate-release products and 4 h after administration of sustained-release products). Serum theophylline levels will not measure dyphylline; specific dyphylline levels may be used to guide therapy.

MUSCARINIC ANTAGONISTS

Ipratropium bromide (Atrovent)

Muscarinic antagonists inhibit the effect of acetylcholine at muscarinic receptors in the airways. These drugs block the contraction of airway smooth muscle and the increase in mucus secretion that occurs as the result of vagal, or parasympathetic, stimulation. The prototypic muscarinic antagonist is **atropine**. While atropine may be very effective in reversing bronchoconstriction in some patients, its use is limited by systemic effects, including dry mouth, urinary retention, tachycardia, loss of visual accommodation, and agitation. **Ipratropium bromide** is a derivative of atropine that can be effective when administered to the airways and has few adverse effects because the drug is very poorly absorbed systemically and does not readily enter the CNS.

Indications: Maintenance treatment of bronchospasm associated with COPD.

Usual dosage: 2 inhalations (36 µg) 4 times/day, with additional inhalations as required, up to 12 inhalations/24 h.

Precautions/contraindications: Use with caution in patients with prostatic hypertrophy, bladder neck obstruction, or narrow-angle glaucoma; contraindicated in patients with known hypersensitivity to atropine or its derivatives.

Side effects/adverse reactions: CNS: Nervousness; **GI:** Nausea, GI distress; **EENT:** Blurred vision, dry mouth, worsening of narrow-angle glaucoma; **Respiratory:** Worsening of symptoms; **GU:** Urinary retention.

Pharmacokinetics: Onset of action: About 15 min, with effects persisting up to 6 h. **Plasma half-life:** About 2 h. **Route of elimination:** Much of dose is swallowed, which leads to fecal excretion. There is little, if any, systemic absorption from the lungs or GI tract.

Interactions: None reported.

Nursing considerations: Monitor respiratory status closely before and during therapy and assess for adverse effects during therapy (see Precautions above).

CROMOLYN SODIUM

Cromolyn sodium (Intal, Nasalcrom)

Cromolyn sodium differs from most asthma medications or bronchodilators in that it is only effective when taken prophylactically. Cromolyn prevents the release of histamine and other bronchoconstricting substances from mast cells in lung tissues. When used prior to exposure, the drug inhibits the immediate and delayed reactions to antigen (or allergy)-induced asthma and exercise-induced asthma. With chronic use, cromolyn sodium may decrease the overall level of bronchial reactivity. The drug has no direct bronchodilator effect and is ineffective in reversing bronchospasm once it occurs.

Indications: Prophylactic management of severe bronchial asthma, prevention of exercise, environmental, or antigen-induced bronchospasm and allergic rhinitis.

Usual dosage: *Asthma*—initially 20 mg, inhaled, 4 times/day (powder or solution) or 1.6 mg (2 inhalations) 4 times/day (aerosol). *Prevention of bronchospasm*—20 mg (powder or solution) or 1.6 mg (aerosol) inhaled not longer than 1 h before exposure to precipitating factor. *Allergic rhinitis*—nasal inhaler, 1 spray (5.2 mg) in each nostril, 3-4 times/day.

Precautions/contraindications: Cromolyn has no use in the management of acute asthma, especially status asthmaticus. Symptoms of asthma may recur if the drug is discontinued or dosage reduced. The aerosol form should be used with caution in patients with coronary artery disease or cardiac dysrhythmias because of the propellant in this preparation; the drug is contraindicated in any patient with hypersensitivity to cromolyn.

Side effects/adverse reactions: Patients may occasionally experience irritation of the throat or trachea, cough, or bronchospasm following inhalation of the drug; transient nasal stinging or sneezing may be experienced by some patients immediately following instillation of the nasal solution.

Pharmacokinetics: Onset of action: Response to the drug generally occurs within 2-4 wks of treatment. **Route of elimination:** Cromolyn acts locally on the nasal and lung mucosa to which it is applied and is poorly absorbed from the GI tract. Following inhalation about 7% is absorbed systemically and excreted unchanged in the bile or urine. The remainder is either exhaled or swallowed and excreted unchanged in the feces.

Interactions: None reported in usual doses.

Nursing considerations: Assess the severity of the patient's symptoms before and during therapy along with the need for concomitant drug therapy (bronchodilators and/or steroids). Instruct the patient not to discontinue prophylactic use of the drug except on the advice of a physician. When the drug is used to prevent bronchospasm, the shorter the interval between administration and exposure to the precipitating factor, the better the results. The dose may be repeated during prolonged exposure or exercise. The drug is administered by inhalation only; the capsules should not be swallowed. Cromolyn sodium may be administered from capsules containing the powder using a special oral inhaler (Spinhaler), from a solution using a power-operated nebulizer (hand-held nebulizers are not suitable), orally with a aerosol inhaler, or with a special nasal inhaler (Nasalmatic). Proper administration is necessary to obtain optimal results. Instruct the patient in the proper administration technique for each preparation of cromolyn sodium, following the manufacturer's directions.

CORTICOSTEROIDS

Even though their precise mechanism of action is not known, corticosteroids have been used for many years to treat asthma and COPD. These drugs do not directly relax airway smooth muscle but decrease airway inflammation when administered to asthmatic patients. Corticosteroids may work by potentiating the effects of beta-receptor agonists or, most probably, by inhibiting or in some way modifying the inflammatory response in airways. Controversy exists concerning the indications and dosages for corticosteroid use in asthma. Corticosteroids may be given to reduce the severity of the acute asthma attack; the dose is then slowly decreased as improvement occurs. Because of side effects, long-term systemic use of corticosteroids is reserved for patients who cannot be adequately managed with bronchodilators. One method of reducing adverse systemic effects is to administer the drug as an aerosol. This method of administration offers effective delivery of the drug to the airways with minimal systemic absorption. With the development of aerosol forms of corticosteroids, which limit the systemic effects, systemic administration is reserved for short-term therapy following acute episodes of bronchospasm and for long-term therapy only in those patients unresponsive to other treatments.

SYSTEMIC CORTICOSTEROIDS

Prednisone
Methylprednisolone

Indications: Bronchial asthma, including status asthmaticus and aspiration pneumonitis.

Usual dosage: *Prednisone*—oral: 30-60 mg/day; *Methylprednisolone*—IV: 1 mg/kg q 6 h. Doses are decreased gradually over a week to 10 days after airway obstruction has improved. When long-term doses are required, alternate-day administration may be helpful in controlling symptoms with fewer side effects than daily administration.

Precautions/contraindications: Use with caution in patients with peptic ulcer, heart disease or hypertension with congestive heart failure, infections, psychoses, diabetes, osteoporosis, glaucoma, or tuberculosis.

Side effects/adverse reactions: Side effects are uncommon with short-term therapy (less than 1 wk) but increase with the duration of therapy. Undesirable effects that may occur include hyperglycemia, sodium retention with edema or hypertension, weight gain, muscle wasting, acne, hypokalemia, peptic ulcer, osteoporosis, increased intraocular pressure, cataract development, psychosis, and exacerbation of infections. Suppression of adrenal function occurs when these drugs are administered over a long period.

Pharmacokinetics: Onset of action: Slow. **Plasma half-life:** *Prednisone*—60 min; *Methylprednisolone*—78-188 min. **Route of elimination:** Metabolized in the liver with renal excretion.

Interactions: Requirement or insulin or hypoglycemic agents may be increased. Phenytoin, phenobarbital, rifampin, and possibly ephedrine may increase metabolism of corticosteroids and reduce the effectiveness of a given dose. Oral contraceptives may inhibit corticosteroid metabolism.

Nursing considerations: Asthmatic children treated for prolonged periods should have periodic eye examinations to detect the development of cataracts. Monitor all patients for development of adverse effects. Patients on long-term therapy must have the drug dose slowly tapered to avoid adrenal insufficiency. Assess all patients for signs of adrenal insufficiency or return of respiratory symptoms during withdrawal of the dose. During periods of stress or severe asthmatic attack, patients recently withdrawn from systemic steroids should have treatment resumed.

AEROSOL CORTICOSTEROIDS

Beclomethasone (Beclovent, Vanceril)
Dexamethasone (Decadron Phosphate Respihaler)
Flunisolide (Aerobid)
Triamcinolone (Azmacort)

Indications: Control of bronchial asthma in conjunction with bronchodilator therapy. Treatment of bronchospasm associated with some chronic lung diseases.

Usual dosage: *Beclomethasone:* 2 inhalations (42 μg/inhalation) 3-4 times/day, up to 12-16 inhalations/day in severe asthma. *Dexamethasone:* 3 inhalations (84 μg/inhalation) 3-4 times/day. *Flunisolide:* 2 inhalations (250 μg/inhalation) twice daily, morning and evening, up to 4 inhalations twice daily. *Triamcinolone:* 2 inhalations (100 μg/inhalation) 3-4 times/day, up to 16 inhalations/day in severe asthma.

Precautions/contraindications: Adrenal insufficiency may occur during transfer from systemic therapy to aerosol steroids or tuberculosis.

Side effects/adverse reactions: Systemic effects (see systemic corticosteroids) are uncommon with long-term inhalation administration. Localized fungal infections involving the mouth, pharynx, or larynx have been reported.

Pharmacokinetics: Onset of action: beneficial effects are seen only with chronic administration. **Route of elimination:** Some degree of systemic absorption occurs following inhalation therapy with metabolism in the lungs or liver and renal or fecal excretion.

Interactions: None reported with aerosol therapy.

Nursing considerations: Treatment is preventive only and is not useful for controlling the acute attack. Patients using inhaled bronchodilators should use the bronchodilators several minutes before corticosteroid administration to improve distribution of inhaled drug in the lungs. Rinsing the mouth with water after administration may reduce or prevent dry mouth and fungal infections. Monitor patients for symptoms of localized fungus infections in the mouth, pharynx, and larynx and instruct patients to notify their physician if persistent sore throat or mouth occurs.

INTRANASAL CORTICOSTEROIDS

Beclomethasone (Beconase nasal inhaler, Vancenase nasal inhaler)
Dexamethasone (Decadron Phosphate Tubinaire)
Flunisolide (Nasalide)

Indications: Relief of symptoms of seasonal or perennial rhinitis in cases of poor response to conventional therapy; allergy or inflammatory nasal conditions or prevention of recurrence of nasal polyps following surgical removal.

Usual dosage: *Beclomethasone:* 1 inhalation (42 μg) in each nostril, 2-4 times/day. *Dexamethasone:* 2 sprays (84μg/spray) in each nostril, 2-3 times/day. *Flunisolide:* 2-4 sprays (50 μg/spray) in each nostril, 2-3 times/day.

Precautions/contraindications: Do not continue therapy beyond 3 wks in the absence of improvement. Use with caution following recent nasal ulcers, injury, surgery, or recurrent epistaxis because nasal corticosteroids may delay local wound healing. Contraindicated in the presence of untreated infections involving the nasal mucosa.

Side effects/adverse reactions: Nasal irritation and dryness. Localized fungal infections of the nose and throat have been reported. Systemic effects (see systemic corticosteroids) are rare unless recommended doses are exceeded.

Interactions: None.

Nursing considerations: Effects are not immediate and may take several days of regular use to become apparent. Instruct the patient to clear nasal passages before use and to use a nasal decongestant before use if nasal passages are blocked.

MUCOKINETIC DRUGS

Mucokinetic drugs are compounds that promote the removal of abnormal or excessive respiratory tract secretions by thinning hyperviscous secretions or promoting ciliary action. They are useful in conditions that result from increased production of respiratory secretions, hyperviscous secretions, reduced ciliary activity, defects in air flow, or reduced cough effectiveness.

MUCOLYTIC DRUGS

Acetylcysteine (Mucomyst)

Mucolytic drugs reduce the thickness and stickiness of pulmonary secretions by breaking links between mucoprotein complexes contained in the secretions. This effect aids in removal of secretions by coughing, postural drainage, or suctioning.

Indications: As an adjunct treatment for abnormal, viscid, or inspissated mucus secretions in chronic bronchopulmonary disease and for pulmonary complications of cystic fibrosis, or atelectasis caused by mucus obstruction. Used as an aid in bronchial studies such as bronchograms and bronchospirometry. (Although not discussed here, acetylcysteine is also used to reduce hepatic injury following acetaminophen overdose.)

Usual dosage: *Nebulization:* 2-20 ml of a 10% solution or 1-10 ml of 20% solution. *Instillation:* 1-2 ml of 10%-20% solution q 1-4 h into trachea.

Precautions/contraindications: Increased volume of secretions may occur. If patient is unable to remove the secretions by cough, adequate suctioning may be needed to maintain an open airway.

Side effects/adverse reactions: Stomatitis, nausea, rhinorrhea; bronchospasm has been reported in a few patients.

Pharmacokinetics: Onset of action: Within 1 min. **Peak effect:** 5-10 min. **Route of elimination:** < 50% of inhaled drug is absorbed through respiratory epithelium; absorbed portion of drug is metabolized in the liver.

Interactions: Incompatible with many drugs when mixed in the same solution.

Nursing considerations: A slight change in solution color may occur in the open bottle but does not affect safety or potency. Solutions of acetylcysteine become discolored and liberate hydrogen sulfide upon contact with rubber and some metals (particularly iron and copper) or when autoclaved. The drug does not react with glass, plastic, aluminum, chromed metal, tantalum, silver, or stainless steel. Nebulizing equipment should be cleaned promptly following use to prevent residues from occluding fine orifices or corroding metal parts. When using dry gas to nebulize, after three fourths of the solution has been nebulized, the remaining portion should be diluted with an equal amount of sterile water to prevent the solution from becoming overconcentrated, which impairs nebulization. Administration may produce a disagreeable sulfurous odor that may be associated with nausea. Nebulization into a face mask may cause stickiness on the face that is easily removed with water. Asthmatic patients should be observed carefully during administration for the development of bronchospasm, and drug administration should be stopped if it occurs.

DILUENTS

Diluents are used to thin the consistency of respiratory secretions to aid in their removal and are administered by ultrasonic nebulizers. Water and saline solutions are used to add moisture to bronchial secretions of patients with chronic respiratory problems. The increased moisture appears to reduce the adhesive properties and viscosity of gelatinous substances in secretions. Inhaled water may be absorbed through the lungs; this must be considered in the patient with a restricted fluid intake. Normal saline (0.9% sodium chloride) exerts the same osmotic pressure as plasma fluids. Hypotonic solutions may provide deeper penetration into the distal airways. Hypertonic solutions (1.8% sodium chloride) are irritants to the respiratory mucosa and help stimulate a productive cough. Large amounts of water are usually encouraged to hydrate the patient and help liquefy secretions if the patient's fluid intake is not restricted.

EXPECTORANTS

Guaifensin
Terpin hydrate
Potassium iodide
Ipecac syrup
Pine tar preparations and others

Expectorants may be of some value in removing pulmonary secretions by liquefying and loosening mucus, soothing bronchial mucosa, and making coughs more productive. Expectorants are included in many

Table 8-1

EXPECTORANTS

Drug	Action*	Side effects/adverse effects	Adult dose
Guaifensin	Increases respiratory tract fluid to reduce viscosity of secretions	May cause GI upset in larger doses	Oral - 200-400 mg q 4 h, maximum of 2.4 g/day
Terpin hydrate	May work by direct stimulation of lower respiratory secretory glands	May cause GI distress if taken on an empty stomach	170 mg 3-4 times/day or 200 mg q 4 h, maximum of 1.2 g/day
Potassium iodide	May increase respiratory tract secretions	Hypersensitivity reactions to iodides may occur, prolonged use leads to thyroid hyperplasia, adenoma, goiter, or hypothyroidism	300-650 mg 3-4 times/ day
Ammonium chloride	No data available	No data available	No data available
Beechwood creosote	No data available	No data available	No data available
Ipecac syrup	No data available	No data available	No data available
Pine tar preparations	No data available	No data available	No data available

*These agents have been classified by the FDA as having insufficient data to establish efficacy.

over-the-counter and prescription cough or upper respiratory preparations, even though there is little evidence of their efficacy. The use of expectorants is primarily based on traditional practice rather than objective evidence of clinical effectiveness. Table 8-1 presents some of the expectorants used, even though they are classified by the FDA as having insufficient data to be classified effective. In addition to drug therapy, humidification of air and adequate fluid intake are important measures to aid in expectoration of respiratory secretions.

ANTITUSSIVES

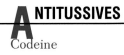
Codeine

Antitussives are effective for providing symptomatic relief of coughing. These drugs should not be used indiscriminately because coughing is a physiologic mechanism for clearing the respiratory tract of secretions and has beneficial effects.

NARCOTIC ANTITUSSIVES

Many narcotics have antitussive, or cough suppressant, properties. The narcotic drugs, in general, inhibit ciliary activity in the respiratory tract, and may cause bronchial constriction in allergic or asthmatic patients. Most of these drugs are used primarily for their analgesic properties; some are often used for their antitussive actions. Codeine has good antitussive activity at doses lower than those required for analgesic effects and has few side effects at the usual antitussive doses. Codeine occupies endorphin receptor sites in the CNS to depress the cough reflex through the cough center in the medulla.

Indications: Suppression of mild to moderate cough due to mechanical or chemical respiratory tract irritation.

Usual dosage: 10-20 mg, q 4-6 h, maximum 120 mg/day.

Precautions/contraindications: With excessive doses, codeine may obscure diagnosis of patients with conditions resulting in pain. Codeine may produce respiratory depression and may increase CSF pressure in the presence of head injury or preexisting increased CSF pressure; it is contraindicated in patients with known hypersensitivity.

Side effects/adverse reactions: Uncommon in the usual oral antitussive doses; most common are nausea, vomiting, sedation, dizziness, and constipation.

Pharmacokinetics: Onset of action: 15-30 min with 4-6 h duration of action. **Plasma half-life:** 2.9 h. **Route of elimination:** Metabolized in the liver and excreted in the urine.

Interactions: May potentiate other CNS depressants; may see excessive effects or other interactions with monoamine oxidase (MAO) inhibitors.

Nursing considerations: Although the abuse potential of codeine is relatively low, psychologic and/or physical dependence and tolerance may develop with prolonged use. Use with caution and monitor closely in patients with a history of drug abuse or dependence. Inform patient to use caution when performing tasks requiring alertness because narcotics may impair physical and mental abilities. Instruct the patient to avoid alcohol and other CNS depressant drugs while taking codeine. Assess the patient for constipation or GI upset during drug therapy.

NONNARCOTIC ANTITUSSIVES

Benzonatate (Tessalon Perles)
Dextromethorphan (Mediquell, Sucrets Cough Control, Hold, Pertussin, and others)
Dextromethorphan and benzocaine (Spec-T, Formula 44 Cough Control Discs, Vick's Cough Silencers)
Diphenhydramine (Beldin, Benylin Cough, Diphen Cough, Valdrene, and others)

The nonnarcotic antitussives lack analgesic properties and are not associated with psychological and/or physical dependence. Benzonatate is related to tetracaine and anesthetizes the stretch receptors in the respiratory tract and pleura to depress the cough reflex. Dextramethorphan controls cough by depressing the cough center in the medulla. Diphenhydramine, an antihistamine, also has antitussive properties.

Indications: Control of nonproductive cough and cough due to colds or allergy.

Usual dosage: *Benzonatate*— 100 mg 3 times/day up to 600 mg/24 h. *Dextromethorphan*— 10-30 mg q 4-8 h, up to 120 mg/24 h; sustained action liquid— 60 mg twice daily. *Dextromethorphan and Benzocaine*— 1-2 lozenges (2.5-10 mg /lozenge) q 1-3 h up to 120 mg/day. *Diphenhydramine*— 25 mg q 4 h up to 150 mg/24 h.

Precautions/contraindications: Not for use in persistent or chronic cough or when cough is accompanied by excessive secretions.

Side effects/adverse reactions: Not for use in chronic cough. *Benzonatate*— sedation, headache, dizziness, constipation, GI disturbances, nasal congestion. *Diphenhydramine:* See Antihistamines.

Pharmacokinetics: Onset of action: 15-20 min.

Interactions: none.

Nursing considerations: benzonatate in the mouth can produce temporary local anesthesia. The capsules should be swallowed without chewing, breaking, or dissolving in the mouth.

ANTIHISTAMINES

Diphenhydramine
Tripelennamine
Chlorpheniramine
Promethazine
Cyproheptadine
Terfenadine and others

Antihistamines do not prevent the release of histamine, bind with, or inactivate histamine. The drugs work by competitively binding with H_1 receptor sites, which antagonizes, to varying degrees, the effects of histamine release. They also have drying, sedative, and anticholinergic effects. The drugs provide symptomatic relief rather than treat the underlying cause of histamine release. Individual response to antihistamines varies considerably. A trial of various antihistamines may be necessary to determine which specific drug provides optimal relief with minimal side effects. Table 8-2 compares antihistamine doses and effects.

Table 8-2

ANTIHISTAMINES: DOSAGE AND EFFECTS

Antihistamine	Dose* (mg)	Dosing interval† (hrs)	Sedative effects‡	Antihistaminic activity‡	Anticholinergic activity‡	Antiemetic effects‡
Ethanolamines						
Diphenhydramine	25 to 50	4 to 6	+++	+ to ++	+++	+++
Carbinoxamine	4 to 8	6 to 8	++	+ to ++	+++	++ to +++
Clemastine	1	12	++	+ to ++	+++	++ to +++
Ethylenediamines						
Tripelennamine	25 to 50	4 to 6	++	+ to ++	±	—
Pyrilamine	25 to 50	6 to 8	+	+ to ++	±	—
Alkylamines						
Chlorpheniramine	4	4 to 6	+	++	++	—
Dexchlorpheniramine	2	4 to 6	+	+++	++	—
Brompheniramine	4	4 to 6	+	+++	++	—
Triprolidine	2.5	4 to 6	+	++ to +++	++	—
Phenothiazines						
Promethazine	12.5 to 25	6 to 24	+++	+++	+++	++++
Trimeprazine	2.5	6	++	+++	+++	++++
Methdilazine	8	6 to 12	+	+++	+++	++++
Piperidines						
Cyproheptadine	4	8	+	++	++	—
Azatadine	1 to 2	12	++	++	++	—
Diphenylpyraline	5§	12§	+	++	++	—
Phenindamine	25	4 to 6	—¶	++	++	—
Miscellaneous						
Terfenadine	60	12	±	++ to +++	±	—
Astemizole	10	24	±	++ to +++	±	—

*Usual single oral adult dose.
†For conventional dosage forms.
‡++++ = very high; +++ = high; ++ = moderate; + = low; ± = low to none.
§Available only in timed release form.
¶Stimulation possible.
©April, 1989 by Facts and Comparisons

Indications: Symptomatic relief of allergic symptoms caused by histamine release, including allergic rhinitis, rhinorrhea, sneezing, oropharyngeal irritation, and conjunctivitis.

Precautions/contraindications: *Phenothiazines*—contraindicated in individuals with CNS depression, jaundice, or bone marrow suppression. Use caution when administering to patients with liver dysfunction, cardiovascular disease, or ulcers. Because of their anticholinergic effects, antihistamines should be used cautiously in patients with narrow-angle glaucoma, prostatic hypertrophy, bladder neck obstruction, or stenosing peptic ulcer. Contraindicated in patients with known sensitivity or taking MAO inhibitors.

Side effects/adverse reactions: CNS: Sedation, dizziness, disturbed coordination and weakness, paradoxic excitement (especially common in children); **GI:** Epigastric distress, nausea, vomiting, constipation, dryness of throat and mouth; **GU:** Dysuria, urinary retention, impotence; **Respiratory:** Thickening of secretions, chest tightness, nasal stuffiness and wheezing; **Other:** Visual disturbances, tinnitus, nervousness, irritability, sweating, chills, and a variety of other minor symptoms.

Pharmacokinetics: Onset of action: Most are well absorbed following oral administration, with onset of effect within 15-60 min. There is little information regarding the pharmacokinetics of most antihistamines.

Interactions: Additive effects may occur when other CNS depressants, including alcohol, are administered. MAO inhibitors may intensify or prolong the anticholinergic effects of antihistamines.

Nursing considerations: Caution patients that the drug may cause drowsiness and sedation, which may disappear after several days of therapy. Selection of antihistamines and doses should be based on the patient's response.

NASAL DECONGESTANTS

Phenylpropanolamine
Pseudoephedrine
Phenylephrine
Epinephrine
Tetrahydrozoline
Ephedrine
Oxymetazoline and others

Nasal decongestants are sympathomimetic amines administered either orally or directly to the nasal membranes. The beneficial effects are the result of alpha-adrenergic stimulation (vasopressor effects) in the nose,

although some of the decongestants also have beta-stimulant effects. Constriction of mucous membranes from alpha stimulation results in improved ventilation, promotes drainage, and reduces the stuffy feeling. The oral preparations are less effective than topical preparations; however, they have a longer duration of effect, cause less local irritation, and generally do not produce a rebound congestion effect. For immediate action the topical preparations are far superior. The vasoconstriction caused by topically applied agents also serves to further reduce systemic absorption of the drug (Table 8-3).

Indications: Temporary relief of nasal and nasopharyngeal congestion associated with colds, upper respiratory allergies, sinusitis, or eustachian tube congestion.

Precautions/contraindications: Use cautiously in patients with hypertension, coronary artery disease, narrow-angle glaucoma, or hyperthyroidism.

Side effects/adverse reactions: Systemic absorption of topical agents may cause stimulation of alpha-adrenergic receptors outside of the nasal mucosa and result in hypertension, tachycardia, hyperglycemia, mydriasis, and CNS stimulation. Vasoconstriction may be followed by vasodilation, which increases congestion or "rebound effect," most commonly seen after prolonged use of topical agents.

Interactions: *Furazoldone, MAO inhibitors* may increase adrenergic effects; *beta-blocking drugs* may result in increased blood pressure and bradycardia; *Guanethidine*, tricyclic antidepressants; *Rauwolfia alkaloids* may increase or decrease effects; *Methyldopa* may cause hypertension; *Phenothiazines* may result in hypotension and tachycardia; *Theophylline* may result in increased GI discomfort.

Nursing considerations: To prevent rebound congestion, topical preparations should not be used on a long-term basis. Most of these products are sold over-the-counter. Be sure to assess the patient for OTC drug use and assess for possible interactions with prescription drug therapy.

ANTIINFECTIVE AGENTS

Penicillin
Nafcillin
Cephalosporin
Tetracycline
Streptomycin
Cefuroxime and others

A variety of antiinfective agents are used to treat respiratory infections. Drug therapy is based on the infecting agent, which is identified whenever possible through the use of cultures. Drug therapy is begun as

Table 8-3

NASAL DECONGESTANTS

Drug	Trade Names*	Route	Usual Adult Dose
Arylalkylamines			
Phenylpropanolamine	Propagest, Sucrets Cold Decongestant Formula,	Oral	25 mg q 4-8 h, 50 mg q 8 h
	Rhindecon	Oral-SR	75 mg q 12 h
Pseudoephedrine	Afrinol Repetabs, Novafed,	Oral	60 mg q 6 h
	Neofed, Sudafed, Sudrin	Oral-SR	120 mg q 12 h
Phenylephrine	Alconefrin, Doktors, Neo-Synephrine, Nostril, Rhinall, Sinex, Sinophen, Vacon	Topical	1-2 sprays or a few drops q 3-4 h (0.125-1% solution)
Epinephrine	Adrenalin	Topical	up to 1 ml/15 min (0.1%)
Ephedrine	Efedron, Vatronol	Topical	2-3 drops q 4 h (0.5%)
Desoxyephedrine			50 mg inhaler
Imidazolines			
Naphazoline	Privine	Topical	2 drops q 3 h (0.5%)
Tetrahydrozoline	Tyzine	Topical	2-4 drops q 3 h (0.05-0.1%)
Oxymetazoline	Afrin, Allerest, Coricidin, Duration, Nostrilla, Sinarest, Sinex	Topical	2-3 drops twice daily (0.025%-0.05%)
Xylometrazoline	Chlorohist-LA, Otrivin	Topical	2-3 drops q 8-10 h (0.5-0.1%)
Cycloalkylamine			
Propylhexedrine		Topical	250 mg inhaler

*Trade names are not complete; many of these products are components in combination products.

soon as cultures are obtained. The patient's response and culture results are then used to modify drug therapy. Table 5-1 on p. 177 presents antiinfective agents used in the therapy of pneumonia. Antiinfectives act either by inhibiting bacterial wall synthesis (e.g., cephalosporins, penicillins) or by directly attacking the ribosomes inhibiting protein synthesis (e.g., aminoglycosides).

Vaccines

PNEUMOCOCCAL VACCINE

Pneumococcal vaccine, polyvalent (Pneumovax 23, Pnu-Imune 23)

The pneumococcal vaccine affords protection against 23 of the most prevalent pneumococcal types, which account for over 90% of all pneumococcal blood isolates. The vaccine stimulates production of antipneumococcal antibodies to prevent pneumococcal disease. The vaccine only provides protection against the types of pneumococci contained in the vaccine. Following administration of the vaccine, healthy individuals generally experience a two-fold or greater increase in antibodies specific for each pneumococcal types in the vaccine. The pneumococcal vaccine is given only once.

Indications: Individuals who are at increased risk for morbidity from respiratory infections, including older persons and those with chronic illness (especially cardiovascular disease and chronic pulmonary disease).

Usual dosage: SC or IM: One 0.5 ml dose.

Precautions/contraindications: Do not administer to patients who have previously received the vaccine. The vaccination should not be administered to individuals with a febrile respiratory illness or active infection unless the potential benefits outweigh the potential risks. Anaphylactic reactions have been reported.

Side effects/ adverse reactions: Local: Up to 90% of patients may experience a mild local reaction, which may include erythema, soreness, swelling, and induration. These reactions generally persist < 48 h; **Systemic:** A low-grade fever lasting < 48 h may occur in

3%-7% of patients. Other systemic reactions that occur less frequently are weakness, myalgia, headache, photophobia, chills, and nausea.

Pharmacokinetics: Onset of action: A protective effect against pneumococcal disease is generally achieved by the third week after immunization.

Interactions: The vaccine may be administered at the same time as influenza vaccine; however, separate syringes and different injection sites should be used. Patients receiving immunosuppressive therapy may not have a satisfactory antibody response to the vaccine.

Nursing considerations: The needle and syringe used must be free of preservatives, antiseptics, and detergents. The vaccine should not be administered IV. Epinephrine should be immediately available in case an anaphylactic reaction occurs.

INFLUENZA VACCINES

Influenza virus vaccine (Fluogen, Fluzone)

Influenza virus vaccines are sterile suspensions prepared from inactivated influenza viruses. The vaccine is available in "whole-virus" (whole-virion) and "split-virus" (subvirion) preparations. Influenza vaccines are formulated annually based on specifications from the U.S. Health Service and contain antigens against those strains that are expected to be prevalent in the forthcoming year. The vaccines provide protection only against those strains, or closely related strains, for which the vaccine is prepared.

Indications: Individuals at high risk for influenza-related complications, including persons with chronic disorders of the cardiovascular or pulmonary systems. Vaccine may also be indicated for health care and other personnel who may transmit the infection to high-risk individuals. Any group or individual who has a need to reduce the chances of acquiring an influenza infection.

Usual dosage: Patients over 12 years of age— one dose (0.5 ml) of whole or split virus. Children should receive only the split-virus preparation because of the lower potential for causing febrile reactions; **age 3-12 years**— 0.5 ml; **age 6-35 months**— 0.25 ml.

Precautions/contraindications: The vaccination should not be administered to individuals with a febrile respiratory illness or active infection unless the potential benefits outweigh the potential risks. Anaphylactic reactions have been reported. Vaccination may not result in seroconversion (evidence of immunity) in all individuals. Sulfites may cause allergic-type reactions in some susceptible individuals.

Side effects/adverse reactions: Local: Soreness at injection site, local erythema; **systemic:** Fever, myalgia,

and other symptoms of toxicity, which generally begin 6-12 h after immunization and persist for 1-2 days, or immediate allergic reactions involving respiratory and skin symptoms. Anaphylactic reactions have been reported. In 1976 an association between that year's influenza vaccine and Guillian-Barrè syndrome was reported. This association has not been noted with subsequent influenza vaccines.

Pharmacokinetics: Onset of action: A protective effect is usually seen within 10-14 days following immunization in most individuals.

Interactions: The vaccine may be administered at the same time as pneumococcal vaccine; however, separate syringes and different injection sites should be used. Patients receiving immunosuppressive therapy may not have a satisfactory antibody response to the vaccine.

Nursing considerations: Influenza vaccines should be refrigerated at 2-8° C. Potency of the vaccine is destroyed by freezing; any vaccine that has been frozen should not be used. Any vaccines remaining after the flu season should be discarded when the next year's influenza vaccine is released. Annual vaccination is required to maintain immunity. The vaccine should be administered by IM injection (preferably in the deltoid muscle). It should not be administered IV. Epinephrine should be immediately available in case an anaphylactic reaction occurs.

References

1. American Cancer Society: Cancer facts and figures—1988, New York, 1988, The Society.
2. American Lung Association: Chronic obstructive pulmonary disease, New York, 1981, The Association.
3. American Lung Association: Occupational lung diseases: an introduction, New York, 1983, The Association.
4. American Public Health Association: Control of communicable disease in man, ed 13, Washington, DC, 1980, The Association.
5. American Thoracic Society: A statement by the Committee of Diagnostic Standards for Nontuberculosis Respiratory Diseases, Am Rev Resp Dis 85:762, 1962.
6. American Thoracic Society: Surveillance for respiratory hazards in the occupational setting, Am Rev Respir Dis 126(5):932, 1982.
7. Association for Practitioners in Infection Control: The APC curriculum for infection control practice, Dubuque, Iowa, 1981, Kendall/Hunt Publishing Co.
8. Barrows JJ: Turning the tide against acute pulmonary edema, Nursing 84 14(3):58-63, 1984.
9. Belshe RB: Viral respiratory disease in the intensive care unit, Heart Lung 15(3):222-226, 1986.
10. Benenson AS, editor: Control of communicable diseases in man, ed 14, Washington, DC, 1985, American Public Health Association.
11. Berkow R, editor: Merck manual of diagnosis and therapy, ed 14, Rahway, NJ, 1982, Merck, Inc.
12. Bernard GR and Bradley RB: Adult respiratory disease syndrome: diagnosis and management, Heart Lung 15(3):250, 1986.
13. Bradley BR: Adult respiratory distress syndrome, Focus Crit Care 14(5):45-59, 1987.
14. Bransetter RD: The adult respiratory distress syndrome, Heart Lung 15(2):155, 1986.
15. Brown LH: The effective cough, Dimen Crit Care Nurse 8(2):77, 1988.
16. Brunner LS and Suddarth DS, editors: Textbook of medical-surgical nursing, ed 6, New York, 1988, JB Lippincott Co.
17. Bullock BI and Rosendahl PP: Pathophysiology: adaptation and alterations in function, ed 2, Boston, 1988, Scott, Foresman & Co.
18. Burrows B: An overview of obstructive lung diseases, Med Clin North Am 65:455, 1981.
19. Campbell ML: Sexual dysfunction in the COPD patient, Dimen Crit Care Nurs 6(2):70-74, 1987.
20. Canobbio MM: Chest x-ray film interpretation, Focus Crit Care 11(2):18-24, 1984.
21. Carrieri VK, Murdaugh C, and Janson-Bjerklie S: A framework for assessing pulmonary disease categories, Focus Crit Care 11(2):10-16, 1984.
22. Carroll PF: Good nursing gets COPD patients out of hospitals, RN July:24-28, 1989.
23. Celentano NL: Mechanical ventilation strategies in adult respiratory distress syndrome, Crit Care Nurs 6(4):71, 1986.
24. Chernecky CC and Ramsey PW: Critical nursing care of the client with cancer, Norwalk, Conn, 1984, Appleton-Century-Crofts.
25. Cherniack RM: Current therapy of respiratory disease, ed 2, Philadelphia, 1986, BC Decker, Inc.
26. Chin R and Pesce R: Practical aspects in management of respiratory failure in chronic pulmonary disease, Crit Care Q 6(2):1, 1983.
27. Connor P, Berg P, Flaherty N, Klem L, Lawton R, and Tremblay M: Two stages of care for pleural effusion, RN February: 30-34, 1989.
28. Cooper D: Sexual counseling of the patient with chronic lung disease, Focus Crit Care 13(3):18-20, 1986.
29. Corbett JV: Laboratory tests and diagnostic procedure with nursing diagnoses, ed 2, Norwalk, Conn, 1987, Appleton & Lange.
30. Cosenza, JJ and Norton LC: Secretion clearance: state of the art form a nursing perspective, Crit Care Nurs 6(4):23-37, 1984.
31. D'Agostino JS: Teaching tips for lungs with COPD at home, Nursing 84 14(2):57, 1984.
32. Darovic GO: Ten perils of mechanical ventilation. . . and how to keep them in check, RN 46(5):37, 1983.
33. Dietary management in chronic pulmonary disease, Columbus, Ohio, 1986, Ross Laboratories.
34. Doenges M, Jefferies MF, and Moorhouse MF: Nursing care plans. In Nursing diagnoses in planning patient care, ed 2, Philadelphia, 1989, FA Davis Co.
35. Donner C and Cooper K: The critical difference: pulmonary edema, Part 1, Am J Nurs 88(1):59, 1988.
36. Dossey BM, Guzzetta CE, and Kenner CV: Essentials of critical care nursing: body-mind-spirit, Philadelphia, 1990, JB Lippincott Co.
37. Dossey B and Passons JM: Pulmonary embolism: preventing it, treating it, Nursing 81 11(3):26-33, 1981.
38. Ehrhardt BS and Graham M: Pulse oximetry: an easy way to check oxygen saturation, Nursing 90 20(3):50, 1990.

39. Ellis EF: Asthma in childhood, J Aller Clin Immunol 72:526, 1983.
40. Erickson RS: Mastering the ins and outs of chest drainage. Part 1, Nursing 89 19(5):37, 1989.
41. Erickson RS: Mastering the ins and outs of chest drainage. Part 2, Nursing 89 19(6) 46, 1989.
42. Farzan S: A concise handbook of respiratory diseases, ed 2, Reston, Va, 1985, Reston Publishing.
43. Fishman AP, editor: Pulmonary diseases and disorders, New York, 1980, McGraw-Hill Book Co.
44. Fowler AA, Hamman RF, and Zerbe GO: Adult respiratory distress syndrome: prognosis after onset, Am Rev Respir Dis 132:472, 1985.
45. Fries JF and Ehrlich GE: Prognosis: contemporary outcomes of disease, Bowie, Md, 1981, The Charles Press Publishers.
46. Fuch PL: Streamlining your suctioning techniques, Nursing 84 145:55-61, 1984.
47. George RB, Light RW, and Matthay RA, editors: Chest physiology, New York, 1983, Churchill Livingstone, Inc.
48. Gettrust KV, Ryan SC, and Engelman DS, editors: Applied nursing diagnosis: guides for comprehensive care planning, New York, 1985, John Wiley & Sons, Publishers, Inc.
49. Goldsmith J, Kamholz SL, Montefusco CM, and Veith FJ: Clinical and experimental aspects of single-lung transplantation, Heart Lung 16(3):231, 1987.
50. Goodnough SC: Reducing tracheal injury and aspiration, Dimen Crit Care 7(6):324-332, 1988.
51. Govoni LE and Hayes JE: Drugs and nursing implications, ed 6, Norwalk, Conn, 1989, Appleton-Century-Crofts.
52. Grossbach I: Troubleshooting ventilator-and patient-related problems. Part 1, Dimen Crit Care Nurs 6(4):58-70, 1984.
53. Hanley MV and Tyler ML: Ineffective airway clearance related to airway infection, Nurs Clin North Am 22(1):35, 1987.
54. Harber P: Value based interpretations of pulmonary function tests, Chest 88(6):874, 1985.
55. Harper RW: A guide to respiratory care: physiology and clinical approaches, Philadelphia, 1981, JB Lippincott Co.
56. Hirsch J and Hannock L, editors: Mosby's manual of clinical nursing practice, St Louis, 1985, The CV Mosby Co.
57. Hoffman LA and Maszkiewicz RC: Airway management: the basics of suctioning, AJN 87(1):40, 1987.
58. Holloway NM: Nursing the critically ill adult, ed 3, Menlo Park, Cal, 1988, Addison-Wesley Publishing Co.
59. Hopp L: Ineffective breathing pattern related to decreased lung expansion, Nurs Clin North Am 22(1):193, 1987.
60. Hudak CM, Gallo BM, and Lohr T: Critical care nursing, ed 4, Philadelphia, 1986, JB Lippincott Co.
61. Hurewitz AN and Bergofsky EH: Pathogenic mechanisms in chronic pulmonary hypertension, Heart Lung 15(4):327-335, 1986.
62. Irwin RS, Rosen MJ, and Braman, SS: Cough: a comprehensive review, Arch Intern Med 137:1186-1191, 1977.
63. Janson-Bjerklie S: Defense mechanisms: protecting the healthy lung, Heart Lung 12:643, 1983.
64. Jaquith S: Chest x-ray interpretation: implication for nursing intervention, Dimen Crit Care Nurs 5(1):10-17, 1986.
65. Karnes N: Don't let ARDS catch you off guard, Nursing 87 17(5):34, 1987.
66. Kim MJ: Ineffective airway clearance and ineffective breathing pattern: theoretical and research base for nursing diagnosis, Nurs Clin North Am 22(1):135, 1987.
67. Kinney MR, Packa DR, and Dunbar SB: AACN's clinical reference for critical-care nursing, ed 2, New York, 1988, McGraw-Hill Book Co.
68. Krull K and Hartswell E: Single-lung allograft: a nursing perspective, Dimen Crit Care Nurs, 8(6):35, 1988.
69. Lewis SM and Collier LC, editors: Medical-surgical nursing, ed 2, New York, 1987, McGraw-Hill Book Co.
70. Luckman J and Sorenson K: Medical-surgical nursing: a psychophysiological approach, ed 3, Philadelphia, 1985, WB Saunders Co.
71. Martin L: Pulmonary physiology in clinical practice: the essentials for patient care and evaluation, St Louis, 1987, The CV Mosby Co.
72. Mayo JM and Hamner JB: A nurse's guide to mechanical ventilation, RN, 50(8):18, 1987.
73. McCance KL and Huether SE: Pathophysiology: the biologic basis for disease in adults and children, St Louis, 1990, The CV Mosby Co.
74. McDonald BR: Validation of three respiratory nursing diagnoses: ineffective airway clearance, ineffective breathing pattern, and impaired gas exchange, Nurs Clin North Am 20(4):697, 1985.
75. Miller LG and Kazemi H: Manual of clinical pulmonary medicine, New York, 1983, McGraw-Hill Book Co.
76. Mims BC: You can manage chest tubes confidently, RN, May 1985.
77. Mitchell RS, Petty TL, and Schwarz MI, editors: Synopsis of clinical pulmonary disease, ed 4, St Louis, 1989, The CV Mosby Co.
78. Niederman MS and Matthey RA: Cardiovascular function in secondary pulmonary hypertension, Heart Lung 15(4):341-351, 1986.
79. Openbrier DR, Hoffman LA, and Wesmiller SW: Home oxygen therapy: evaluation and prescrip-

tion, Am J Nurs 88(2):192-197, 1988.

80. Phipps W, Long B, and Woods N: Medical-surgical nursing: concepts and clinical practice, St Louis, 1983, The CV Mosby Co.

81. Price SA and Wilson LM: Pathophysiology: clinical concepts of disease processes, ed 2, New York, 1982, McGraw-Hill Book Co.

82. Rakel RE: Conn's current therapy, Philadelphia, 1987, WB Saunders Co.

83. Ralph ED: Infections of the lower respiratory tract. In Mandell LA and Ralph ED, editors: Essentials of infectious disease, Boston, 1985, Blackwell Scientific Publications.

84. Respiratory disorders, Springhouse, Penn, 1984, Springhouse Corp.

85. Reynolds HY and Merrill WW: Airway changes in young smokers that may antedate chronic obstructive disease, Med Clin North Am 65:667, 1981.

86. Rifas E: Teaching patients to manage acute asthma: the future is now, Nursing 83 13(4):77, 1983.

87. Roberts S: Pulmonary tissue perfusion, altered: emboli, Heart Lung 16(2):128-138, 1987.

88. Rosen P, editor: Emergency medicine: concepts and clinical practice, St Louis, 1983, The CV Mosby Co, pp 774-789.

89. Scanlan CL: Egan's fundamentals of respiratory therapy, ed 5, St Louis, 1990, The CV Mosby Co.

90. Seidel HM, Ball JW, Dains JE and Benedict WG: Mosby's guide to physical examination, ed 2, St Louis, 1991, Mosby–Year Book Inc. (In press.)

91. Shapiro BA, Harrison RA, and Trout CA: Clinical application of respiratory care, ed 3, Chicago, 1985, Year Book Medical Publishers.

92. Shively M and Clark A: Continuous monitoring of mixed oxygen saturation: an instrument for research, Nurs Res 35(1):56-58, 1986.

93. Smith L and Thier S: Pathophysiology: the biological principles of disease, Philadelphia, 1981, WB Saunders Co.

94. Snukst-Torbeck G, Werhane MJ, and Schraufnagel, DE: Treatment of tuberculosis in a nurse-managed clinic, Heart Lung 16(1):30-33, 1987.

95. Stevens J and Raffin R: Adult respiratory distress syndrome—etiology, mechanism, and management, Postgrad Med 60:505, 1984.

96. Stratton CW: Bacterial pneumonias—an overview with emphasis on pathogenesis, diagnosis, and treatment, Heart Lung 15(3):226-243, 1986.

97. Tatum VD and Light RW: Approach to the diagnosis of secondary pulmonary hypertension: the chest roentgenogram as a diagnostic tool, Heart Lung 15(4):352-357, 1986.

98. Taylor JD: Lung cancer and acute respiratory failure: respiratory stressors. In Respiratory problems, Springhouse, Penn, 1987, Springhouse Corp.

99. Thompson JM, McFarland GK, Hirsch JE, Tucker SM, and Bowers AC, editors: Mosby's manual of clinical nursing, ed 2, St Louis, 1989, The CV Mosby Co.

100. Thorn GW, et al: editors: Harrison's principles of internal medicine, ed 11, New York, 1986, McGraw-Hill Book Co.

101. Traver GA: Ineffective airway clearance: physiology and clinical application, Dimen Crit Care Nurs 4(4):198-208, 1985.

102. Tucker S, Canobbio M, Paquette EV, and Wells MF: Patient care standards: nursing process, diagnosis, and outcomes, ed 4, St Louis, 1988, The CV Mosby Co.

103. U.S. Department of Health and Human Services/ Public Health Services/CDC: 1983 tuberculosis statistics: states and cities, March 1985.

104. Veith FJ, Kamholz SL, Mollenkopf FP, and Montefusco CM: Lung transplantation 1983, Transplantation 35(4), 1983.

105. Vincent JE: Medical problems in the patient on a ventilator, Crit Care Q 6:33, 1983.

106. Waldbott G: Health effects of environmental pollutants, ed 2, St. Louis, 1978, The CV Mosby Co.

107. Wallach J: Interpretation of diagnostic tests. Boston, 1986, Little, Brown & Co.

108. Wannamaker LW, Rammelkamp CH, and Top FH, Sr.: Streptococcal infections. In Wehrle PF and Top FH, Sr, editors: Communicable and infectious diseases, ed 9, St Louis, 1981, The CV Mosby Co.

109. Wanner A and Sackner MA: Pulmonary disease, Boston, 1983, Little, Brown & Co.

110. Weiss EB: Bronchial asthma, Clin Symp 27:39, 1975.

111. Westra B: "I can't breathe," Nursing 84 14(5):34-39, 1984.

112. Whitcomb ME: The lung: normal and diseased, St Louis, 1982, The CV Mosby Co.

113. Wollschlager CM and Khan FA: Secondary pulmonary hypertension: clinical features, Heart Lung 15(4):336-340, 1986.

114. Woodin LM: Your patient with a pneumothorax, Nursing 82 12(11):50-56, 1982.

115. Woodruff ML: Pulmonary thromboembolism: risk factors, pathophysiology, and management, Dimen Crit Care Nurs 4(4):52-63, 1984.

116. York K: Clinical validation of two respiratory nursing diagnoses and their defining characteristics—ineffective airway clearance and ineffective breathing patterns, Nurs Clin North Am 20(4):657-667, 1985.

Index

RESPIRATORY RESOURCES

ORGANIZATIONS AND AGENCIES

**American Association of Critical
Care Nurses (AACN)**
One Civic Plaza, Suite 330
Newport Beach, CA 92660
(714) 644-9310

**American Cancer Society,
National Headquarters**
1599 Clifton Road NE
Atlanta, GA 30329
(404) 320-3333

**American Lung Association,
National Headquarters**
1740 Broadway
New York, NY 10019
(212) 315-8700

**Asthma and Allergy Foundation
of America**
1717 Massachussetts Avenue NW,
Suite 305
Washington, DC 20036
(202) 265-0265

**Asthma Care Association
of America**
PO Box 568
Spring Valley Road
Ossining, NY 10562
(914) 762-2110

Canadian Lung Association
75 Alberta, Suite 908
Ottawa, Ontario K1P 5E7
(613) 237-1208

**Cancer Information Line and
Antismoking Helpline**
(800) 4-CANCER
(800) 638-6070—Alaska
(800) 524-1234—Hawaii; in Oahu,
dial direct.

Cystic Fibrosis Foundation
6931 Arlington Road
Bethesda, MD 20814
(301) 951-4422
(800) FIGHT CF

Lung Disease Hotline
(800) 222-LUNG
(303) 398-1477—Colorado

National Cancer Institute
9000 Rockville Pike
Building 31, 10A24
Bethesda, MD 20892
(800) 4-CANCER
(301) 496-5583

**National Heart, Lung, and
Blood Institute**
9000 Rockville Pike
Building 31, 4A21
Bethesda, MD 20892
(301) 496-4236
Information Center—(301) 951-3260

**National Institute of Allergies
and Infectious Diseases
NIAID/NIH**
9000 Rockville Pike
Building 31, Room 7A32
Bethesda, MD 20892
(301) 496-5717

**National Jewish Center for
Immunology and Respiratory
Medicine**
1400 Jackson Street
Denver, CO 80206
(303) 388-4461
(800) 222-5864

SOME LEADING STOP-SMOKING PROGRAMS

Many organizations, private companies, and public health agencies sponsor smoking-cessation programs. Here are some leading ones. Some programs associated with non-profit organizations are either free or charge a nominal to moderate fee.

Freedom From Smoking: Behavioral change program developed by the American Lung Association (ALA) and conducted by local ALA affiliates at certain scheduled times. Contact your local ALA affiliate.

**American Lung Association
National Headquarters**
1740 Broadway
New York, NY 10019

Fresh Start Program: A four-session class (either twice a week for two weeks or once a week for four weeks), led by a trained ex-smoker to help you figure out your smoking patterns, set a date for quitting, learn techniques of stress management and how to keep from returning to smoking once you have quit. Conducted by local American Cancer Society units, listed in white pages of local telephone directories.

American Cancer Society
90 Park Ave.
New York, NY 10016
(212) 599-8200

Plan to Stop Smoking: Sponsored by the Seventh-day Adventist Church and organized by churches in communities. Contact the Seventh-day Adventist Church in your area.

Seventh-day Adventists
12501 Old Columbia Pike
Silver Spring, MD 20904
(301) 680-6000

BOOKS

Asthma

The Allergy Encyclopedia, edited by The Asthma & Allergy Foundation of America and Craig T. Norback, New York: New American Library, 1981.

Asthma: The Complete Guide to Self-Management, Allan M. Weinstein, M.D., New York: McGraw-Hill, 1987.

Asthma and Allergies: An Optimistic Future, Patrick Young, Washington: U.S. Department of Health and Human Services, 1980, 179 pages. NIH Publication No. 80-388. Based on the report of the Task Force on Asthma and Other Allergic Diseases. For sale by the Superintendent of Documents, U.S. Government Printing Office, Washington, DC 20402.

Asthma and Hay Fever, Alan Knight, New York: Arco Publishing, 1981.

Asthma: The Facts, Donald J. Lane and Anthony Storr, New York: Oxford University Press, 1979.

Asthma: Stop Suffering, Start Living, M. Eric Gershwin and E.L. Klingelhofer, Reading, MA: Addison-Wesley, 1986.

Breathe Easy:An Asthmatic's Guide to Clean Air, Stanley Reichman, New York: Thomas Y. Crowell, Co., 1977.

Breathing Exercises for Asthma, Karen R. Butts, Springfield, IL: Charles C Thomas, 1980. For professionals and parents of asthmatic children.

Children With Asthma: A Manual for Parents, Dr. Thomas F. Plaut, Amherst, MA: Pedi-Press, 1983. Mail order from PediPress, 125 Red Gate Lane, Amherst, MA 01002.

Living With Your Allergies and Asthma, Theodore Berland, New York: St. Martin's Press, 1983.

Speaking of Asthma, Dr. Dietrich Nolte, New York: Delair, 1980.

Cystic Fibrosis

Alex: The Life of a Child, Frank Deford, New York: Viking, 1983.

CF in His Corner, Gail Radley, New York: Four Winds Press, 1984.

Child in a White Fog, Jann D. Jansen, New York: Vantage Press, 1982.

Faith, Hope and Luck, a Sociological Study of Children Growing up with a Life threatening Illness, Charles Waddell, Washington, DC: University Press of America, 1983.

The Time of Her Life, Meg Woodson, Grand Rapids, MI: Zondervan Publishing, 1982.